Machine Learning and Deep Learning in Medical Data Analytics and Healthcare Applications

Biomedical and Robotics Healthcare

Series Editors:
Utku Kose, Jude Hemanth, Omer Deperlioglu

Artificial Intelligence for the Internet of Health Things
Deepak Gupta, Eswaran Perumal and K. Shankar

Biomedical Signal and Image Examination with Entropy-Based Techniques
V. Rajinikanth, K. Kamalanand, C. Emmanuel and B. Thayumanavan

Mechano-Electric Correlations in the Human Physiological System
A. Bakiya, K. Kamalanand and R. L. J. De Britto

Machine Learning and Deep Learning in Medical Data Analytics and Healthcare Applications
Om Prakash Jena, Bharat Bhushan, Utku Kose

For more information about this series, please visit: https://www.routledge.com/ Biomedical-and-Robotics-Healthcare/book-series/BRHC

Machine Learning and Deep Learning in Medical Data Analytics and Healthcare Applications

Edited by

Om Prakash Jena, Bharat Bhushan, and Utku Kose

CRC Press
Taylor & Francis Group
Boca Raton   London   New York

CRC Press is an imprint of the
Taylor & Francis Group, an **informa** business

First edition published 2022
by CRC Press
6000 Broken Sound Parkway NW, Suite 300, Boca Raton, FL 33487-2742
and by CRC Press
2 Park Square, Milton Park, Abingdon, Oxon, OX14 4RN

CRC Press is an imprint of Taylor & Francis Group, LLC

Library of Congress Cataloging-in-Publication Data

Names: Jena, Om Prakash, editor. | Bhushan, Bharat, editor. | Kose, Utku, 1985- editor.
Title: Machine learning and deep learning in medical data analytics and
healthcare applications / edited by Om Prakash Jena, Bharat Bhushan, Utku Kose.
Description: First edition. | Boca Raton : CRC Press, 2022. | Series: Biomedical and robotics
healthcare | Includes bibliographical references and index. | Summary: "The book incorporates
the many facets of computational intelligence, such as machine learning and deep learning, to
provide groundbreaking developments in healthcare applications. It discusses theory, analytical
methods, numerical simulation, scientific techniques, analytical outcomes, and computational
structuring"-- Provided by publisher.
Identifiers: LCCN 2021043580 (print) | LCCN 2021043581 (ebook) | ISBN 9781032126876 (hardback) |
ISBN 9781032127644 (paperback) | ISBN 9781003226147 (ebook)
Subjects: LCSH: Medical technology. | Medical care--Technological innovations. |
Robotics in medicine.
Classification: LCC R855.3 .M33 2022 (print) | LCC R855.3 (ebook) |
DDC 610.285--dc23/eng/20211103
LC record available at https://lccn.loc.gov/2021043580
LC ebook record available at https://lccn.loc.gov/2021043581

ISBN: 978-1-032-12687-6 (hbk)
ISBN: 978-1-032-12764-4 (pbk)
ISBN: 978-1-003-22614-7 (ebk)

DOI: 10.1201/9781003226147

Typeset in Times LT Std
by KnowledgeWorks Global Ltd.

Contents

Preface

The most astonishing difference between computers and humans lies in the fact that computers need to be programmed in order to respond to any event whereas humans learn from their past experience. However, with the advent of machine learning (ML) and deep learning (DL), it is possible for computers to learn from their experiences. Recent advances in ML/DL algorithms are impervious to large-scale technological disruptions and have transformed numerous industries such as governance, transportation, manufacturing, and healthcare. These techniques have shown tremendous results in varied healthcare-related tasks such as brain tumor segmentation, medical image reconstruction, lung nodule detection, classification of lung diseases, and medical image recognition. Furthermore, the exponentially growing volume of biomedical big data generated due to health data collection through digital health wearables, genomic sequencing, and electronic health records (EHRs) is another matter of concern. ML/DL schemes have a proven ability to extract actionable knowledge from these large health datasets. ML models can also contribute toward improving the quality of care, enhancing patient safety, and mitigating the overall healthcare costs. Extraction of appropriate data would be extremely beneficial in resolving serious medical conditions to a significant extent. ML/DL approaches can be used to extract certain attributes, and the trained model can be used to make proper diagnoses and prognoses from available medical data and photographs. These can also ease the identification of high-risk patients, early detection of lung cancer, detection of abusive and fraudulent health insurance claims, and diagnosis of respiratory ailments from chest X-rays. ML and big data strategies are used to build predictive diagnostic systems on collected data. However, designing and implementing an effective diagnostic system remains a difficult task due to a variety of issues such as stability, accessibility, scalability, safety, development standards, and technologies. This book covers the fundamentals of ML and DL in the healthcare domain where these models are used to train the system and implicitly extract positive solutions. The main aim of this book is to highlight the role of ML/DL algorithms in improved healthcare diagnostic systems, processing EHRs, medical signal analysis, and consequently enhance the overall quality of life by enhancing disease diagnosis and life expectancy. Further, this book endows varied communities with its innovative advances in theory, modeling, statistical analysis, analytical approaches, analytical results, numerical simulation, computational structuring, and case studies related to applications of ML/DL models in the healthcare domain.

Editors

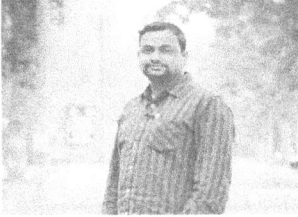

Dr. Om Prakash Jena (PhD) is currently working as an Assistant Professor in the Department of Computer Science, Ravenshaw University, Cuttack, Odisha, India. He has ten years of teaching and research experience in the undergraduate and postgraduate levels. He has published several technical papers in international journals, conferences, and edited book chapters of reputed publications. He is a member of IEEE, IETA, IAAC, IRED, IAENG, and WACAMLDS. His current research interest includes database, pattern recognition, cryptography, network security, artificial intelligence, machine learning, soft computing, natural language processing, data science, compiler design, data analytics, and machine automation. He has many edited books to his credit, published by Wiley, CRC Press, Bentham Publication, and is also the author of two textbooks under Kalyani Publisher. He also serves as a reviewer committee member and editor of many international journals.

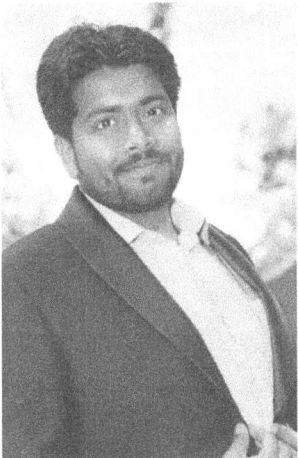

Dr. Bharat Bhushan (PhD) is an Assistant Professor of Department of Computer Science and Engineering (CSE) at School of Engineering and Technology, Sharda University, Greater Noida, India. He is an alumnus of Birla Institute of Technology, Mesra, Ranchi, India. He received his Undergraduate Degree (B-Tech in Computer Science and Engineering) with Distinction in 2012, received his Postgraduate Degree (M-Tech in Information Security) with Distinction in 2015, and his Doctorate Degree (Ph.D. Computer Science and Engineering) in 2021 from Birla Institute of Technology, Mesra, India. He has earned numerous international certifications such as CCNA, MCTS, MCITP, RHCE, and CCNP. In the last 3 years, he has published more than 80 research papers in various renowned international conferences and SCI-indexed journals including Wireless Networks (Springer), Wireless Personal Communications (Springer), Sustainable Cities and Society (Elsevier), and Emerging Transactions on Telecommunications (Wiley). He has contributed with more than 25 book chapters in various books and has edited 11 books from the most famed publishers like Elsevier, IGI Global, and CRC Press. He has served as a reviewer/editorial board member for several reputed international journals. In the past, he worked as an assistant professor at HMR Institute of Technology and Management, New Delhi, and Network Engineer in HCL Infosystems Ltd, Noida. He has passed GATE exams for successive years and gained the highest percentile of 98.48 in GATE 2013. He is also a member of numerous renowned bodies including IEEE, IAENG, CSTA, SCIEI, IAE, and UACEE.

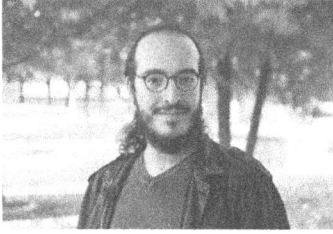

Dr. Utku Kose (PhD) received the BS degree in 2008 in Computer Education at Gazi University, Turkey as a faculty valedictorian. He received his MS degree in 2010 from Afyon Kocatepe University, Turkey in the field of computer and his DS/PhD in 2017 from Selcuk University, Turkey in the field of computer engineering. Between 2009 and 2011, he worked as a Research Assistant in Afyon Kocatepe University. Following this, he has also worked as a Lecturer and Vocational School Vice-Director at Afyon Kocatepe University between 2011 and 2012, as a Lecturer and Research Center Director in Usak University between 2012 and 2017, and as an Assistant Professor in Suleyman Demirel University between 2017 and 2019. Currently, he is an Associate Professor in Suleyman Demirel University, Turkey. He is published in more than 100 publications including articles, authored and edited books, proceedings, and reports. He is also on the editorial boards of many scientific journals and serves as one of the editors of the Biomedical and Robotics Healthcare book series by CRC Press. His research interest includes artificial intelligence, machine ethics, artificial intelligence safety, optimization, the chaos theory, distance education, e-learning, computer education, and computer science.

Contributors

Amira Hassan Abed
Department of Information Systems
   Center
Egyptian Organization for
   Standardization & Quality
Cairo, Egypt

C. B. Abhilash
Indian Institute of Information Technology
Dharwad, India

K. Balakrishnan
Indian Institute of Information
   Technology
Tiruchirappalli, Tamil Nadu, India

Shawli Bardhan
Indian Institute of Information Technology
Una, India

Loubna Bouhachlaf
Faculty of Science
Mohammed V University
Rabat, Morroco

Azedine Boulmakoul
FSTM
Casablanca, Morocco

Aju D
Vellore Institute of Technology
Vellore, India

K. T. Deepak
Indian Institute of Information Technology
Dharwad, India

Kuldeep Dhama
Division of Pathology
ICAR-Indian Veterinary Research
   Institute
Bareilly, India

R. Dhanalakshmi
Indian Institute of Information Technology
Tiruchirappalli, India

Souad El Hajjaji
Faculty of Science
Mohammed V University
Rabat, Morroco

Ahmed A. Elngar
Faculty of Computers and Artificial
   Intelligence
Beni-Suef University
Beni-Suef, Egypt

Yousef Farhaoui
T-IDMS Faculty of Sciences and
   Techniques Errachidia
Moulay Ismail University
Meknes, Morocco

Manasi Gyanchandani
Department of CSE
MANIT
Bhopal, India

Abubakar Kamagata Hamisu
P P Savani University
Kosamba, Gujarat, India

Rajendra Hegadi
Indian Institute of Information Technology
Dharwad, India

Hassan Homayoun
Quantitative MR Imaging and
   Spectroscopy Group, Research Center
   for Cellular and Molecular Imaging
Tehran University of Medical Sciences
Tehran, Iran

Om Prakash Jena
Department of Computer Science
Ravenshaw University
Cuttack, India

Sushitha Susan Joseph
Vellore Institute of Technology
Vellore, India

Jasleen Kaur
P P Savani University
Kosamba, Gujarat, India

Utkarsh Mahadeo Khaire
Department of CSE
MANIT
Bhopal, India

Nilay Khare
Indian Institute of Information Technology
Dharwad, India

Aziz Mabrouk
FSTM
Tetouan, Morocco

Jamal Mabrouki
Faculty of Science
Mohammed V University
Rabat, Morroco

Kavi Mahesh
Indian Institute of Information Technology
Dharwad, India

Ashima Sindhu Mohanty
GIET University
Gunupur, Odisha, India

Ranjan K. Mohapatra
Department of Chemistry
Government College of Engineering
Keonjhar, India

Behzad Soleimani Neysiani
Department of Research and Development
Ava Aria Information Company
Demis Holding
Isfahan, Iran

Madhumita Pal
Electronics Science and Engineering
    C. V. Raman Global University
Bhubaneswar, India

Priyadarsan Parida
GIET University
Gunupur, Odisha, India

Smita Parija
Electronics Science and Engineering
    C. V. Raman Global University
Bhubaneswar, India

Krishna Chandra Patra
GIET University
Gunupur, Odisha, India

B. Rajitha
Motilal Nehru National Institute of
    Technology Allahabad
Prayagraj, India

Mithun Singh Rajput
School of Pharmacy
Devi Ahilya Vishwavidyalaya
Indore, India

Nitin Singh Rajput
Vellore Institute of Technology
Vellore, India

G. V. Eswara Rao
Motilal Nehru National Institute of
    Technology Allahabad
Prayagraj, India

Purnima Dey Sarkar
Department of Medical Biochemistry
M.G.M. Medical College
Indore, India

Prashant Sengar
Indian Institute of Information
    Technology
Una, India

Essam M. Shaaban
Faculty of Computers & Artificial
    Intelligence
Cairo, Egypt

Bhawna Swarnkar
Department of CSE
MANIT
Bhopal, India

Ruchi Tiwari
Department of Veterinary Microbiology
    and Immunology
College of Veterinary Sciences
DUVASU
Mathura, India

1 Common Data Interface for Sustainable Healthcare System

C. B. Abhilash, K. T. Deepak,
Rajendra Hegadi, and Kavi Mahesh

CONTENTS

DOI: 10.1201/9781003226147-1

1

1.1 INTRODUCTION

People are well connected in more places than ever and actively participate in digital healthcare activities in the current generation. Healthcare professionals look for deeper health insights and actionable information like making better decisions and efficiently improving patient record information at lower costs. The current healthcare scenario is expected to be digitized. People regularly connect to their different health gadgets and regularly monitor their health activities. Digital healthcare enables the healthcare ecosystem to have a huge amount of connected data for regular monitoring. The proposed high-level integration architecture is the open architecture that provides services in compliance with data standards and has a capability that inspires new healthcare application developers to design next-gen connected health and wellness systems like digital gadgets that connect across the healthcare devices, unlike other open architecture. In the current scenario, we see a patient present at the emergency department. We don't know anything about them even though they might have a lot of electronic records (R. Bayer et al. 2015). Knowing them as digital citizens, we take care of them on time and at a lesser cost. The connected healthcare system supports these features and enables the individual's data or health record to be accessible at any point in time for the health ecosystem's concerned stakeholders. So there is a necessity that automation and integration are necessary. We have found that our automated systems are often much siloed (T. Benson et al. 2016).

It is a long-term challenge to make the health entities interoperable. When health data and related information are standalone systems, they need to be connected to serve the purpose for which they had been originally designed or intended. To achieve interoperability, the databases are gradually deployed in a distributed architecture and the subsequent federation by reusing resources to build a knowledge-based system. But this can be well implemented by incorporating standards in healthcare systems. With the wide opportunity of semantic technology, we can incorporate interoperability (B. Hu et al. 2006).

In the federated system approach, various databases are put together to exchange and communicate the data. But this can be achieved with certain constraints in design and usage. In a semantic-based approach, the meaning of the information that needs to be integrated is considered when integrating the database schema with respective row and column names. Thus, it is the syntactic approach of integration.

The amount of data in the healthcare ecosystem keeps growing. Patient data is generated by various health stakeholders like physicians, laboratories, medical devices, research facilities, and now even from in-home data sources such as personal fitness devices. Sharing this data across so many disparate systems is critical to ensuring the successful care of individual patients and improving overall population health.

In G. Alterovitz et al.'s (2015) study, the authors report a typical case system from ontology mapping. A similar integration algorithm and data will produce different results. The results are arbitrary, as evidenced in the formatting and annotation, which make the result difficult to reuse. And, this makes semantic integration difficult to apply.

The healthcare stakeholder's data is available in different formats, and systems match the data generally by matching the strings. Each system has its data structure, so it is preferred to have a standard methodology for data translation and exchange. The standard-based translation for data interchange is recommended (T. Benson et al., 2016). The source and target system both need to understand and interpret the data in the same way. This chapter discusses the existing data integration techniques available in the healthcare domain. We propose a novel methodology that intelligently integrates all healthcare applications with minimal change configurations to the existing data and structure. The proposed methodology follows the metadata approach. A 12-digit unique ID is generated considering the respective stakeholders' predefined district and talk code, and appended by an identification code and the unique random number. The unique ID is stored as metadata information in a separate server for interoperable operations. The open-source tools are available to consume or send data in fast health interoperability resources (FHIR), HL7v2 easily. We can write code to handle data in any custom format as well. Also, the proposed model uses different integration techniques with different functionalities as defined in the common data interface (CDI) layer.

This paper describes developing a novel method for having unified access to health information in the healthcare ecosystem.

This work proposes a unique CDI layer that fits the existing system architecture to adapt the data standards to achieve interoperability. Section 1.2 illustrates the related work considering semantics and other healthcare attributes. Section 1.3 discusses the various healthcare data standards required to achieve interoperability. Finally, in Section 1.4, the methodology is discussed, along with a case study considering the patient registration process. Our proposed method uses a well-established natural language processing technique to match the patient records with the unique ID.

1.2 RELATED WORK

In this section, the previous literature is reviewed, with regard to semantic interoperability and healthcare standards. This paper aims to study the existing interoperable approaches to enhance the health care ecosystem. With FHIR, the health data is exchanged as resources using the XML code format. As artificial intelligence (AI) and machine learning (ML) technologies (K. Paramesha et al. 2021) continue to break through the restrictions of scientific drug research, ML is preferable for sentiment analysis (SA) for user-generated drug reviews. Many neurolinguistic programming (NLP) techniques can benefit from ML's unique learning style. Having this as the main objective, it becomes obvious that existing literature had to be reviewed in order to understand the process for introducing the proposed CDI layer.

1.2.1 SEMANTIC INTEROPERABILITY AND SEMANTIC INTEROPERABILITY IN EHR

Semantic interoperability is achieved when the data is exchanged across the interfaces with the required data interpretation in an unaltered way (S. Schulz et al. 2013). Data sharing is interoperable, allowing systems to exchange information about electronic health records (EHR) and the possibility of changing the healthcare system using ontology (A. Kiourtis et al. 2019). It can automatically integrate information between multiple users and systems to improve feedback efficiency to query terms and ensure that the feedback is true and clear regardless of the data representation (J. D. Heflin et al. 2000). Web ontologies can be used to integrate data and semantic interoperability from medical data because they use existing health standards to access patient records. In addition, the location of data instances is consistent with medical terminology (D. Teodoro et al. 2011).

EHR is a digital representation of a patient's health record, including medical treatment, diagnosis, treatment plan, and medical history. This is a systematic way to store this information and provide it to all parties under each party's authorization. Therefore, EHR adopted a prototype-based approach that enables clinical decision support system (CDSS) tools to make decisions about patient care (R. Bayer et al. 2015).

Assuming that the EHR is patient-centric, it is not an institution. It has a long-term care record, including the various medical care that the patient has received, and the medical treatments, plans, and prognostic instructions followed. The EHR prototype provides a simplified process for the flow of information between clinicians without interpreting information in the existing system. The terms used in the system are not universally defined; they may be specific to a particular system developer's specific prototype. As a result, integrating this information between different prototypes constitutes a limitation (S. Garde et al. 2007).

1.2.2   Fast Health Interoperability Resources

The FHIR standard provides flexibility when developing ontologies by introducing resource description framework (RDF) vocabulary to be used in framework development. This is accomplished while preserving semantic interoperability in EHR. To support CDS tools for precision medicine, genomic data must be linked to phenomena variants in a patient's EHR, which is done using the FHIR standard. EHR that comply with substitutable medical applications and reusable technologies (SMART) can be used to obtain clinical data for use in patient diagnosis, medication selection, and care course prediction (G. Alterovitz et al. 2018).

FHIR has built-in modules like administration, clinical module, diagnostic medicine, medications, and clinical reasoning, which can be used to map the ontology framework to avoid information mismatch. The purpose of ontology has to be properly defined so that the output can be properly derived. The best approach is to base the ontology on the FHIR standard, which has all the modules mentioned above. For precision dosing, proper data mapping is required to achieve interoperability (G. Alterovitz et al. 2020).

The federated health information model (FHIM) (The Open Group Healthcare Forum 2015) is advancing the healthcare interoperability by using standards. In this digital era, health and healthcare are privileged to be managed via technology. However, the process of transforming healthcare information often feels stuck in a time warp. For example, consider a case where patient X suffers from multiple health problems like diabetes, heart disease, low back pain, obesity, and depression. When patient X experiences moderate chest pain, he visits the cardiologist. The concerned healthcare provider asks patient X to provide the health conditions, insurance, and basic demographic details of patient X. This continues as and when patient X visits all types of care providers. The problem is that while patient X's information is already stored at the cardiologist center, it is not accessible or shareable with the diabetic care provider. Interoperability is the approach to solve this problem to avoid delay and provide the necessary information at the right time to the right.

1.2.3 EXISTING SYSTEMS

Semantic interoperability can be achieved by incorporating healthcare standards (U. Batr et al. 2014). The author has compared various standards and their implications to achieve semantic interoperability. Choosing the best adoptable standard is very important. HL7 is used widely as a messaging model.

In Pijush Kanti et al.'s (2019) study the author discusses the "V's" of healthcare big data where volume, velocity, variability, validity, variety, veracity, viability, vulnerability, and visualization of data are described. To achieve the efficient use of big data in healthcare, incorporating standards is very much required. EHR require data across healthcare applications using standards-based methods by which seamless data exchange can be done.

HealthSuite (Philips, USA, 2018) is a cloud-based open digital platform that offers users continuous, personalized health care. The kit includes functions for analysis, sharing, and processing. Healthcare service coordination. The analysis section employs ML algorithms as well as various predictive analysis technologies. Shared functionality is essentially multi-device platform interoperability. Orchestration, in essence, achieves workflow synchronization, such as Tasks and so on (D. P. Pijush Kanti et al. 2019).

Watson health (IBM) is a complete software package developed by IBM that can help all aspects of health. It has AI and ML capabilities that can help diagnose and treat diseases effectively and reduce hospital staff and patient care staff. Watson can understand the patient's medical history and ask for all possible new drugs or technologies on the market, thus saving the doctor's time checking all the literature.

A fully integrated system with the Internet of Healthcare Things (IoHT) framework can be used remotely to assist medical experts in diagnosing and treating skin cancer (A. Khamparia et al. 2020). According to the performance index evaluation, the proposed framework outperforms other pre-trained architectures regarding accuracy, recall, and accuracy of detecting and classifying skin cancer from skin lesion images.

Even though internet of health things (IoHT) has a very complex architecture due to the connectivity of a wide range of devices and services in the system, it can be incorporated into the healthcare system for data collection and real-time monitoring. This paper presents a brief overview of urban IoT systems designed to support smart cities and advanced communication technologies (A. K. Rana et al. 2019).

Random Forest algorithm is a well-known decision tree-based ensemble method that tries to increase the system accuracy and can be applied to classification and regression applications. It has excellent data adaptability and can solve the "large p, small n" problem. Moreover, it shows how functions interact with one another and how they are related (P. Sudhansu Shekhar et al. 2021)

ML in healthcare can improve health information management and health information exchange to improve work processes (P. Pattnayak et al. 2021), modernize them, make clinical data more accessible, and improve the accuracy of health information. Most notably, it improves information processing efficiency and transparency.

A CDSS based on an expert system will be a better solution because it will perform both ML functions. In addition, an expert system can assist medical staff in diagnosing diseases when experienced doctors are unavailable in rural and remote areas (N. Panigrahi et al. 2021). This is achieved by using interoperability.

1.3 TERMINOLOGIES IN THE HEALTHCARE ECOSYSTEM

There are several challenges when working with healthcare data. First, the data can be transmitted in any number of formats. For example, HL7v2 or some completely customized format. Second, sharing the data in different formats between systems and integrating them is difficult and time-consuming.

The second challenge is that, even if the data is in the same format, it is represented differently by the various systems that use this data. There are several coding systems such as LONIC, SNOMED, ICD-10. So sharing results that are coded differently within systems is challenging since translation is required to integrate. It is necessary to have one standard, or a mapping engine that works between standards should be developed.

1.3.1 Standardizing Healthcare Data

S. Schulz et al. (2019) seek classification in a report titled "Medical Data Standards." They clarify relevant, language-driven concepts to define the types of data standards in healthcare. Also, the authors describe four concepts that characterize various aspects of clinical data, as outlined below (ISO/TR 20514:2005).

1.3.1.1 Referencing Terminology

Referencing terminology is the set of unique, human-understandable, unambiguous, standardized labels for terms is referred to as a reference term that is, the term used as a reference.

1.3.1.2 Syntax

Syntax is the standard that specifies the required order of composition when anatomical terms and various restrictions, such as "acute," "distal," "left and right," are used in clinical narratives.

1.3.1.3 Semantics

Semantics is the study of meaning. Semantic standards are concerned with the real-world meanings of various terminology codes.

1.3.1.4 Pragmatics

Pragmatics is the study of how things work; it makes use of terminology in specific clinical settings or contexts. Although various resources may contain medical terminology, such as "asthma," context is required to differentiate resources and descriptions of "suspicious" asthma. For example, asthma is classified as "severe." Furthermore, resources containing the term asthma may be a laboratory test for asthma, so pragmatics is important. Therefore, it is necessary to specify that the resource is an asthma test.

These are useful in understanding the healthcare terminology system. The most common and standard terminology is ontology. The healthcare system's widely used ontology is Systematized Nomenclature of Medicine – Clinical Terms (SNOMED–CT).

1.3.2 Fast Health Interoperability Resources

The FHIR is an HL7 standard for exchanging information between systems. It can support multiple formats defined in its packages like JSON & XML. FHIR uses Restful API to exchange resources across different nodes. About the representation formats (T. Benson et al., 2016).

It follows the CRUD method:

- **Create:** It creates new resources in a server-provided location.
  - This is done by the HTTP Post method: POST [service_url]/[type_of_resource]
- **Read:** It accesses the current content of the specified resource.
  - This is done by the HTTP GET method: GET [service_url]/[type_of_resource]/id
- **Update:** It creates a new version of a resource for the existing resource. Also, it will update the existing ID with resource information.
  - This is done by the HTTP PUT method: PUT [service_url]/[type_of_resource]/id
- **Delete:** It deletes the existing resource.
  - This is performed by: HTTP DELETE method: DELETE [service_url]/[type_of_resource]/id

1.3.3 FHIR as API

FHIR includes descriptions of API specifications. For instance, Restful API is used as an architectural style. As an open internet for data exchange, the FHIR standard specifies the HTTP Web protocol. This style is unique. Naturally, the decision will differentiate between the server and the client. FHIR-compliant clients provide lightweight applications that use FHIR data, and FHIR provides this data. Security, threads, multiple representations, search and indexing, and persistence are all addressed by the server. FHIR-compliant clients and servers use FHIR resources for data transmission and exchange data following FHIR API specifications.

1.3.4 COMMON DRUG CODES FOR INDIA (CDCI)

The CDCI is categorized into two types by the national resource center for EHR standards, Pune, India (NRC):

- Common Drug Codes for India (Terminology Integrated Package).
- Common Drug Codes for India (Flat Files Package).

The CDCI Terminology Integrated Package is a set of files that integrate with the standard SNOMED–CT terminology files and content for use in any data entry, analysis, or record exchange systems that adhere to certain EHR standards (HER Standards).

This enables standardized coding of medicinal products for clinical care and enables linkages to terminology and use in clinical data, data retrieval, data analytics, etc.

Common Drug Codes for India (Flat Files Package) is introduced to support standardized coding and sharing of drug codes without the need to integrate the complete terminology. The existing system integration can be incorporated by using this option and provide their data such as batch code or packages for customized use.

1.3.5 EHR STANDARDS

The EHR standards, indicated in Table 1.1, is the standards that is openly available at national resource center repository. The standard digital healthcare system should incorporate the following EHR standard for interoperability.

1.4 METHODOLOGY

Healthcare architecture has been proposed over time by many researchers in our methodology we propose an innovative middleware that is responsible for achieving interoperability in adherence to the existing system architecture of healthcare applications. The adherence to the existing system may vary with minor configurations and add-ons. This section proposes the novel CDI layer, which can be implemented as middleware architecture to the existing system. The methodology is illustrated considering the case study of patient registration and data access mechanism. The novel CDI layer generates a 12-digit unique number that follows the standard approach. The health unique number is illustrated in Figure 1.6. With the unique CDI ID, the system can identify the patient, the health facility, and all stakeholders of the healthcare ecosystem. This flexibility of identification makes the system more efficient and easier to adopt.

TABLE 1.1
EHR Standards by NRC

S. No.	Type	Standard Name	Intended Purpose
1	Identification & Demographics	ISO/TS 22220:2011 Health Informatics – Identification of Subjects of Health Care	Basic identity details of patient
2		MDDS – Demographic (Person Identification and Land Region Codification) version 1.1	Complete demographic for interoperability with E-Governance systems
3	Patient Identifiers	UIDAI Aadhaar	Preferable identifier where available
4		Local Identifier	Identifier given within institution/clinic/lab
5		Government Issued Photo Identity Card Number	Identifier used in conjunction with local in absence of Aadhaar
6	Architecture Requirements	ISO 18308:2011 Health Informatics - Requirements for an Electronic Health Record Architecture	System architectural requirements
7	Functional Requirements	ISO/HL7 10781:2015 Health Informatics - HL7 Electronic Health Records-System Functional Model Release 2 (EHR FM)	System functional requirements
8	Reference Model and Composition	ISO 13940 Health informatics - System of Concepts to Support Continuity of Care	Concepts for care, actors, activities, processes, etc.
9		ISO 13606 Health informatics - Electronic Health Record Communication (Part 1 through 3)	Information model architecture and communication
10		openEHR Foundation Models Release 1.0.2	Structural definition and composition
11	Terminology	SNOMED – Clinical Terms (SNOMED–CT)	Primary terminology
12	Coding System	Logical Observation Identifiers Names and Codes (LOINC)	Test, measurement, observations
13		WHO Family of International Classifications (WHOFIC) including ICD, ICF, ICHI, ICD-O	Classification and reporting
14	Imaging	Digital Imaging and Communications in Medicine (DICOM) PS3.0-2015	Image, waveform, audio/video
15	Scanned or Captured Records	JPEG lossy (or lossless) with size and resolution not less than 1024px x 768px at 300dpi	Image capture format
16		ISO/IEC 14496 – Coding of Audio-Visual Objects	Audio/Video capture format
17		ISO 19005-2 Document Management – Electronic Document File Format for Long-Term Preservation – Part 2: Use of ISO 32000-1 (PDF/A-2)	Scanned documents format

(Continued)

TABLE 1.1   (Continued)
EHR Standards by NRC

S. No.	Type	Standard Name	Intended Purpose
18	Data Exchange	ANSI/HL7 V2.8.2-2015 HL7 Standard Version 2.8.2 – An Application Protocol for Electronic Data Exchange in Healthcare Environments	Event/Message exchange
19		ASTM/HL7 CCD Release 1 (basis standard ISO/HL7 27932:2009)	Summary Records exchange
20		ISO 13606-5:2010 Health informatics – Electronic Health Record Communication – Part 5: Interface Specification	EHR archetypes exchange [Also, refer to openEHR Service Model specification]
21		DICOM PS3.0-2015 (using DIMSE services & Part-10 media/files)	Imaging/Waveform Exchange
22	Other Relevant Standards	Bureau of Indian Standards and its MHD-17 Committee	Standards Development Organizations (SDOs)
23		ISO TC 215 set of standards	
24		IEEE/NEMA/CE standards for physical systems and interfaces	
25	Discharge/ Treatment Summary	Medical Council of India (MCI) under regulation 3.1 of Ethics	Composition as prescribed
26	E-Prescription	Pharmacy Practice Regulations, 2015 Notification No. 14-148/ 2012- PCI as specified by Pharmacy Council of India	Composition as prescribed
27	Personal Healthcare and medical Device Interface	IEEE 11073 health informatics standards and related ISO standards for medical devices	Device interfacing
28	Data Privacy and Security	ISO/TS 14441:2013 Health Informatics – Security & Privacy Requirements of EHR Systems for Use in Conformity Assessment	Basis security and privacy requirements
29	Information Security Management	ISO/DIS 27799 Health informatics – Information Security Management in Health using ISO/IEC 27002	Overall information security management
30	Privilege Management and Access Control	ISO 22600:2014 Health informatics – Privilege Management and Access Control (Part 1 through 3)	Access control
31	Audit Trail and Logs	ISO 27789:2013 Health informatics – Audit trails for Electronic Health Records	Audit trail
32	Data Integrity	Secure Hash Algorithm (SHA) used must be SHA-256 or higher	Data hashing
33	Data Encryption	Minimum 256-bits key length	Encryption key
34		HTTPS, SSL v3.0, and TLS v1.2	Encrypted connection
35	Digital Certificate	ISO 17090 Health informatics – Public Key Infrastructure (Part 1 through 5)	Digital certificates use and management

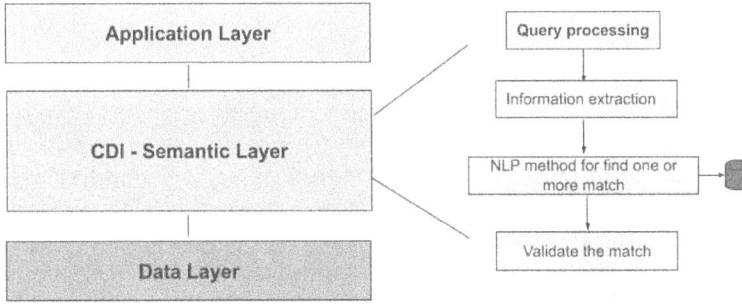

FIGURE 1.1 High-level interoperable architecture.

1.4.1 HIGH-LEVEL ARCHITECTURE

The high-level architecture of the proposed CDI layer is represented in Figure 1.1. It consists of three layers, the data layer at the bottom where federated databases are connected and, above, the CDI semantic layer that processes the user query and extracts the relevant information about the user mentioned in the query. The information extraction is purely based on the natural language processing techniques discussed in our further work. The processing will generally follow searching and matching text patterns with the stored metadata information (P. Young et al. 2003). The semantic search algorithm will be used to relay the meaning of the search text considering the context. Also, semantic string match operations can be performed. The top layer of the architecture is the application layer, where the user interface is provided for different applications. Semantic interoperability would imply that a unified representation of all clinical terminologies is implemented, but this is quite difficult in practice because clinical practice is highly diversified, with new terms being created regularly, necessitating constant evolution of standards. Certain physical and logical illustrations in EHR may have similar meanings and be semantically indistinguishable (D. P. Pijush Kanti et al. 2019). This makes clinical data exchange more than just a data structure with clear terminology and alignment. As a result, the system must recognize, process, and similarly calculate semantically equivalent data.

1.4.2 HIGH-LEVEL REPRESENTATION OF CDI LAYER

Following the existing healthcare data integration systems, our proposed CDI layer is a middleware that fits the existing system architecture with minimalistic configurations. The CDI is used as a medium of data exchange in XML format, using the HL7 standard. The CDI layer can be used in federated systems where data needs to be transferred or exchanged seamlessly. The CDI middleware is introduced with minimal changes to the existing application to capture data. Figure 1.1 shows the high-level representation of the CDI with its functionalities as suggested by the National Digital Health Mission – digital blueprint by Ministry of Health and Family Welfare, Government of India. The proposed methodology helps you avoid these problems by intelligently integrating all healthcare applications without modifying the existing data and structure. Open-source tools are available to consume or send data in FHIR, HL7v2 easily. Also, we can write code to handle data in any custom format.

Additionally, data aggregation functionality for reports generation, these reports are required by the administration authority for monitoring and other needs. The CDI layer has a semantic algorithm that is rule-based, and transformations are defined to match the data source with the available metadata information stored in the CDI server database. An FHIR resource repository is also included to store all FHIR resources with the built-in data transformations. You can transform all HL7 messages or any other custom data to FHIR and store all data in one central location if required.

Furthermore, CDI for healthcare includes data anonymization, consent manager, health locker, health information exchange, and health analytics. Using the stored CDI ID, the messages are immediately interpreted, making it clear what each piece of data means. However, this chapter mainly focuses on the specific CDI functionality, which is indicated in Figure 1.2.

1.4.3 COMMON DATA INTERFACE FUNCTIONALITY

The CDI layer functionality is to enable communication between the system and applications. The data about a patient or facility can be extracted across applications by making it interoperable in the federated environment. The CDI acts as middleware and fits the existing healthcare system with minimalistic configurations. As indicated in the figure, the CDI is an independent entity and operates between the application and data layers. In this chapter, we illustrate one specific functionality of CDI: user data retrieval and storage process.

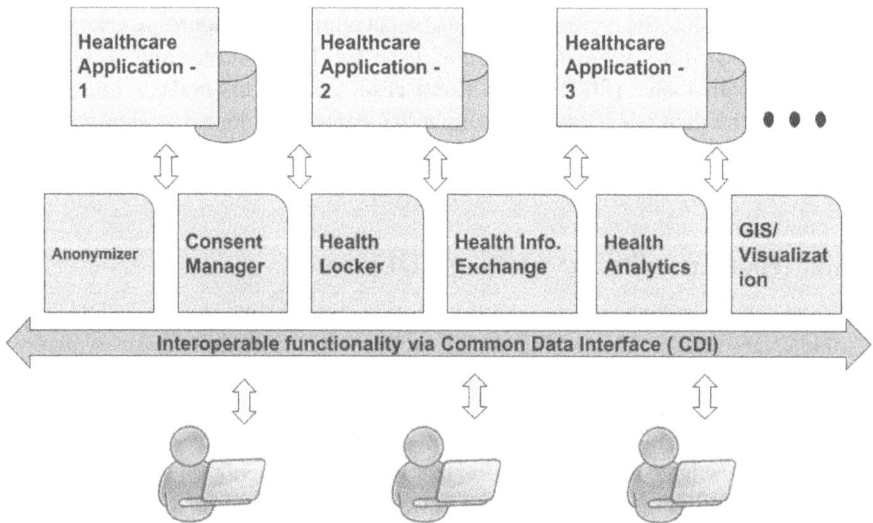

FIGURE 1.2   Interoperable functionality representation.

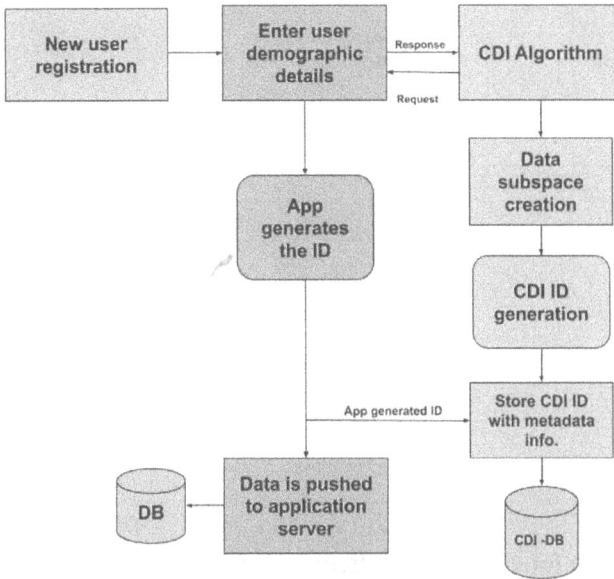

FIGURE 1.3 CDI – new user registration process.

Figure 1.3 shows the new user registration process via a CDI. The registration process follows the regular data flow. However, the CDI algorithm via API fetches the user demographic details and process the demographic details to create the data subspaces. The figure illustrates the data subspaces creation and mapping process. Further, the data subspaces are assigned with a unique CDI ID as defined in the section. Finally, the CDI ID, data subspaces, and application-generated user ID are stored in the CDI server for further processing.

The assumption of a new and existing user is as follows:

- **New user:** Refers to newly introduced to the healthcare application. No previous health records.
- **Existing user:** Refers to all stakeholders who have registered to at least one healthcare application.

The detailed process of the CDI algorithm is indicated considering new and existing patient scenarios.

1.4.3.1 New Patient Registration

Step 1: Fetch user demographic data.
Step 2: Create data subspace of demographic data.
Step 3: Assign unique CDI ID for data subspace.
Step 4: Get the corresponding application user ID and link it to CDI ID.
Step 5: Store the CDI ID along with data subspace and application user ID.

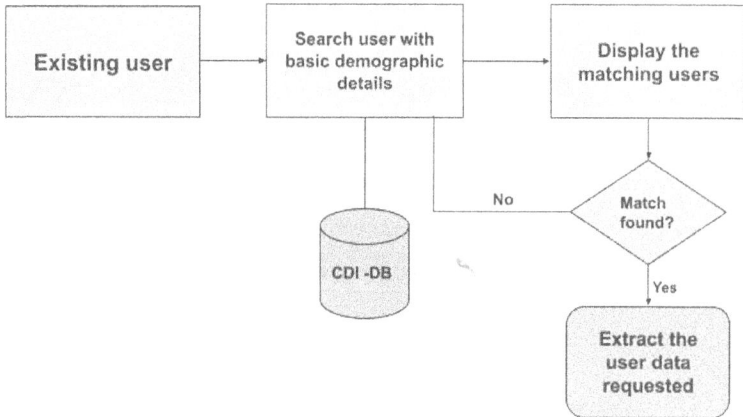

FIGURE 1.4   Existing user registration process.

1.4.3.2   Search for an Existing Patient in Application Database

Patients who have made more than one visit to any health facility fall under the existing patient category. In the existing scenario of the healthcare system, patient data is stored in multiple databases. All of these applications work in a silo. We can make these applications interoperable under certain conditions by introducing the proposed CDI layer to its architecture. The application's interoperability is via the CDI layer, with the existing patient's metadata information in its server repository. The data flow of this process is as indicated in Figure 1.4.

1.4.3.3   Existing Patient Information Extraction Process

> **Step 1:** Input the user query (with demographic data).
> **Step 2:** Semantic search operation for data subspace match.
> **Step 3:** Match found – proceed with step 4, else repeat step 1.
> **Step 4:** Extract user details considering various applications.

1.4.3.4   Searching for Patient Data in a Federated System

In healthcare, patient data is generated from a variety of healthcare applications. With the advancement of technologies (K. Paramesha et al. 2021), we generate enormous amounts of data with health gadgets. When these applications work and function in a silo, the main challenge is integration. To make these applications talk to each other for data exchange, we need to make them interoperable. The best and feasible solution is to adopt the healthcare standards discussed in the earlier sections. But in the present scenario, the existing healthcare applications have already been developed and been in use for a long time. These have many data repositories, so we need a smart and innovative approach to handle the existing data and make it interoperable. We are proposing a middleware-based approach with this vision. This CDI is yet to be implemented and tested. However, it is compatible with new and existing data processing. The technology behind this is purely based on semantic interoperability.

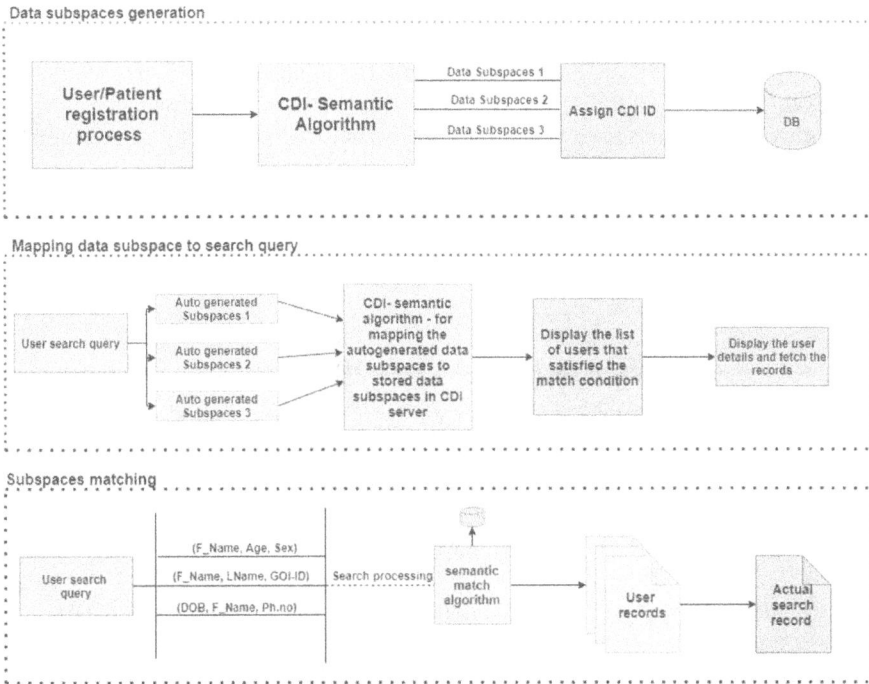

FIGURE 1.5 Data subspace generation and processing in CDI layer.

The data subspaces are generated as shown in Figure 1.5. The patient demographic details are fetched using the API interface between the health applications and the CDI server.

With the demographic details, using the combination technique, the data is categorized into subspaces. Further, these subspaces are assigned with the unique system-generated CDI ID number. The data subspaces are the reference data that are generated considering the patient demographic details. Further, as indicated in Figure 1.5, patient data is processed. The patient data extraction starts with the user query that is further processed to generate data subspace based on the query's parameters. Then, the match for the auto-generated subspaces from the user query is searched with the CDI server repository with the metadata information. Once the match is found, the data is extracted based on the application selected by the same. A detailed illustration of the same is indicated in Figure 1.5.

1.4.3.5 Use Case

Consider a scenario where we need to find the patient data across an application database. Let's assume the patient is PX121, and he is registered with many health care providers. When a query is entered to search for his clinical records, the request is processed via the CDI layer, which uses the semantic search technique proposed in Section 1.4. Accordingly, the list of matching patient information is listed for user selection. The workflow of the same is illustrated in Figure 1.5.

1.4.4   CDI SUBSPACE CREATION

The subspace for the data is created based on the number of attributes available. For example, suppose set A has "n" elements, then several subspaces of A are 2^n. Figure 1.5 indicates the subspace generation mechanism in detail. For example, consider a case where the following attributes of patients are captured:

- **P_name:** Patient's name.
- **DOB:** Patient's date of birth.
- **Gender:** Patient's gender.

GIVEN A SET A{P_NAME, DOB, GENDER}

Cardinality of **n(A) = 3**
Total Subspace of **A = 8**
i.e. S_1{P_name} S_2{DOB} S_3{gender} S_4{P_name, DOB} S_5 {P_name, gender}
S_6 {P_name, DOB, gender} S_7{gender, DOB} S_8{$^\phi$}

Now consider the power set, that is, all subspaces of the given set A, denoted as P(A).

P(A) = set of all possible subspaces of A
$P(A) = 2^A = \{S_1, S_2, S_3, S_4, S_5, S_6, S_7, S_8\}$
$P(A) = 2^A = \{\{P\_name\}$ S_2{DOB} S_3{gender} S_4{P_name, DOB} S_5 {P_name, gender}
S_6 {P_name, DOB, gender} S_7{gender, DOB} S_8{$^\phi$}}

Further P(A) is given as the input to the semantic algorithm for finding the best match of patient record.

The semantic search is very useful for retrieving the most relevant result from the data repository. The approach of NLP makes this task easier. The context-based analysis in NLP verifies the unique CDI ID code and accordingly processes the search result. For instance, if we need to search for a hospital in a particular district, the search query first identifies the district code by checking for the facility code and then processing the query request. Once the facility is identified as the hospital, the search is done only for the repository about the hospital databases.

General workflow:

Step1: Identify the district and taluk code.
Step2: Verify the facility identification code – **"understand the query intent."**
Step3: Search operation based on the intent – patient/hospital/lab etc.
Step4: Understand the conceptual similarity.
Step5: Validate the data to match.

TABLE 1.2
Indicating the Metadata Table Format of CDI Server DB

Index	CDI ID	Subspace Data	App1ID	App2ID	App3ID	App4ID	...
1	231312002316	xxxxxxxxx	12xxxx	23xxx	Axxx2	FxxxH2	-
2	481311022381	Xxxxxxxxx	13xxxx	-	-	SxxxF7	-
...	...	...	...	...	...	...	...

1.4.5 CDI ID Process and Reference Model

The CDI layer will have a data repository. All the healthcare stakeholder information is stored in the format shown in Table 1.2.

Table 1.2 shows the sample data attributes and their values, and "..." (three dots) signifies that it has many records. We have indicated only two records for our illustration. Patients can be registered with one or many healthcare applications. For example, consider row 2 in Table 1.2: patient with CDI ID 481311022381 is registered with health application 1 and application 4. So when we query to obtain his details, the query is processed with this application only. The CDI ID is a unique number generated by the CDI server with the corresponding patient ID of various applications. Metadata is stored in the CDI server.

1.4.6 CDI ID Format

Generating a unique ID is an important aspect of any application integration. Unfortunately, having the common ID across the application is not possible considering the current healthcare system architecture and design. So we propose a novel method for generating the unique ID for operating the CDI layer. The CDI ID is used as a unique ID for making applications interoperable.

1.4.6.1 Novel Unique ID Design

Figure 1.6 represents the 12-digit unique number generation mechanism to be followed by the CDI layer.

The unique ID comes with twelve (12) digit length and has three segments as indicated in figure. In the first segment, each district and taluk are mapped with a

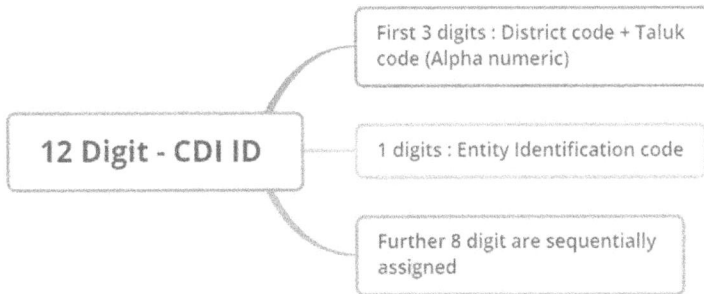

First 3 digits : District code + Taluk code (Alpha numeric)

12 Digit - CDI ID

1 digits : Entity Identification code

Further 8 digit are sequentially assigned

FIGURE 1.6 CDI ID format.

three-digit alphanumeric number which is predefined in the system and automatically assigned based on patient's demographic data. The next segment is the identification code. The detailed identification code types are represented in Figure 1.7. The identification code is useful in reducing the search mechanism in the CDI server. With the identification code, the algorithm can identify the respective facility and reduce the search operations. The identification code is generally used to indicate

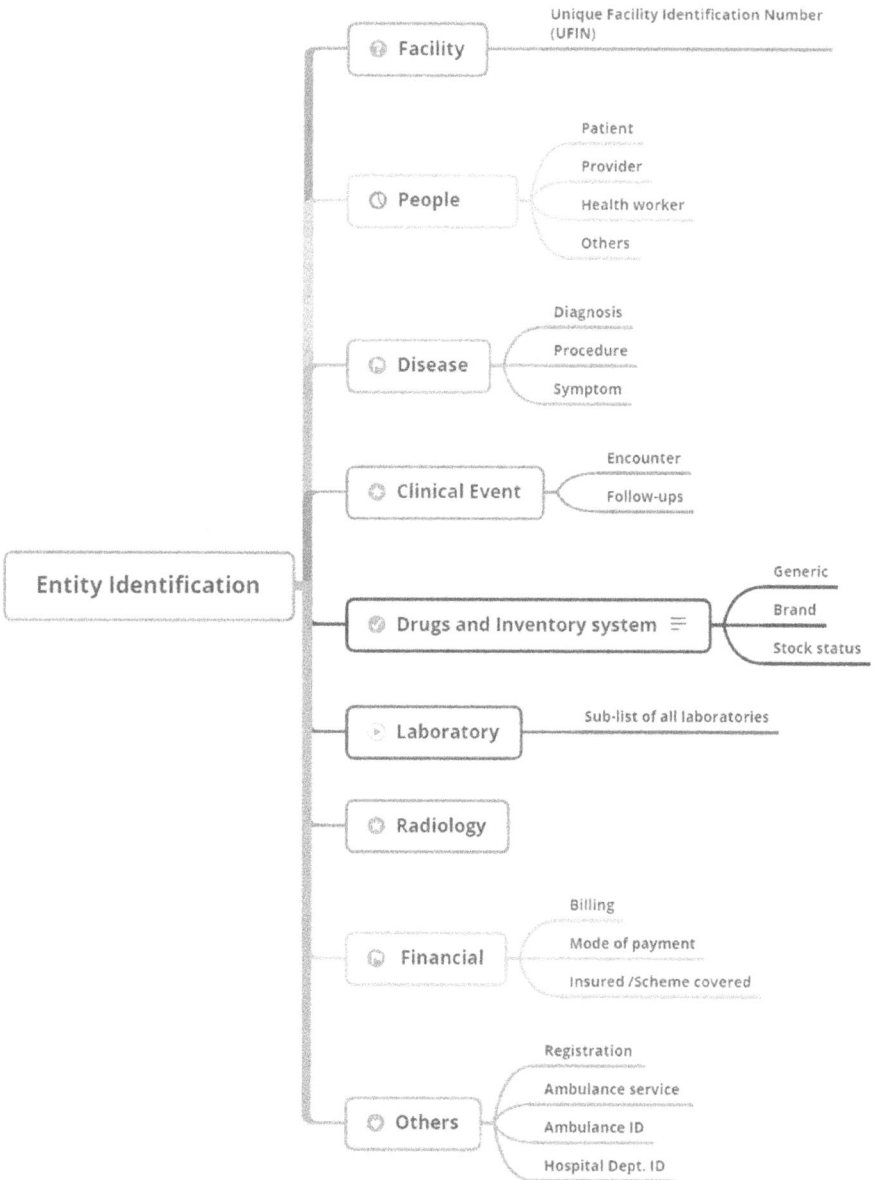

FIGURE 1.7   Types of facilities in the healthcare ecosystem.

the particular stakeholders referred to in the healthcare ecosystem. This is important to identify each entity or service of the healthcare system uniquely for efficient, interoperable operation. The identification code can indicate whether the CDI ID is a person or a disease, or a lab. This feature will generate the aggregated information referring to two different entities of the same district and taluk. The remaining eight digits is a sequential number that is assigned. The combination of district + taluk + facility identification + sequential number = unique CDI ID.

Referring to Figure 1.6, the unique ID has one segment which indicates the entity identification code. The various elements of healthcare ecosystem will be identified using the entity segment. It is one-digit length.

1.5   DISCUSSION AND CONCLUSION

This chapter illustrates the semantic interoperability and methodology of incorporating interoperability using CDI middleware. First, the approach for what is available and what needs to be incorporated is constructed. Second, this chapter aims to answer how interoperability can be achieved without altering the existing silo systems, including how data is structured for interoperable function and how unique IDs can be used for interoperability. The initial discussion is about the existing healthcare system and the available healthcare standards for interoperability, while the third part explains the CDI layer and its importance in achieving interoperability for sustainable healthcare.

Connected healthcare improves doctor and patient communication by reducing the existing hurdles for which interoperability plays a major role. The high-level architecture also aims to support health analytics like prediction based on the aggregated data generated by different healthcare applications. The connected healthcare system is a means to analyze the schemes and facilities, and it measures the healthcare program's outcome. The ultimate goal is to define scalable architecture with middleware that handles the interoperable operations. This chapter aims to improve the digital healthcare system by the connected approach that will eventually lead to interoperable and sustainable healthcare systems. In our ongoing work, an attempt is made to connect the patient health records using semantic interoperability. Further, we are yet to use the semantic mapping of local terms to standard terminologies using ontology-based methodology.

1.6   FUTURE ENHANCEMENT

The system will be completely interoperable only when all laboratories collaborate with clinical providers to adopt and use standardized vocabularies/terminologies. This will impact broader public health activities and costs associated with using electronic information systems. The limitation of this chapter is incorporating standard vocabularies to CDI layer functionality. The ontology-based approach can be used to achieve the same in further work. Also, the data in the CDI server can be represented in the semantic net formats by which more relevant and search results can be drawn.

ACKNOWLEDGMENTS

This work is supported in part by the Department of Health and Family Welfare Services, Government of Karnataka, India. We also thank the E-Health section of KHFWS for continuous support and encouragement in this work. Finally, we would like to thank two anonymous reviewers and editors of this chapter for commenting on earlier versions of this chapter.

REFERENCES

Aggarwal, M., and M. Madhukar (2017) IBM's Watson analytics for health care: A miracle made true. In: Cloud Computing Systems and Applications in Healthcare. IGI Global, 117–134. 10.4018/978-1-5225-1002-4.ch007

Alterovitz, G., D. Dean, C. Goble, M. R. Crusoe, S. Soiland-Reyes, A. Bell et al. (2018) Enabling precision medicine via standard communication of HTS provenance, analysis, and results. PLoS Biol 16(12): e3000099. https://doi.org/10.1371/journal.pbio.3000099

Alterovitz, G., B. Heale, J. Jones, et al. (2020) FHIR Genomics: Enabling standardization for precision medicine use cases. NPJ Genomic Medicine 5(13). https://doi.org/10.1038/s41525-020-0115-6

Alterovitz, G., J. Warner, P. Zhang, Y. Chen, M. Ullman-Cullere, D. Kreda, I.S. Kohane (2015) SMART on FHIR Genomics: Facilitating standardized clinico-genomic apps. Journal of the American Medical Informatics Association 22(6):1173–78. https://doi.org/10.1093/jamia/ocv045

Batra, U., S. Mukherjee, A. Nandal, S. Sachdeva (2014) Explorative study of healthcare data interchange standards. Journal of Theoretical and Applied Information Technology 63(2): 420–430.

Bayer, R., J. Santelli, R. Klitzman (2015) New challenges for electronic health records: Confidentiality and access to sensitive health information about parents and adolescents. JAMA 313(1):29–30. https://doi.org/10.1001/jama.2014.15391

Benson, T, G. Grieve (2016) Principles of health interoperability. Health Information Technology Standards. London, Springer-Verlag. https://doi.org/10.1007/978-3-319-30370-3_2

Dutta Pramanik, P. K., S. Pal, M. Mukhopadhyay (2019) Healthcare big data: A comprehensive overview. In: Intelligent Systems for Healthcare Management and Delivery 2019:72–100. https://doi.org/10.4018/978-1-5225-7071-4.ch004

Garde, S., P. Knaup, E.J. Hovenga, and S. Heard (2007) Towards semantic interoperability for electronic health records. Methods of Information in Medicine 46(03):332–43.

Heflin, J. D., and J. Hendler (2000) Semantic interoperability on the web. Proceedings of Extreme Markup Languages 2000.

Hu, B., Y. Kalfoglou, H. Alani, D. Dupplaw, P. Lewis, N. Shadbolt (2006) Semantic metrics. In: Staab S., Svátek V. (eds) Managing knowledge in a world of networks. EKAW 2006. Lecture Notes in Computer Science, vol 4248. Berlin, Heidelberg, Springer. https://doi.org/10.1007/11891451_17

ISO/TR 20514:2005 (2005) Health informatics – Electronic health record – Definition, scope, and context by ISO/TC 215, Multiple. Distributed through American National Standards Institute, 1–27.

Khamparia, A., P. K. Singh, P. Rani, D. Samanta, A. Khanna, B. Bhushan (2020) An internet of health things-driven deep learning framework for detection and classification of skin cancer using transfer learning. Transactions on Emerging Telecommunication Technologies: e3963. https://doi.org/10.1002/ett.3963

Kiourtis, A., S. Nifakos, A. Mavrogiorgou, and D. Kyriazis (2019) Aggregating the syntactic and semantic similarity of healthcare data towards their transformation to HL7 FHIR through ontology matching. International Journal of Medical Informatics 132:104002. doi: 10.1016/j.ijmedinf.2019.104002.

MedLine Plus (2018) High blood pressure. Retrieved, 19 April 2018. https://medlineplus.gov/highbloodpressure.html

NRC. EHR Standards for India. Retrieved, 2020 https://nrces.in/standards/ehr-standards-for-india#standards_at_a_glance

The Open Group Healthcare Forum (2015) Enhancing health information exchange with the FHIM: Introduction, evaluation, suggestions, and next steps, White Papers in Healthcare, 20.

Paramesha, K., H. L. Gururaj, O. P. Jena (2021) Applications of machine learning in biomedical text processing and food industry. In: Sachi Nandan Mohanty, G. Nalinipriya, Om Prakash Jena, Achyuth Sarkar (eds) Machine Learning for Healthcare Applications. Wiley [Online]. https://doi.org/10.1002/9781119792611.ch10

Panigrahi, N., I. Ayus, O. P. Jena (2021) An Expert System-Based Clinical Decision Support System for Hepatitis-B Prediction & Diagnosis. Wiley [Online]. https://doi.org/10.1002/9781119792611.ch4

Patra, S. S., O. P. Jena, G. Kumar, S. Pramanik, C. Misra, K. N. Singh (2021) Random Forest algorithm in imbalance genomics classification. In: Rabinarayan Satpathy, Tanupriya Choudhury, Suneeta Satpathy, Sachi Nandan Mohanty, Xiaobo Zhang (eds) Data Analytics in Bioinformatics: A Machine Learning Perspective. Wiley, [Online]. https://doi.org/10.1002/9781119785620.ch7

Pattnayak, P., O. P. Jena (2021) Innovation on machine learning in healthcare services – An introduction. In: Sachi Nandan Mohanty, G. Nalinipriya, Om Prakash Jena, Achyuth Sarkar (eds) Machine Learning for Healthcare Applications. Wiley [Online]. https://doi.org/10.1002/9781119792611.ch1

Philips (USA) (2018). "A Cloud-based Platform: Purpose-built for Healthcare". Retrieved July 24, 2017, from http://www.usa.philips.com/healthcare/innovation/about-health-suite

Pijush Kanti D. P.,, S. Pal, and M. Mukhopadhyay (2019) Healthcare big data: A comprehensive overview. Intelligent Systems for Healthcare Management and Delivery : 72–100.

Rana, A. K. et al. Machine learning methods for IoT and their future applications (2019) International Conference on Computing, Communication, and Intelligent Systems (ICCCIS) (2019): 430–34.

Schulz, S., C. Martínez-Costa (2013) How Ontologies Can Improve Semantic Interoperability in Health Care. Lecture Notes in Computer Science. Heidelberg, Springer International Publishing.

Schulz, S., R. Stegwee, C. Chronaki (2019) Standards in healthcare data. In: Kubben P, Dumontier M, Dekker A. (eds) Fundamentals of Clinical Data Science. Cham, Springer. https://doi.org/10.1007/978-3-319-99713-1_3

Teodoro, D., R. Choquet, D. Schober, G. Mels, E. Pasche, P. Ruch, C. Lovis (2011) Interoperability driven integration of biomedical data sources. Studies in Health Technology and Informatics 169:185–9.

Young, P., N. Chaki, V. Berzins, Luqi (2003) Evaluation of middleware architectures in achieving system interoperability. Rapid Systems Prototyping Proceedings, 14th IEEE International Workshop, 108–116.

2 Brain–Computer Interface
Review, Applications and Challenges

Prashant Sengar and Shawli Bardhan

CONTENTS

2.1 INTRODUCTION

A BCI provides an interface between the brain and the computer. Also called a mind–machine interface or brain–machine interface, it does not require the use of muscles to interact with a computer. It instead employs sensors attached directly to the brain to transfer those signals to a computer. BCI has found its application in medical fields where these devices are used by patients in locked-in state to communicate with their caretakers. A number of BCI devices are also used to augment and/or assist motor functions including the use of prosthesis [1]. The main advantage of using BCI-based devices is that they work even if the patient faces nervous damage due to the fact that the signals are not transmitted through nerves to the prosthetic implant, but rather through the BCI device directly from the brain. Recently, BCI is finding its use in various other non-medical fields including authentication, controlling robots or other moving devices, and also communication [2–4]. It also faces challenges in protecting the privacy of users and reducing the cost of hardware used.

The natural way for humans to communicate is by using their muscles by either making gestures, creating sound using their throat and other muscles, or other means. The person communicated to watches the actions or listens to the sounds and

DOI: 10.1201/9781003226147-2

deciphers the message communicated. The process consists of the brain generating electrical signals which are then sent to the muscle group which has to perform the action, via the nervous system.

A similar process is followed when a person wants to communicate with a computer using a keyboard or a mouse or another input device. This can be called human–computer interaction. This is improved using other input devices like a microphone and camera through which a person can speak or issue commands using their voice or facial expressions. This can further be improved if we send the brain's electrical signals directly to the computer. This communication process is referred to as the brain–computer interface.

One of the first definitions of BCI, given by Jonathon R. Wolpaw in 1999, is [5]:

> A brain-computer interface (BCI) is a communication or control system in which the user's messages or commands do not depend on the brain's normal output channels. That is, the message is not carried by nerves and muscles and furthermore, neuromuscular activity is not needed to produce the activity that does carry the message.

A more recent definition given by the same author is as follows [6]:

> A BCI is a system that measures central nervous system (CNS) activity and converts it into artificial out-put that replaces, restores, enhances, supplements, improves natural CNS output and thereby changes the ongoing interactions between the CNS and its external or internal environment.

BCI works by first acquiring the brain signals, then extracting the intentions of those signals and then translating those signals to commands to the BCI application. An illustration of a BCI system is shown in Figure 2.1. This was presented by Jack Vidal in 1973.

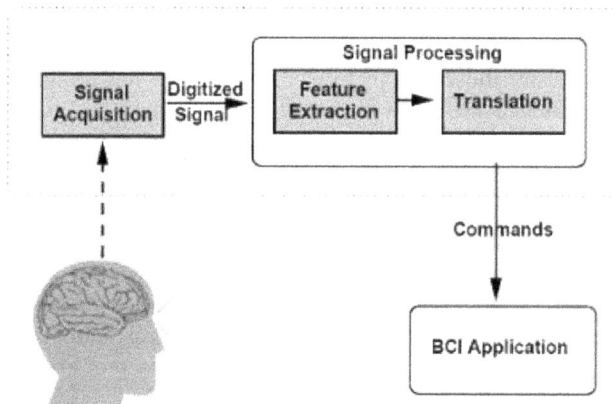

FIGURE 2.1   Brain–computer interface [see [7]].

2.1.1 Phases of a BCI

The following sections can be said as the phases of a BCI.

2.1.1.1 Signal Acquisition

The human brain communicates to other parts of the body with the help of electrical signals which produce electric and magnetic fields. To know what the brain intends to do, we first have to measure those signals. There are three types of methods of signal acquisition which follow the similar technique of placing sensors at or near those parts of the brain which generate the specific kinds of signals that we wish to listen to. There are three suitable techniques to acquire the signals by recording the electrical or magnetic fields using suitable devices:

1. **Invasive methods:** In invasive methods of signal acquisition, the electrodes are placed on the surface of cortex by surgical methods. These methods offer a great resolution but suffer from a number of disadvantages. Apart from the issues due to surgery, the electrodes once placed cannot be moved to another part of the brain to measure other signals. Therefore, invasive methods are restricted to being used in tests on animals and medical usage by a few patients.
2. **Partially invasive methods:** This involves placing the recording device on the surface of the cortex. This has lower signal strength but prevents scarring of the brain tissue.
3. **Non-invasive methods:** For a more widespread and easier use of BCI, it is necessary to remove the surgical aspect of it. Non-invasive methods of signal acquisition place electrical rods at the scalp to measure the signal. It has poor signal strength in comparison to the other invasive methods, but it can always be improved to have a decent resolution. It also makes the implementation easier versus needing a surgery to place the signal acquiring electrodes.

The most common method is recording the electrical signals from the brain called electroencephalography. Since electrical fields also produce magnetic fields, it is possible to measure the magnetic fields similarly by a process called magnetoencephalography.

- **Electroencephalography (EEG):** In EEG, we record the brain activity of a person by measuring the electrical signals produced. In this method, electrodes are placed on the scalp of the subject. The main advantage of EEG is that it offers high temporal resolution [8]. One of the disadvantages of EEG is the amount of noise that can be present in the generated signal. To reduce the environmental noise, gels are being used which are applied on the scalp. Since wet gels dry up after some time, better dry electrodes with low impedance are being developed with similar or even better signal-to-noise ratio [9]. Electrodes are also safe in the long term as well.

- **Magnetoencephalography (MEG):** In MEG, we record the brain activity of a person by measuring the magnetic fields produced. It has a great spatial resolution, but the device needs to be kept very close the brain surface since the magnetic fields generated by neurons are very small in magnitude.
- **Functional Magnetic Resonance Imaging (fMRI):** In fMRI, the oxygen levels of the brain are measured during any activity. It results in high spatial resolution. It offers great insight into which parts of the brain are active during a particular activity.

2.1.1.2   Feature Extraction

After acquiring the signal, the next step is extracting the features from the signal. Removing noise and artifacts, smoothening the signal is required because noise gets added and dampened due to muscular activity while recording the signals. Different methods such as linear, adaptive, and spatial filtering are used for the same.

2.1.1.3   Signal Classification

After extracting the features of the signals, they are used in classification to convert them into actions. Different machine learning algorithms like the linear discriminant analysis (LDA), Hidden Markov Model, k-NN are used in the step for the classification process.

The field of BCI is getting popular with recent efforts from the private company Neuralink to get BCI devices into the mainstream. Focusing on the recent developments in the field of BCI, the first objective of this chapter is to demonstrate a comprehensive survey related to recent advancement of BCI. The second objective includes the popular application areas of BCI along with the issues and challenges related to the application and methodologies. In summary. the paper contains the details of recent advancements in the area of BCI systems and their applications. Relating to the recent developments, the paper describes the issues and challenges of BCI which requires further developments.

The remaining of this chapter is organized as follows: Section 2.2 contains the review related to the recent studies on BCI with Table 2.1 summarizing the literature reviewed, Section 2.3 summarizes the application areas of BCI, and Section 2.4 focused on the recent issues and challenges present in BCI development. Finally, the conclusion and future work are presented in Section 2.5.

2.2   REVIEW WORK

There has been a lot of work during the past few years in the field of BCI to build cost-effective and accurate devices for the common usage.

In 2015 Martin Spuler [10] in his study tried to create a system to allow users to control the mouse and keyboard directly using BCI, thus enabling them to control arbitrary applications. A 32-channel EEG setup was used to measure the electrical signals and extended the Tubingen c-VEP software to allow direct control over mouse and keyboard input. There have been applications for painting, browsing, and other uses but the BCI system could only control that single dedicated application.

TABLE 2.1

Literature Review on BCI

Publication Year & Reference	Objective	Methods	Data	BCI Setup and Software	Results
2013 [19]	To control an artificial arm to grab and move a target to a final location using motor imagery	Subjects imagined different movements recorded EEG signal sent to application to move the robotic arm	2 healthy participant, 1 post-stroke patient	Neuroscan cap (64 channels) JACO arm, BCI2000	Vertical arm claw accuracy: 24.7%, horizontal arm claw accuracy: 12%
2015 [10]	To allow users to control mouse and keyboard using BCI	c-VEP based system with 32 visual stimuli	Not mentioned	32 channel EEG setup Tubingen C-VEP BCI	Controlling the PC using mouse and computer
2016 [1]	To control a prosthetic arm using an EEG based BCI	NeuroSky headset to record brain EEG waves, MATLAB's® ThinkGear module for processing. Transmitted to the microcontroller for control	One user	Neurosky headset MATLAB®	Flexion and extension of fingers of prosthetic arm using BCI signals
2016 [11]	Classification of left and right movement	Discrete Wavelet Transform to extract features from signals, SVM to classify	NUST dataset Male, Right-handed Age – 21 years	Not mentioned	Possible to classify brain waves as intending to move right or left hand
2017 [26]	To create a hybrid non-invasive BCI to control devices	ANN based classification for SSVEP based EEG channels and microcontroller sensor to record neurophysiological changes	5 persons with no medical condition Age – 25–35 years 5 spinal cord injury patients Age – 45–80 years	Not mentioned	Average classification accuracy of 74% and information transfer rate (ITR) of 27 bits/min
2018 [9]	Comparing dry and wet electrodes-based EEG systems	Two sessions, one each using wet and dry EEG system, for 27 participants	27 participants in 2 recording sessions	Wet electrodes, wired Dry electrodes, wireless	Dry EEG can record electrophysiological signals without any sufficient decrease in quality
2018 [20]	Classification of BCI data using CNN	Feature extraction using filter-bank common spatial patterns	2008 BCI competition IV-2a EEG dataset	Not mentioned	Average accuracy of 74.46

(Continued)

TABLE 2.1 (Continued)
Literature Review on BCI

Publication Year & Reference	Objective	Methods	Data	BCI Setup and Software	Results
2018 [21]	Study of a multi-modal feedback based BCI	AV feedback using velocity control vector, decoding by Kalman filter	16 participants over 3 sessions	64-channel acquisition system	Audio Video feedback accuracy: 68.3%
2019 [17]	To create a BCI system to allow free communication	CA SSVEP based BCI speller with asynchronous communication	17 participants with no BCI experience	Not mentioned	Classification accuracy of 96% and 88% for 2 participants
2019 [18]	Controlling an arm using computer vision and BCI	In a clean workspace, users asked to grasp an object using BCI with CV guided robots	11 healthy participants, accuracy tested on 5 of them	UR5 robot	Average success rate of 73.74%,70.94%, 35.62% over 3 sessions
2019 [22]	Assessing effects of complex visual stimuli on P300 BCI	Participants shown specific stimuli collections: flashing letters, neutral pictures, emotional pleasant pictures, emotional unpleasant pictures	23 volunteers controlled 4 spellers	BCI2000	99.64% accuracy (highest) for Emotionally Pleasant Pictures (EPP), ITR of 46.07 bits/min
2019 [31]	Use BCI to control AR based smart home	SSVEP based BCI, along with eye tracking, looked at an object to select it	12 participants went through 36 trials	HoloSSVEP, g.Nautilus head-set	89.3% accuracy for EyeTracking and BCI combined system
2020 [23]	EEG image classification using deep neural network	Deep convolutional neural network for extraction of features	Physionet dataset	Not mentioned	Classification accuracy of 68.72%
2020 [24]	3D Robot arm control using EEG signals	Multi-directional convolution neural network	15 participants, 11 male, 4 female Age: 25–31 years	JACO arm, 64 electrodes cap BrainAmp	60% success rate
2020 [25]	EEG classification using personalization-based design	Stacked long short-term memory	4 participants	Low cost, off-the-shelf EEG headset	0.975 classification accuracy

In their study about identifying hand movement using BCI, Pattnaik et al. [11] demonstrated how one could implement left- and right-hand movement classification from the EEG signals recorded. They showed that these waves can be divided into constituent alpha, beta, and delta waves by various sampling methods such as discrete wavelet transform, and these could be used as the feature vector for classifiers in support vector machines (SVMs).

Seo-Hyun Lee et al. [12] in their work on imagined speech and visual imagery in 2019 tried to create an application that could detect what the user wanted to speak using BCI. They compared imagined speech (imagining the literals of the word to be spoken) and visual imagery (imagining the object when trying to speak that word). They used a 64-channel EEG cap to measure the brain signals and employed multiclass classification of more than 10 classes in both paradigms.

In the study based on authenticating users in a virtual reality (VR)-based environment, Sukun Li et al. [13] studied whether active portions of the brain are influenced by the presence of VR and use it for authentication. In the study, 32 participants were shown a video in a VR and non-VR setup and their brain signals were recorded and analyzed to authenticate them. The best classification accuracy was achieved up to 80.91%. It was demonstrated that a BCI could be used to recognize a user even in a virtual environment.

In the study based on a gaming system using a steady state visually evoked potential BCI (SSVEP-BCI), Nayak et al. [14] designed an SSVEP-based computer game based on Jewel Quest. They used a 32-channel Neuroscan system for recording brain signals and tried to improve rare target classifications characterized by class imbalance and overlap.

Bahman et al. [15] in their research to control a robot in 2019 designed a P300-based BCI system using a low-priced EEG headset. They recorded brain signals using a 14-channel Emotiv Epoc-EEG headset (shown in Figure 2.2) and created a graphical user interface (GUI) (shown in Figure 2.2) over BCI2000 to give directions. The study showed impressive results with 93.3% accuracy while detecting the direction. This paves the way for low cost BCI devices for regular usage.

There was another study in 2015 by Arunkumar et al. [3]. They used a NeuroSky BCI headset (shown in Figure 2.3) in their study to detect brain waves to control a robot wirelessly. The study was aimed at locked-in patients to control a robot using their attention level and eye blinks.

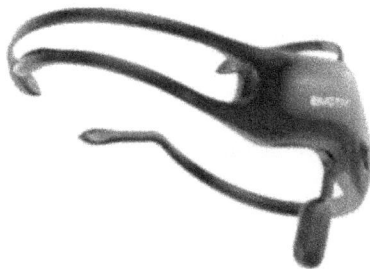

FIGURE 2.2   Emotiv Headset.

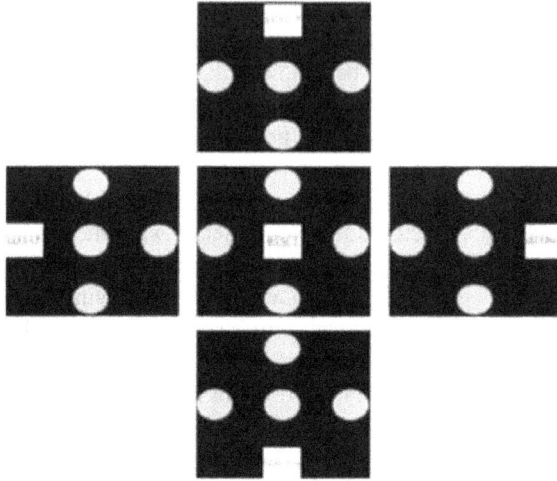

FIGURE 2.3   GUI designed for robot control [see [15]].

In their study on prosthetic arm control using BCI, Bright et al. [1] attempted to create a BCI for controlling an artificial arm. They too used a NeuroSky headset to record brain EEG waves, and used MATLAB®'s ThinkGear module for processing. These commands are then sent over to the microcontroller which controls the arm. They were able to control the movement of fingers by contracting and expanding them. The researchers plan to upscale this system to support full range of motion of the arm.

Kama et al. [9] in their work in 2018 compared EEG systems with dry and wet electrodes. They worked with the same 27 participants with both dry and wet electrodes on different days. They were able to conclude that both types of electrodes give comparable results and that dry electrodes do not compromise the quality of EEG signals when compared to wet electrodes. Thus, they could be used at most of the places instead of wet electrodes. They are also preferred for the low preparation effort (Figure 2.4).

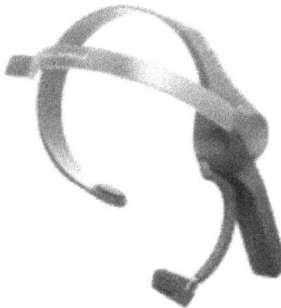

FIGURE 2.4   NeuroSky MindWave Sensor.

In their study to control a smart home using eye movements, Putze et al. [16] worked on a BCI-based AR system. They used an SSVEP-based BCI, along with a binocular eye tracker, where the participants selected an object by gazing at it. BCI tracking had lower accuracy than when it was combined with eye tracking, which had an accuracy of 89.3%.

Renton et al. [17] in their study on human communication using BCI introduced a system for free communication between participants without any fixed phrases or cues. They created an asynchronous two-user messaging interface that allowed the users to freely communicate. With high accuracy ranging from 88% to 96%, the researchers mention that the focus of communication-based BCI setups should be on usability rather than speed.

In the study to compare BCI-based systems with augmented BCI to control a synthetic arm, Xu et al. [18] implemented a system that uses computer vision coupled with BCI for controlling a robot arm. The BCI system was based on motor-imagery and it had a good success rate of more than 70%. They noted that the unsuccessful trials were due to poor guidance while using BCI. The researchers also mention that one of the reasons for such high accuracy was that they had only one object in the workspace.

In the study to control a prosthetic arm using EEG-based BCI, Baxter et al. [19] tried to create a convenient system for controlling an artificial arm. The participants imagined moving their left and right hands to move the respective arms. Similarly, other such visualized movements were used by the BCI system to map a specific hand movement. They had significant success with the system having an accuracy of 24.7% and 12% in vertical and horizontal arm claw movement, respectively.

Sakhavi et al. [20], in their work to classify BCI information, utilized convolutional neural networks to create a new classification framework. Most of the previous classification frameworks were solely based on energy values and neglected temporal information which was utilized by the researchers in this study. They used filter-bank common spatial patterns for feature extraction and achieved an accuracy of 74.46%.

In their study of BCI systems with audio-visual (AV) feedback, Brumberg et al. [21] researched multimodal feedback on real-time speech synthesis using BCI. Three different groups received only one of visual, audio, or both audio and video feedback of their BCI synthesized speech. They noticed that the AV feedback had the highest accuracy of 68.3% compared to 47.2% and 50.1% of video only and audio only feedback respectively.

In their study on a P300 based BCI speller, Fernández et al. [22] assess P300 based spellers which work with complex visual stimuli. Participants were flashed with visual stimuli which included pictures which were emotionally pleasing or unpleasing. Emotionally pleasant pictures were detached in P300 BCI with an accuracy of 99.64%. Such picture sets could thus be used for visual P300-based BCI applications.

In their study to classify chessboard EEG images, Fadel et al. [23] used a deep convolutional neural network (DCNN) along with long short-term memory. They extracted spatial, frequency, and temporal features to classify them into one of either four different motor imagery classes or rest class. They had a classification accuracy of 68.72% compared to SVM's 64.64% accuracy.

Jeon et al. [24] developed a system to control three-dimensional movement of a robotic arm using a deep learning methodology which used a multi-directional convolution neural network. Over several trials with 11 participants, they used motor imagery to move the robotic arm. With a success rate of 60%, they demonstrated how deep learning also finds a role in motor imagery.

In their work in 2020, Wu et al. [25] developed a deep learning-based EEG classification framework. This uses a personalization module over long short-term memory structure to achieve high classification accuracy. The research demonstrated the use of pre-processing and personalization for better classification of individual EEG data which can be further used in applications.

2.3   APPLICATIONS

BCI has been useful in a lot of medical cases from allowing patients in locked-in state to communicate with their caretakers, to controlling wheelchairs and robots. A lot of applications and games have also been developed to induce relaxation and lower stress levels of the person wearing the BCI device. There are a lot of non-medical uses of BCI too, including authentication, communication, and entertainment.

There has been a lot of work to create BCI devices to control the movements of robots, including those based on P3000 potentials using an EEG headset [15]. This work by Bahman et al. [15] was attempted at high real-time accuracy using an EEG headset which was not very expensive. It can be useful for patients who cannot use a remote control for next-gen robot caretakers. Another such application was devised where the applicants tried to use their brain to control a robot arm. It was based on motor imagery and used a small setup [19].

A hybrid BCI (hBCI) system combines a BCI with other physiological or technical signals. hBCI systems have been used as a prosthesis in patients with spinal cord injury. The prosthesis was shown to be used for moving hands, and grasping and releasing objects. It is majorly suited for patients who have a damaged hand but with shoulder and elbow capable of movement. [27].

A lot of use cases of BCI from the medical field also find their place in various non-medical use cases. One of these is the attention-enhancing ball game [28]. The authors propose an EEG-based game where the user uses his/her attention to play. It is shown that it is able to increase the attention levels of the player using the feedback mechanism, taking advantage of the plastic nature of the brain. The game also features multiple difficulty levels for the user to enhance his/her attention level by training over a number of days.

There have also been attempts to create games using BCI as one of the input modalities along with keyboard, mouse, and joystick. Little similar to [28], Pope et al. in [29] also looked at the application of BCI to help kids with ADHD to improve their attention levels by using neuro feedback.

Another attempt to use hybrid BCI in a well-known game is found in [30] where a game similar to Jewel Quest is designed using BCI. It used SSVEP-based target classification without a cascading menu, thus, decreasing the time required to play.

Using other devices along with BCI has improved the classification accuracy as seen with [31] having an aim to control a home based on augment reality (AR) using

BCI. The system presented in the study does not require training and is easy to set up as well.

Another such application was seen in [18] where the researchers used a computer-guided system along with motor imagery-based BCI which allow the participants to move a robotic arm and grab an object.

One of the most interesting uses of BCI in non-medical fields is its use in authentication. Since the brain EEG activities of each person are unique, it can be used as an authentication method for unlocking devices and at other places where a pin or a password is required [13]. [20] has shown that it is possible to detect brain waves even in VR environments as in physical environments and hence it is possible both to confirm the user's authenticity and that he/she is in a virtual environment. It was also trialed to authenticate people in VR applications and it turned out to be very successful [13].

Another exciting prospect is controlling a computer without any peripheral device except the BCI. There have been successful attempts earlier to control a specific application using BCI such as the P300 speller which created a new application for typing using brain signals. Martin Spuler [10] has already shown a method to control any arbitrary application using brain signals. An application was developed to control the mouse and keyboard using the BCI based EEG signals. Other attempts such as [31] have created complete user systems integrating a browser, file manager, and other applications.

Another application of BCI is communication. This is complex, exciting, and unnerving at the same time. Various methods have been proposed for brain-to-brain communication, including connecting multiple animal brains to create an organic brain network [32]. It has also been shown that both visual imagery and imagined speech can be used in BCI applications to communicate using brain signals [12]. In the early stages, it is employed for patients with a disabled neurological system for communicating with their caretakers with a fixed set of words. Even for non-medical usage, it can be a game-changing idea. Another such method is explored in [21] where the user is given feedback on their synthesized BCI speech in real time to improve the user speech.

A lot of BCI spellers do not actually test on free communication but on guided cues and fixed phrases or words. In [17], the researchers tried to challenge the status quo by experimenting with free communication between different participants. They have also applied cross-classification, where the trained template from other users' experience could be used. This would completely eliminate training and users would be able to start communicating using BCI without any extra setup time.

2.4 ISSUES AND CHALLENGES

The current BCI technology faces a lot of hurdles before it could be brought to widespread use by the general public. First is the required hardware; BCI devices are still very cumbersome for regular usage and are expensive. Though there has been work in this area with new generation devices to measure brain waves such as commercially available devices like the NeuroSky headset, it will be some time before these devices will be used more commonly.

Another challenge that the field faces and which prevents a more widespread usage is the variable nature of the brain waves. Each person's brain waves are unique. Although the identifying features are the same, people have different mental abilities and attention spans. The data set for most of the studies is small with only a small number of participants are a part of them. Extensive testing is necessary to improve the techniques and to study them on a wider audience.

There is also the issue of privacy with BCI applications. BCI applications are allowed to read all the brain signals read by the headset. This could lead to the leak of information to authentic-looking, malicious applications which could later lead to awful consequences. Improving this aspect of BCI is also essential with its studies in the field of authentication. With newer applications every day, it is becoming easier to exploit someone who is not wary of such attacks [33].

There are also ethical considerations when trying to communicate using brain signals or when researchers try to create an organic computer by connecting multiple brains through the means of BCI. These questions need detailed discussion to reach a consensus.

2.5 CONCLUSION

BCI is an exciting field. With regular new advancements in machine learning, we are close to achieving the reality of communicating directly with the brain and doing many more such tasks without utilizing any muscles [34–47].

It has found applications in remote-controlling robots, wheelchairs, and prosthetic arms and legs thus helping immensely those who for any reason are not able to move their complete body or some specific parts of the body. BCI spellers and applications which allow the user to control the computer without peripheral devices also find use for many such patients suffering from diseases affecting their motor skills.

Other than applications specifically targeted for patients, there has been work lately on studies for other uses. Using brain waves for authentication and communication demands huge efforts in the future for these to be brought in publicly. The use of templates lifted from other users' experiences is also being attempted so that there is no training required before using the application. This brings in the issue of ease of use which is an important aspect when we talk about have widely accepted BCI.

Many such applications have already materialized, although in simpler forms, as seen above, but researchers keep on improving existing works. Along with the advancements, we also face the challenges that plague the field. One of the biggest issues that challenges the adoption of BCI is the price of the hardware used. Similarly, there is hesitancy in using BCI devices because of the privacy challenges. There are also the ethical considerations which must be kept in mind while working in the field.

REFERENCES

[1] Bright, Dany, Amrita Nair, Devashish Salvekar, and Swati Bhisikar. "EEG-based Brain Controlled Prosthetic Arm." *2016 Conference on Advances in Signal Processing (CASP)*, 2016. doi:10.1109/casp.2016.7746219

[2] Yousefi, Fares, Hoshang Kolivand, and Thar Baker. "SaS-BCI: A New Strategy to Predict Image Memorability and Use Mental Imagery as a Brain-based Biometric Authentication." *Neural Computing and Applications*, 2020. doi:10.1007/s00521-020-05247-1

[3] Stephygraph, L R, N Arunkumar, and V. Venkatraman. "Wireless Mobile Robot Control through Human Machine Interface Using Brain Signals." *2015 International Conference on Smart Technologies and Management for Computing, Communication, Controls, Energy and Materials (ICSTM)*, 2015. doi:10.1109/icstm.2015.7225484

[4] Soman, Sumit, and B K Murthy. "Using Brain Computer Interface for Synthesized Speech Communication for the Physically Disabled." *Procedia Computer Science* 46 (2015): 292–8. doi:10.1016/j.procs.2015.02.023

[5] Wolpaw, Jonathan R, Niels Birbaumer, Dennis J McFarland, Gert Pfurtscheller, and Theresa M Vaughan. "Brain–Computer Interfaces for Communication and Control." *Clinical Neurophysiology* 113, no. 6 (June 2002): 767–91. doi:10.1016/s1388-2457(02)00057-3

[6] Wolpaw, Jonathan R, and Elizabeth Winter Wolpaw. "Brain–Computer Interfaces: Something New under the Sun." In *Brain–Computer Interfaces Principles and Practice*, 3–12. Oxford University Press, 2012. doi:10.1093/acprof:oso/9780195388855.003.0001

[7] Vidal, J.. "Real-time detection of brain events in EEG." In *Special Issue on BiolSignal Processing and Analysis*. IEEE Proc, 1977. 633–664.

[8] Ramadan, Rabie A., and Athanasios V. Vasilakos. "Brain Computer Interface: Control Signals Review." *Neurocomputing* 223 (2017): 26–44. doi:10.1016/j.neucom.2016.10.024

[9] Kam, Julia W Y, Sandon Griffin, Alan Shen, Shawn Patel, Hermann Hinrichs, Hans-Jochen Heinze, Leon Y. Deouell, and Robert T. Knight. "Systematic Comparison between a Wireless EEG System with Dry Electrodes and a Wired EEG System with Wet Electrodes." *NeuroImage* 184 (January 2019): 119–29. doi:10.1016/j.neuroimage.2018.09.012

[10] Spuler, Martin. "A Brain-Computer Interface (BCI) System to Use Arbitrary Windows Applications by Directly Controlling Mouse and Keyboard." In *2015 37th Annual International Conference of the IEEE Engineering in Medicine and Biology Society (EMBC)*. IEEE, 2015. doi:10.1109/embc.2015.7318554

[11] Pattnaik, Prasant Kumar, and Jay Sarraf. "Brain Computer Interface Issues on Hand Movement." *Journal of King Saud University – Computer and Information Sciences* 30, no. 1 (January 2018): 18–24. doi:10.1016/j.jksuci.2016.09.006

[12] Lee, Seo-Hyun, Minji Lee, Ji-Hoon Jeong, and Seong-Whan Lee. "Towards an EEG-Based Intuitive BCI Communication System Using Imagined Speech and Visual Imagery." *2019 IEEE International Conference on Systems, Man and Cybernetics (SMC)*. IEEE, 2019. doi:10.1109/smc.2019.8914645

[13] Li, Sukun, Sonal Savaliya, Leonard Marino, Avery M. Leider, and Charles C. Tappert. "Brain Signal Authentication for Human-Computer Interaction in Virtual Reality." *2019 IEEE International Conference on Computational Science and Engineering (CSE) and IEEE International Conference on Embedded and Ubiquitous Computing (EUC)*. IEEE, 2019. doi:10.1109/cse/euc.2019.00031

[14] Nayak, Tapsya, Li-Wei Ko, Tzyy-Ping Jung, and Yufei Huang. "Target Classification in a Novel SSVEP-RSVP Based BCI Gaming System." *2019 IEEE International Conference on Systems, Man and Cybernetics (SMC)*. IEEE, 2019. doi:10.1109/smc.2019.8914174

[15] Bahman, Shafie, and Mohammad B. Shamsollahi. "Robot Control Using an Inexpensive P300 Based BCI." *2019 26th National and 4th International Iranian Conference on Biomedical Engineering (ICBME)*. IEEE, 2019. doi:10.1109/icbme49163.2019.9030408

[16] Putze, Felix, Dennis Weiss, Lisa-Marie Vortmann, and Tanja Schultz. "Augmented Reality Interface for Smart Home Control Using SSVEP-BCI and Eye Gaze." *2019 IEEE International Conference on Systems, Man and Cybernetics (SMC)*. IEEE, 2019. doi:10.1109/smc.2019.8914390

[17] Renton, Angela I., Jason B. Mattingley, and David R. Painter. "Optimising Non-Invasive Brain-Computer Interface Systems for Free Communication between Naïve Human Participants." *Scientific Reports* 9, no. 1 (December 2019). doi:10.1038/s41598-019-55166-y

[18] Xu, Yang, Cheng Ding, Xiaokang Shu, Kai Gui, Yulia Bezsudnova, Xinjun Sheng, and Dingguo Zhang. "Shared Control of a Robotic Arm Using Non-Invasive Brain–Computer Interface and Computer Vision Guidance." *Robotics and Autonomous Systems* 115 (May 2019): 121–29. doi:10.1016/j.robot.2019.02.014

[19] Baxter, Bryan S., Andrew Decker, and Bin He. "Noninvasive Control of a Robotic Arm in Multiple Dimensions Using Scalp Electroencephalogram." *2013 6th International IEEE/EMBS Conference on Neural Engineering (NER)*. IEEE, 2013. doi:10.1109/ner.2013.6695867

[20] Sakhavi, Siavash, Cuntai Guan, and Shuicheng Yan. "Learning Temporal Information for Brain-Computer Interface Using Convolutional Neural Networks." *IEEE Transactions on Neural Networks and Learning Systems* 29, no. 11 (November 2018): 5619–29. doi:10.1109/tnnls.2018.2789927

[21] Brumberg, Jonathan S., Kevin M. Pitt, and Jeremy D. Burnison. "A Noninvasive Brain-Computer Interface for Real-Time Speech Synthesis: The Importance of Multimodal Feedback." *IEEE Transactions on Neural Systems and Rehabilitation Engineering* 26, no. 4 (April 2018): 874–81. doi:10.1109/tnsre.2018.2808425

[22] Fernández-Rodríguez, Álvaro, Francisco Velasco-Álvarez, María Teresa Medina-Juliá, and Ricardo Ron-Angevin. "Evaluation of Emotional and Neutral Pictures as Flashing Stimuli Using a P300 Brain–Computer Interface Speller." *Journal of Neural Engineering* 16, no. 5 (September 11, 2019): 056024. doi:10.1088/1741-2552/ab386d

[23] Fadel, Ward, et al. "Chessboard EEG Images Classification for BCI Systems Using Deep Neural Network." *Bio-Inspired Information and Communication Technologies Lecture Notes of the Institute for Computer Sciences, Social Informatics and Telecommunications Engineering*, 2020, 97–104. doi:10.1007/978-3-030-57115-3_8

[24] Jeong, Ji-Hoon, et al. "Brain-Controlled Robotic Arm System Based on Multi-Directional CNN-BiLSTM Network Using EEG Signals." *IEEE Transactions on Neural Systems and Rehabilitation Engineering*, 28, no. 5 (2020): 1226–38. doi:10.1109/tnsre.2020.2981659

[25] Wu, Di, Huayan Wan, Siping Liu, Weiren Yu, Zhanpeng Jin, and Dakuo Wang. "DeepBrain: Towards Personalized EEG Interaction through Attentional and Embedded LSTM Learning." arXiv.org, April 14, 2021. https://arxiv.org/abs/2002.02086.

[26] Chai, Rifai, Ganesh R. Naik, Sai Ho Ling, and Hung T. Nguyen. "Hybrid Brain–Computer Interface for Biomedical Cyber-Physical System Application Using Wireless Embedded EEG Systems." *BioMedical Engineering OnLine* 16, no. 1 (January 7, 2017). doi:10.1186/s12938-016-0303-x

[27] Muller-Putz, G., Leeb, R., Tangermann, M., Hohne, J., Kubler, A., Cincotti, F., ... Millan, J. del R. (2015). "Towards Noninvasive Hybrid Brain–Computer Interfaces: Framework, Practice, Clinical Application, and Beyond." *Proceedings of the IEEE*, 10, no. 6, 926–43. doi:10.1109/jproc.2015.2411333

[28] Shenjie, Sun, Kavitha P. Thomas, K.G. Smitha, and A.P. Vinod. "Two Player EEG-Based Neurofeedback Ball Game for Attention Enhancement." *2014 IEEE International Conference on Systems, Man, and Cybernetics (SMC)*. IEEE, 2014. doi:10.1109/smc.2014.6974412

[29] Pope, A. T. and Palsson, O. S. (2001), "Helping Video Games Rewire 'Our Minds'", *Langley Research Center Research Report*, Hampton, VA, http://ntrs.nasa.gov/archive/nasa/casi.ntrs.nasa.gov/20040086464_2004090499.pdf. Accessed 14 April 2011.

[30] Nijholt, Anton, Danny Plass-Oude Bos, and Boris Reuderink. "Turning Shortcomings into Challenges: Brain–Computer Interfaces for Games." *Entertainment Computing* 1, no. 2 (April 2009): 85–94. doi:10.1016/j.entcom.2009.09.007

[31] He, Shenghong, Yajun Zhou, Tianyou Yu, Rui Zhang, Qiyun Huang, Lin Chuai, Madah-Ul- Mustafa, et al. "EEG- and EOG-Based Asynchronous Hybrid BCI: A System Integrating a Speller, a Web Browser, an E-Mail Client, and a File Explorer." *IEEE Transactions on Neural Systems and Rehabilitation Engineering* 28, no. 2 (February 2020): 519–30. doi:10.1109/tnsre.2019.2961309

[32] Pais-Vieira, Miguel, Gabriela Chiuffa, Mikhail Lebedev, Amol Yadav, and Miguel A L Nicolelis. "Building an Organic Computing Device with Multiple Interconnected Brains." *Scientific Reports* 5, no. 1 (July 9, 2015). doi:10.1038/srep11869

[33] Landau, Ofir, Aviad Cohen, Shirley Gordon, and Nir Nissim. "Mind Your Privacy: Privacy Leakage through BCI Applications Using Machine Learning Methods." *Knowledge-Based Systems* 198 (June 2020): 105932. doi:10.1016/j.knosys.2020.105932

[34] Patra, Sudhansu Shekhar, Om Praksah Jena, Gaurav Kumar, Sreyashi Pramanik, Chinmaya Misra, and Kamakhya Narain Singh. "Random Forest Algorithm in Imbalance Genomics Classification." *Data Analytics in Bioinformatics: A Machine Learning Perspective* (2021): 173–90.

[35] Pattnayak, Parthasarathi, and Om Prakash Jena. "Innovation on Machine Learning in Healthcare Services–An Introduction." *Machine Learning for Healthcare Applications* (2021): 1–15.

[36] Panigrahi, Niranjan, Ishan Ayus, and Om Prakash Jena. "An Expert System-Based Clinical Decision Support System for Hepatitis-B Prediction & Diagnosis." *Machine Learning for Healthcare Applications* (2021): 57–75.

[37] Paramesha, K., H. L. Gururaj, and Om Prakash Jena. "Applications of Machine Learning in Biomedical Text Processing and Food Industry." *Machine Learning for Healthcare Applications* (2021): 151–167.

[38] Bardhan, Shawli, Mrinal Kanti Bhowmik, Tathagata Debnath, and Debotosh Bhattacharjee. "RASIT: Region shrinking based Accurate Segmentation of Inflammatory areas from Thermograms." *Biocybernetics and Biomedical Engineering* 38, no. 4 (2018): 903–917.

[39] Bardhan, Shawli, and Mrinal Kanti Bhowmik. "2-Stage classification of knee joint thermograms for rheumatoid arthritis prediction in subclinical inflammation." *Australasian Physical & Engineering Sciences in Medicine* 42, no. 1 (2019): 259–77.

[40] Shawli Bardhan, Satyabrata Nath, Tathagata Debnath, Debotosh Bhattacharjee, and Mrinal Kanti Bhowmik, "Designing of an Inflammatory Knee Joint Thermogram Dataset for Arthritis Classification Using Deep Convolution Neural Network", *Quantitative InfraRed Thermography Journal (to be published by Taylor & Francis).* doi:10.1080/17686733.2020.1855390

[41] Shawli Bardhan, and Sukanta Roga. "Feature Based Automated Detection of COVID-19 from Chest X-Ray Images." In *Emerging Technologies During the Era of COVID-19 Pandemic*, 348 (2021): 115–31, Springer, doi:10.1007/978-3-030-67716-9_8

[42] Shawli Bardhan, and Sukanta Roga. "Edge Feature Based Classification of Breast Thermogram for Abnormality Detection." In *Advances in Mechanical Engineering*, 511–17. Springer, Singapore, 2020. doi:10.1007/978-981-15-3639-7_61

[43] Sukanta Roga, Shawli Bardhan, Dilip H. Lataye. "Air Pollution Monitoring using Blue Channel Texture Features of Image." *International Conference on Deep Learning, Artificial Intelligence and Robotics Applications (ICDLAIR-2019)*, Springer, MNIT, Jaipur, 2020. doi:10.1007/978-3-030-67187-7_15

[44] Shawli Bardhan, Samarpita Debnath, and Mrinal Kanti Bhowmik. "Classification of IR Image Based Inflammatory Pain Diseases Using Statistical Pattern Analysis Approach." *International Journal of Computational Intelligence & IoT* 1, no. 2 (2018). https://ssrn.com/abstract=3354550

[45] Shawli Bardhan, Satyabrata Nath, and Mrinal Kanti Bhowmik. "Evaluation of background subtraction effect on classification and segmentation of knee thermogram." In *2017 8th International Conference on Computing, Communication and Networking Technologies (ICCCNT)*, 1–7. IEEE, 2017. doi:10.1109/ICCCNT.2017.8204011

[46] Mrinal Kanti Bhowmik, Shawli Bardhan, Kakali Das, Debotosh Bhattacharjee, and Satyabrata Nath. "Pain related inflammation analysis using infrared images." In *Thermosense: Thermal Infrared Applications XXXVIII*, 9861:986116. International Society for Optics and Photonics, SPIE, 2016. doi:10.1117/12.2223425

[47] Shawli Bardhan, Mrinal Kanti Bhowmik, Satyabrata Nath, and Debotosh Bhattacharjee. "A review on inflammatory pain detection in human body through infrared image analysis." In *2015 international symposium on advanced computing and communication (ISACC)*, 251–257. IEEE, 2015. doi:10.1109/ISACC.2015.7377350

3 Three-Dimensional Reconstruction and Digital Printing of Medical Objects in Purview of Clinical Applications

Sushitha Susan Joseph and Aju D

CONTENTS

DOI: 10.1201/9781003226147-3

3.1   INTRODUCTION

Three-dimensional printing has made a significant impact on the manufacturing industry. It is a quickly developing revolutionary technology that is receiving considerable interest from both the scientific community and academicians with users from various domains like aerospace, military, engineering, architecture, chemical industry, and automotive and medical fields. Three-dimensional printing, also known as additive manufacturing technology, easily produces designs of composite internal structure and architecture when compared to conventional methods. The automobile and aerospace industries have been using 3D printing technology for more than 30 years. Medical and pharmaceutical fields started using this technology on the recent development of novel biodegradable materials. Today the technology is rapidly expanding and has extensive applications in the clinical field ranging from personalized implants to protective equipment.

The history of medical 3D printing begins with the invention of stereolithography by Chuck Hull in 1983. In 1988 the first bioprinting was performed using the technique of micro positioning of cells. In the early 1990s dental implants and custom prosthetics were 3D printed for medical purposes. In 1999 first laser-assisted bioprinting came into existence. In due course, technological advancement supported the development of organs from human cells which required the support of 3D printed scaffolds in 2001. In 2002 the 3D Bioplotter, using extrusion-based bioprinting, came into reality followed by the development of the inkjet printer in 2003. Further evolution of technology aimed complete functioning organ without scaffold and this became a reality in 2004. The year 2008 witnessed the first 3D printed prosthetic leg. Vascular constructs without scaffold were fabricated in 2009. In 2012 articular cartilage and artificial liver were bioprinted. Fabrication of tubular structures using coaxial technology was performed in 2015. In 2016 a cartilage model was produced using a tissue integrated organ printer. Eventually in 2019 Brazilian researchers successfully 3D printed a mini-liver which performs all the functions of a liver. There is a rapid increase in the speed of development of 3D printing technologies in the medical field.

Doctors mostly rely on two-dimensional (2D) X-ray, CT, and MRI images to acquire the perception of pathologies. There is a need to view and understand the pathology and structural relationship prior to surgery. Three-dimensional reconstruction helps by enhancing understanding and visualization which means surgery can be planned more accurately. The emergence of 3D printing provides haptic qualities to models. Complex surgical procedures require guidance to obtain esthetical results. When compared to conventional learning, a 3D printed model can be used to analyze complex cases, practice surgical procedures, and teach medical students and patients.

There has been an increasing demand for organ transplantation in the medical field which resulted in the emergence of tissue engineering. In tissue engineering, scaffold fabrication using conventional techniques, like solvent casting and particle leaching, electrospinning, and gas foaming, results in restrictions in design flexibility. When compared to traditional techniques, 3D organ printing provides design flexibility and automation. The necessity for enhanced visualization and tactile properties has given rise to 3D printed anatomical models, patient-specific guides, and custom-made prosthetics. Three-dimensionally printed personalized drugs have the capability of providing accurate dosage suitable for each patient, boosting drug absorption, and controlling the cell distribution and extracellular matrix for drug testing.

This chapter provides detailed summary of the utilization of 3D reconstruction and 3D printing technologies in the medical field. A brief overview of printing techniques such as selective laser sintering (SLS), selective laser melting (SLM), selective electron beam melting (SEBM), laser-induced forward transfer (LIFT), nanoparticle jetting (NPJ), and binder jetting (BJ) used for manufacturing is provided. The specific characteristics and clinical applications of biometals such as stainless steel, titanium, tantalum, cobalt chromium alloy, magnesium, iron, and zinc used in 3D printing is discussed. Moreover, the application of 3D printing in medical education, surgical training and practice, personalized implants, prostheses, surgical tools and bioprinting, pharmaceutical industry, personal protective equipment is brought into focus. Furthermore, the software, advantages, disadvantages, and limitations associated with 3D reconstruction and 3D printing are explored.

The organization of this chapter is as follows. Section 3.2 provides information on the techniques used for 3D reconstruction of different organs. Further, Section 3.3 explains the workflow of medical 3D printing process. Current 3D printing technologies used for manufacturing various components are discussed in Section 3.4. Section 3.5 provides an overview of the biometals used in 3D printing process. Section 3.6 gives a brief description of how 3D printing is being utilized in medical applications. The challenges and future perspectives of 3D reconstruction and printing are discussed in Section 3.7, followed by concluding remarks in Section 3.8.

3.2 LITERATURE REVIEW

Three-dimensionally reconstructed models are being utilized in diagnostic and prognostic decision making by medical practitioners. The patient-specific reconstructed model helps in the surgical management by improving the confidence of surgeons while handling complex cases (Lamadé et al. 2000). Customization, which provides great value in the medical field, is the greatest advantage of 3D printing. There is a reduction in the use of unnecessary resources with a minimum number of parts being used, and parts that require frequent modifications can be printed at low cost. When compared to traditional manufacturing of implants, speed and repeatability of 3D printing is good. Various approaches that have been put forth for the 3D reconstruction of organs and 3D printing in the literature are discussed in this section.

Marching Cubes is the standard algorithm which performs 3D reconstruction by isosurface extraction. Medical visualization heavily utilizes isosurface creation of digitized images obtained from CT and MRI scans. Brain tumor reconstruction, as performed by Arakeri and Reddy (2013), using Marching cubes helps in the visualization and volume computation. Detection and reconstruction of breast cancer by Marching Cubes (Gnonnou and Smaoui 2014) helps the oncologist to visualize the tumor and determine its spread. Three-dimensional reconstruction of the heart (Nugroho, Basuki, and Sigit 2016) with a combination of Marching Squares and Marching Cubes helps to identify the abnormalities of the heart. Coronary artery disease is a cardiovascular disease that is diagnosed by computed tomography angiography. Kigka et al. (2018) developed semi-automated methodology that minimizes user interaction for the 3D reconstruction of coronary arteries including lumen, plaques, and outside walls. The method proposed by Yoo (2011) uses triangular Beizer patches for interpolation of the triangles generated by Marching Cube algorithm in order to reconstruct the human bone obtained from a CT scan.

Brain tumor reconstruction using Delaunay's triangulation combined with the maximizing volume method (Tawbe et al. 2008) was proposed to study the development of brain tumors. Human rib cage reconstruction by statistical shape models (Dworzak et al. 2010) helped in the interval studies of a particular disease. Guo et al. (2011) proposed the method of an immune sphere-shaped support vector machine that was successful in reconstructing the irregular surface of the brain. The method of one class support vector machine proposed by Lecron et al. (2013) provides advantage over the traditional Gaussian distribution for the 3D reconstruction of spine in a scoliotic patient. Duan et al. (2015) proposed the partial least square regression method for the complex 3D craniofacial reconstruction.

(Abdelazeem et al. 2020) proposed a combination of comparative digital holography and holographic projection for the 3D reconstruction and assessment of brain tumor progression. Automatic 3D reconstruction and visualization using augmented and virtual reality (Chen, He, and Jia 2020; González Izard et al. 2020) was developed to aid radiologists and as an effective tool for teaching anatomy. Security assisted sparse aware convolution neural network with dictionary learning was introduced by More et al. (2020). This method achieves good visual quality of images and uses Internet of Healthcare Things (IoHT). The method proposed by (Zhang et al. 2020) combines deep learning with IoHT and introduces advanced ray casting for 3D reconstruction. The main advantage of the method is the increased efficiency in reduced time and memory cost. The study of integrating cinematic rendering in anatomy conducted by Binder et al. (2021) suggests that the method is effective and is beneficial in anatomical education. Yin et al. (2021) developed slip interface imaging for 3D reconstruction and performed classification of meningiomas. The power of generative adversarial networks (Pradhan et al. 2020; Pennarossa et al. 2021) and convolution neural network (Ng et al. 2020; Karayegen and Aksahin 2021) was utilized in 3D reconstruction and in tracking the progression of brain tumors.

With the emergence of 3D printing, there is progress in the area of tissue engineering and bioprinting. The team of surgeons working on separating conjoined twins (Inserra et al. 2020) used 3D printed ribcage modeling, bone modeling, color-coded skin and internal organs which substantially reduced operating times along with the risk for the patients. Moreover, preoperative planning using the 3D reconstructed anatomical models revealed the connection between two hearts and aided in the surgeons' technical preparations. In 2017 3D printed ovaries restored the ovarian function in infertile mice when the scaffolds are follicle seeded with vascularization (Laronda et al. 2017). Cyborg beast (Zuniga et al. 2015) is the 3D printed prosthetic hand developed for children which aims at reducing the cost of prosthetics, making it available to children from low income families. The Food and Drug Administration (FDA) perspective of additively manufactured products (Di Prima et al. 2016) discusses 3D printing in medicine. The FDA centers handle different products. The Center for Device and Radiological Health (CDRH) reviews medical devices, drugs, and biologics. The Center for Drug Evaluation and Research (CDER) reviews 3D printed drugs. The Center for Biologics Evaluation and Research (CBER) reviews bioprinting products.

The power of Internet of Things (IoT) can be combined with 3D printing to compensate for the limitations and challenges in the medical field (Haleem, Javaid, and Vaishya 2020; Khamparia et al.; Goyal et al. 2021). Three-dimensional printing provides solutions to organ transplantation and the 3D printed organs increase patients' longevity. In order to transmit and store data, sensors and actuators can be integrated with these organs which can trace the organ's lifeline. This gives doctors information regarding the time to transplant the organ again (Sharma et al. 2020). Similarly, 3D printed pacemakers integrated with IoT can be used to track patient conditions. Surgeries performed with the help of surgical robots provide freedom of hand movement and customized 3D printed surgical tools reduce risks by providing more accurate results (Jindal, Gupta, and Bhushan 2019; Kumar et al. 2020).

Artificial intelligence (AI) has the potential to influence healthcare. AI together with 3D printing contributes to hyperrealism by obtaining realistic renderings during surgical training (Engelhardt et al. 2018). During the design stage, 3D printing, when combined with machine learning (ML) approaches of hierarchical clustering and support vector machines (SVM), helps the novice designers to enhance the decision making process (Maidin, Campbell, and Pei 2012; Yao, Moon, and Bi 2017). AI provides solutions to the process planning problem in 3D printing through improving the slicing acceleration (A. Wang et al. 2017) and path optimization (Fok et al. 2016). The technique of using conformal geometric algebra with ML (Pillai and Megalingam 2020) and the Random Forest algorithm based on decision trees (Patra et al. 2021) successfully identified and reconstructed a tumor. ML techniques highly influence the healthcare field (Pattnayak and Jena 2021) and organizations benefit from these expert systems (Panigrahi, Ayus, and Jena 2021; Paramesha, Gururaj, and Jena 2021).

3.3 MEDICAL 3D PRINTING WORKFLOW

The mathematical basis of 3D printing is Fubini's theorem which states that an object of n dimensions can be represented as a spectrum of layers of shapes of (n−1) dimensional layers (Anastasiou et al. 2013). Three-dimensional printing proves that it is possible to print 3D shapes of a real-world object as layers of 2D planes. According to Fubini's theorem, suppose M and N are complete measures of spaces and $f(a,b)$ is $M \times N$ measurable. If,

$$\int_{M \times N} |f(a,b)| \, d(a,b) < \infty \tag{3.1}$$

where the integral is taken with respect to a product measure on the space over $M \times N$, then

$$\int_{M} \left(\int_{N} f(a,b) db \right) da = \int_{N} \left(\int_{M} f(a,b) da \right) db = \int_{M \times N} f(a,b) d(a,b) \tag{3.2}$$

The first and second integrals are iterated integrals with respect to M, N respectively and the third one is an integral with respect to the product of M, N.

The process of 3D printing an object from medical images consists of several steps. The initial step is the data acquisition in the form of diagnostic scans, followed by segmentation on the scans to extract the desired region of interest. Then 3D reconstruction provides the volume representation of the segmented part in 3D display. Optimization of anatomical geometry data is performed with computer-aided design (CAD) software. Then this model is transformed into a standard tessellation or triangle language (STL) file, after which it is sliced into digital layers. The output file is then imported to the 3D printer and the suitable biomaterials and printing parameters of the printer are determined. The printer builds the model by depositing material first on the bottom layer and then depositing layers one after the other on the bottom layer. The printed model undergoes further refinement such as cleaning and polishing to obtain the desired part. Figure 3.1 depicts the various steps involved in developing a 3D printed object.

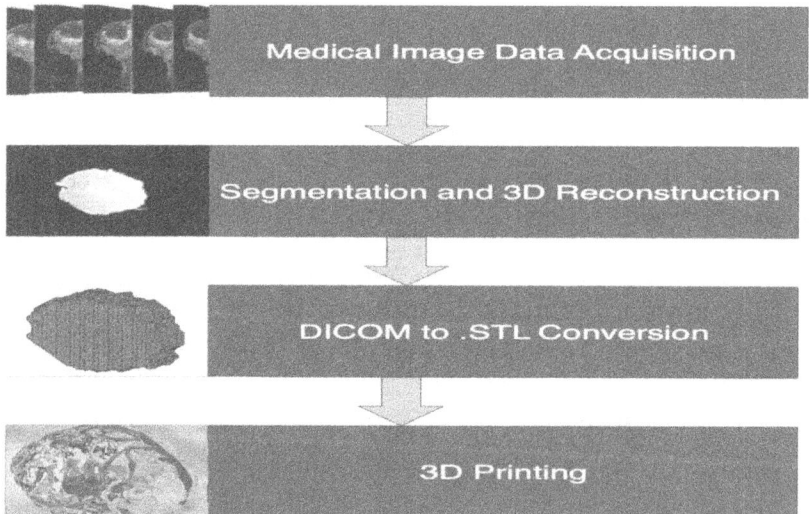

FIGURE 3.1   Steps in developing 3D printed physical object.

Digital data and technology have transformed the imaging field. Medical imaging is at the heart of the healthcare field as it helps in the reliable early detection and diagnosis of disease as well as in medical communication. The commonly used imaging modalities for obtaining diagnostic scans are MRI, CT, positron emission tomography (PET), and ultrasound. The acquired images are in the standard DICOM format. Two-dimensional segmentation extracts the particular region of interest from the whole scan and the 3D reconstruction creates a reference to form a physical model.

The most commonly used technologies for 3D reconstruction are ray casting, splatting, shear warp, and texture mapping. Ray casting was developed in 1980s and 1990s and involves rays being cast from the eye or viewpoint across the image plane and dataset. Instead of selecting the closest point, the ray splits the volume for the interpolation of color and opacity. Merging of the interpolated values produces the visibility on the image plane. Consider a model which has volume with density $D(a,b,c)$ and is penetrated by ray S. For each point along the ray, there is an illumination $I(a,b,c)$ reaching the point (a,b,c) from the source of light. The intensity of the ray depends on this value, phase function H, and the local density $D(a,b,c)$. The density function is given along the ray as $D(a(t),b(t),c(t)) = D(t)$ and the illumination from light source as $I(a(t),b(t),c(t)) = I(t)$. The illumination spread along S from a point distance t along the ray can be defined as $I(t)D(t)H(\cos\theta)$ where θ is the angle between S and M, where M is the light vector. Ray casting computes volume rendering integral $V_\lambda(x,r)$, the amount of light of wavelength λ, coming from ray direction r, at the point of location x as in equation (3.3). L_λ is the light of wavelength λ reflected at position s in the direction of r. The color $L(s_i)$ and opacity $o(s_i)$ are calculated in the interval i, and the interval width Δs.

$$V_\lambda(x,r) = \sum_{i=0}^{H/\Delta s} L_\lambda(s_i) o(s_i) . \prod_{j=0}^{i-1}\left(1-\alpha(s_j)\right) \tag{3.3}$$

where

$$L_\lambda(s_i) = L_\lambda(i\Delta s) \text{ and } o(s_i) = o(i\Delta s) \tag{3.4}$$

Splatting is faster than ray casting and works on the principle of the feed forward method. The idea behind splatting is to project the voxel onto the image plane and the projection depends on the color and opacity of the voxel. Further computation determines the part of the image plane to be included for each thrown voxel. Splatting computes $V_\lambda(x,r)$ as in (3.3) with the values of $L_\lambda(s_i)$ and $o(s_i)$ computed as follows:

$$L_\lambda(s_i) = \frac{\int_{i\Delta s}^{(i+1)\Delta s} L_\lambda(s)ds}{\Delta s} \text{ and } o(s_i) = \frac{\int_{i\Delta s}^{(i+1)\Delta s} \alpha(s)ds}{\Delta s} \tag{3.5}$$

Shear warp is a process that eliminates the computational expense involved in arbitrary rotations of volume rendering. The main process in the shear warp algorithm is to create shearing slices from volume data by translating and scaling each slice, obtaining the intermediate image by combining the slices in fore end to rear end sequence, transforming the intermediate image to the final image by warping it. Shear warp computes $V_\lambda(x,r)$ as in (3.3) with $L_\lambda(s_i)$ and $o(s_i)$ computed as in ray casting but with an extra constraint Δs, which depends on view direction as follows.

$$\Delta s = \sqrt{\left(\frac{dx}{dz}\right)^2 + \left(\frac{dy}{dz}\right)^2 + 1} \qquad (3.6)$$

Texture mapping technique reduces the complexity involved in mathematical model-based 3D reconstruction. Role played by computer graphics hardware is important in texture mapping. The object is loaded into the texture memory and the graphics hardware rasterizes it into a polygon on the screen. The major drawback of this method is that swapping is required when there is a large dataset that cannot fit into the main memory and it requires expensive hardware too. Texture mapping computes volume rendering integral $V_\lambda(x,r)$, as does ray casting as per equations (3.3) and (3.4).

The digital model obtained using reconstruction is converted to STL format which is an automated process in 3D printers. Software such as Magics can rectify the errors associated with. STL file conversion. In order to add the feature details such as color and surface texture, additive manufacturing format and 3D manufacturing format can be used. Then the STL file is sliced by the specialized software to obtain the layer-by-layer 3D printed object. The software tools that are available for segmentation and 3D reconstruction of medical data are 3D Doctor, Analyze, 3DVIEWNIX, MeVisLab, Seg3D, 3D Slicer, InVesalius, Osirix Lite, and ImageJ. The software tools used for 3D printing are Materialise Mimics and RepRap.

3.4 THREE-DIMENSIONAL PRINTING TECHNOLOGIES

Three-dimensional printing is very promising for clinical applications as it gives rise to extensive fabrication of personalized and customized implants. When compared to conventional manufacturing, 3D printing has the ability to manufacture components with complex geometries in reduced steps. Although several 3D printing technologies with their own characteristics are available, some of the latest commonly used manufacturing technologies in medical applications are discussed in this section. Choosing the right technology to manufacture the component depends on the particular application.

3.4.1 SELECTIVE LASER SINTERING

SLS is an additive layer manufacturing process where thermal energy fuses regions of a powder bed to build 3D parts. This is a rapid prototyping technique with the capability to process materials such as metals, polymers, ceramics, and composites. The metallurgical mechanism used in this process is liquid-phase sintering. SLS entails selective usage of a laser, usually a carbon dioxide laser, to create a layer-by-layer prototype from a thin powder base. The thin powder particles cohere and harden when a laser beam is applied. With the help of a beam deflection arrangement, every surface is examined pursuant to its corresponding cross section of sliced CAD data. The accumulation of consecutive powder layers is achieved using a powder deposition system. The molding process of SLS is simple as it does not require any support structures and is suitable for the fabrication of complicated shapes (Yap et al. 2015). The limitation of this method is in the post-processing involved in improving the surface quality of the manufactured parts. Current advances of SLS provide the capacity to manufacture low-stiffness scaffolds which benefits the production of cardiac tissue (Bahraminasab 2020).

3.4.2 SELECTIVE LASER MELTING

SLM is considered to be a subclass of SLS as it is developed based on SLS. SLM uses high-power density lasers, high-quality powder paving, and advanced metallurgical operations that fully melt powders for the additive manufacturing of metals (Pattanayak et al. 2011). SLM is executed in a vacuum or argon- or nitrogen-protected build chamber to reduce oxidation during the build process. SLM technology makes objects with good dimensional accuracy and surface roughness, devoid of any intermediate binding or processes. As the metal powder is fully melted, the manufactured parts have high densities, excellent mechanical properties, and metallurgically bonded structures that do not demand post-processing. A large combination of materials including metals, polymers, metal-polymer, metal-ceramic compounds can be fabricated using SLM which has applications in forming dental restorations (van Noort 2012), femoral implants (Wang et al. 2016), and orthopedic surgery templates (Zhang et al. 2017). The SLM technique is expensive and is relatively slow in terms of printing speed.

3.4.3 SELECTIVE ELECTRON BEAM MELTING

SEBM is a powder-based additive manufacturing methodology. Like the SLM process, which uses laser beam as heat source, SEBM uses high-energy electron beams as a heat source to fuse metal particles. The high-power electron beam can work at high temperatures and velocities enabling the application of novel melting strategies. The feasible material diversity of SEBM is limited to metals and alloys, which are conductive materials. The vacuum environment is essential for preventing the oxidation of metal powder in the course of liquid phase melting and to preserve the energy and cutting ability of electrons. In comparison with other technologies, SEBM provides thick microstructure formation and high efficiency with no support for the molding process. Although SEBM has the advantage of simultaneous production of multiple parts, post-processing of finished parts and expensive equipment are its limitations. SEBM finds application in 3D printing of acetabular cups, femoral knee implants, and intramedullary rods (Murr et al. 2012) while the formation of orthopedic implants faces the challenge of optimization of finished implant surface.

3.4.4 LASER-INDUCED FORWARD TRANSFER

LIFT is an additive direct printing technology which does not need metal powder, with its principle of operation different from traditional 3D printing. The high focusing pulsed laser displayed on the solid donor film results in printing a small fraction of material onto the receiver layer. LIFT is capable of printing inks in a broad range of viscosities and of any particle size, preserving all the functionality of the materials. The strength of LIFT lies in its capability to print metals and oxides, ceramics, polymers, biomolecules, and alive cells. Based on LIFT, mesenchymal stem cells were printed for the construction of scaffold-free autologous grafts. DNA strands, antigens, immunoglobulins, enzymes, human osteosarcoma cells, and stem cells have also been 3D printed using LIFT.

3.4.5 NANOPARTICLE JETTING

NPJ is a newly evolved technology that uses liquid ink for wrapping metal powders. The nanoparticles obtained by smashing large metal pieces are given as input into a binder that creates a regular printing ink. The suspensions of powdered material in the ink avoids the need for sieving as in powder-based techniques and the ink released through the nozzle enables fine detail printing. Extreme temperatures inside the system cause the liquid to vaporize leaving behind smooth parts made from the building material. The advantage of NPJ is that it provides a good surface finish and precision with simple operations which are safe too. High resolution of parts is obtained at low cost. In comparison with traditional 3D printing, the parts obtained by NPJ have a low temperature tolerance. Hearing aids, surgical tools, crowns, and bridges are the commonly manufactured objects using NPJ.

3.4.6 BINDER JETTING

BJ is a quickly developing additive manufacturing technology in which powder material is deposited into a layer and the required shape of the layer is obtained by selective joining using a polymeric liquid binder. Then the printed metal part undergoes subsequent sintering in order to achieve the vital mechanical strength. This technology uses a thermally controlled sintering process and involves low-cost operations. Metallic materials, ceramics, and composite materials are commonly used materials in the BJ process. BJ finds application in the manufacturing of medical models such as the heart, ankle, backbone, knee, and pelvis (Salmi 2016).

3.5 BIOMETALS FOR 3D PRINTING

The current market experiences ample collection of natural, synthetic and hybrid materials which leads to substantial growth in the availability of diverse biomaterials (Ige, Umoru, and Aribo 2012). In the medical and healthcare field, each patient is distinctive which gives rise to the necessity of personalized medical applications. Biomaterials are natural or man-made substances that are designed to reside in a biological environment. Selection of the material to be used in medical application depends on factors such as whether the material property is apt for the medical application and the host reaction to the implants regardless of the nature of the reaction is known as biocompatibility. Based on biocompatibility, biomaterials are classified into bioinert and biodegradable. Biologically inert or bioinert materials are ones which do not initiate an adverse response from the host and are suitable for long-term implantations. Biodegradable materials are designed to degrade in the body over a specific implantation period such that degradation performs a particular function. A perfect biomaterial should be biologically compatible, easily printable, and mimic real tissue.

Metals and their alloys are broadly used in the 3D printing of hard tissues as implants and fixtures due to their high strength and ductility (Frazier 2014). Permanent metallic implants obtained from surgical stainless steel (316L), cobalt-chromium (CoCr) alloys, titanium (Ti) alloys, and tantalum (Ta) have applications in fracture fixation, angioplasty, and bone remodeling (Saini et al. 2015). This is owing to their good mechanical properties and long-term stability. Although low corrosion, friction, and wear are observed in these materials, there are possibilities of metal degradation resulting in the liberation of unwanted metallic ions leading to local tissue damage, inflammatory reactions such as osteolysis, or systemic damage such as metal hypersensitivity (Farahani, Dubé, and Therriault 2016). Moreover, permanent metallic implants used in orthopedic applications require a costly and invasive second surgery for removal or adjustment. In order to overcome these problems, implants made of degradable biometals were developed. Biodegradable biometals such as magnesium (Mg), iron (Fe), and zinc (Zn) alloys are used in orthopedic and cardiovascular applications.

3.5.1 STAINLESS STEEL

Stainless steel is composed of chromium, nickel, and molybdenum with chromium in high amount. Conventional stainless steel and Ni-free stainless steels are the two types of stainless steels used in biomedical applications. Although Ni has the property of high corrosion resistance, it decreases stress corrosion as well as biocompatibility. Therefore, in order to maintain low Ni content, nitrogen is alloyed with Ni-free stainless steel. Both conventional stainless steel and Ni-free stainless steels are used for manufacturing of stents while conventional stainless steel is used in load bearing purposes. To provide support, stainless steel is largely used in bone fracture treatments in the form of screws, fracture plates, pins and orthopedic implants. Stainless steel is used to fabricate durable implant trials and 3D dental implants.

3.5.2 TITANIUM ALLOY

Titanium and Ti-based alloys are superior to stainless steel for their high ratio strength. Major amounts of orthopedic implants use Ti6Al4V (Ti-64) and commercially pure titanium (CP–Ti). Three-dimensional printing technology is successful in manufacturing implants with porous microstructures. Porous titanium possesses the advantages of low weight and lower mechanical modulus compared to solid titanium (<20 GPa vs. 110 GPa), resistance to corrosion, high surface area, and relatively high mechanical strength. Porous titanium alloy implants reduce the stress shielding effect, initiate human bone tissue development, and build a powerful contact with tissues and implants. Three-dimensionally printed Ti-based porous implants develop an enhanced osteointegration effect which provides favorable stability and long life to the implants (Shi et al. 2019). There are many surgical resections that success-fully place 3D printed titanium implants, including mandibular prosthesis (Gadia, Shah, and Nene 2018), heel prosthesis (Imanishi and Choong 2015), cervical cage for spinal fusion (Spetzger et al. 2017), metacarpal prosthesis (Punyaratabandhu et al. 2017), and vertebral body (Wei et al. 2020).

3.5.3 Tantalum

Tantalum (Ta) has been widely used in 3D printing due to its ideal biocompatibility and anti-corrosion property. Tantalum substantially stimulates bone ingrowth, cell proliferation, and osteointegration. The widespread acceptance of tantalum prod-ucts was previously hindered by its costly manufacturing process and impotence to build modular implants. In several studies, porous tantalum has been shown to have the benefits of possessing less elastic modulus, substantial surface area, and good pore connectivity which makes it apt for orthopedic and dental applications. Three-dimensionally printed porous tantalum implants are employed as joint prosthesis in total knee arthroplasty (Wang et al. 2020), hip arthroplasty (Hailer 2018), spine fusion surgery (Patel et al. 2020), trabecular metal material in dental implants (Bencharit et al. 2014), and knee joint cushions. However, tantalum's high melting point of 3017°C makes it difficult for the 3D printing equipment to work with tantalum powder. Moreover, porous scaffolds exhibit low fatigue resistance. In order to overcome these difficulties, many studies have been conducted to fabri-cate solid or porous Ta using new techniques such as laser engineered net shaping (Balla et al. 2010), spark plasma sintering (Dudina, Bokhonov, and Olevsky 2019), and selective laser melting (Thijs et al. 2013). Coating of Ta on Ti using laser engineered net shaping improved osteointegration properties while strength and ductility was improved using spark plasma sintering. Selective laser melting was successful in improving the ductility and osteoconductive properties, and normal-ized fatigue strength.

3.5.4 Cobalt-Chromium Alloy

Cobalt-chromium (Co-Cr) alloys are superalloys with cobalt and chromium as major constituents. These biomaterials have biocompatibility with superior mechanical properties such as good wear-corrosion resistance and fatigue resistance (Niinomi, Narushima, and Nakai 2015). They have high strength and can be exposed to high temperature conditions making it feasible for 3D printing of orthopedic implants, dental prosthetics, and cardiovascular stents. Furthermore, exhaustive studies on the mechanical property, biocompatibility, and microstructure of SLM-fabricated Co-Cr alloys have proved their capability as promising substances for manufacturing 3D printed dental and maxillofacial prosthetics (Pillai et al. 2021). Porous Co-Cr scaf-folds reduce stress shielding, minimize elastic modulus, and provide implant longev-ity by good osteointegration stability (L. Wang et al. 2017). Co-Cr alloy exhibits increased ceramic–metal bond strength, excellent electrochemical stability, and microstructure homogeneity. Three-dimensionally printed Co-Cr alloy shows the desirable property of decreased release of metal ions in dental prosthodontics by corrosion degradation.

3.5.5 MAGNESIUM

Biodegradable magnesium (Mg) and its alloys are the most promising candidates for use in orthopedic, cardiology, respirology, urology implants as they eliminate the effects of stress shielding and second implant removal surgery. Magnesium and its alloys have similar density, stiffness, compressive yield strength, and elastic modulus to human bone making it ideal to be used in load-bearing implants. Magnesium alloys are biosafe and biocompatible, and they accelerate growth and healing of bone by osteoblastic cell proliferation and differentiation. The orthopedic applications of magnesium are bone screws, rods, and plates. Magnesium alloys are used as cardiovascular stents (Erbel et al. 2007), tracheal stents (Luffy et al. 2014), and urinary implants (Zhang et al. 2016). In spite of the challenges involved in processing magnesium alloys due to their flammability, the requisite of 3D printed products composed of Mg alloys is increasing. Research studies showed that wire arc additive manufacturing can extract the good mechanical properties of magnesium (Han et al. 2018; Gneiger et al. 2020). Porous magnesium and magnesium alloy scaffold meet the functional requirement of the ideal bone substitute (Yazdimamaghani et al. 2017).

3.5.6 IRON

Iron (Fe) and Fe-based materials are favorable candidates for producing biodegradable implants due to their strength, good mechanical characteristics, and medium corrosion process. Iron is a non-toxic metal and the ions discharged during degradation can be held by the body which allow pure Fe stents to be fixed into porcine aorta (Peuster et al. 2006).The first metal used in 3D printing of bio functional scaffolds was an iron-based metal (Do et al. 2015). Development of iron-manganese (Fe-Mn) alloys with enhanced degradation rate and good mechanical properties offers high efficiency in biomedical applications (Schinhammer et al. 2010). Studies show that Fe-Mn, Fe-Mn-Ca, and Fe-Mn-Mg alloys all exhibit cytocompatibility. Porous iron scaffolds prepared by topological design using direct metal printing (DMP) has the potential to be used in orthopedic applications as they promote bone regeneration (Li et al. 2018).

3.5.7 ZINC

Zinc is a vital trace element in the human body. Zinc possesses the properties such as good antibacterial activity and negligible toxicity, and the degradation rate is in the middle of iron and magnesium. These properties along with biocompatibility and biodegradability make zinc and its alloys promising materials to serve as dental implants and vascular stents. Studies have been carried out on fabricating 3D printed zinc using SLM (Demir, Monguzzi, and Previtali 2017).

3.6 APPLICATIONS OF 3D PRINTING IN HEALTHCARE

Three-dimensional printing is able to produce realistic representations of normal and pathological variations. The advancements in 3D printing technology help to save and enhance lives with the power to produce custom-made products and equipment. Three-dimensional printing technology has various kinds of applications in the medical field, including as a tool for medical education, in surgical training and practice, for manufacturing personalized implants, prostheses, surgical tools and bioprinting, in pharmaceutical industry, and for producing personalized protective equipment. Figure 3.2 depicts the applications of 3D printing in healthcare.

3.6.1 MEDICAL EDUCATION

Standard anatomy training of medical students is carried out using cadavers which involves difficulties such as cost, availability of cadaver, adding formalin preservatives, and ethical issues (Hsieh et al. 2018). The advent of 3D printing has paved the way for using models in anatomy training with adequate haptic feedback and moderate cost. They provide better interpretation of anatomical features of a disease state preoperatively (Matthews et al. 2009). Three dimensional printed models of the nervous system (Tam et al. 2018), heart (Z. Wang et al. 2017), skull (Chen et al. 2017), spine (Li et al. 2015), ventricular system (Yi et al. 2019), and thoracic aorta (Garcia et al. 2018) have been used in training of medical students. Multicolored 3D printed models have the power to better interpret the normal and diseased anatomy, are

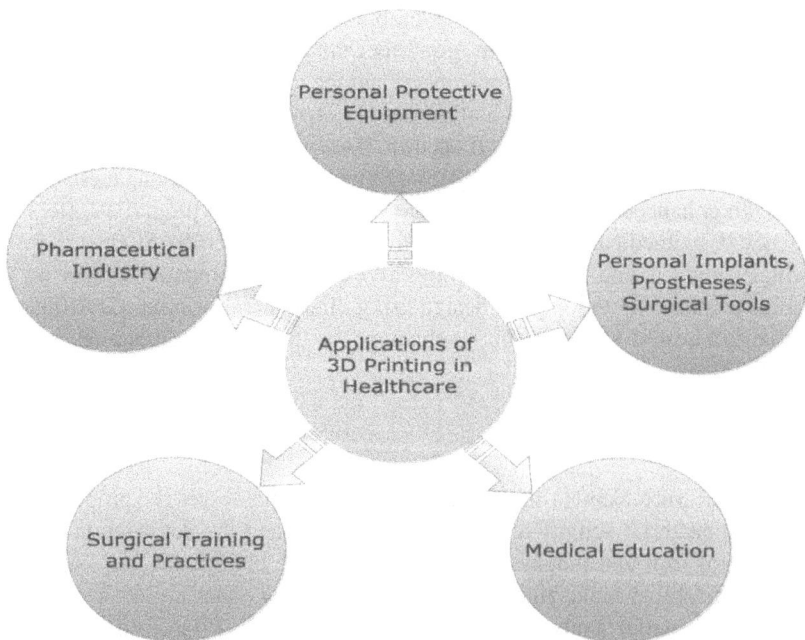

FIGURE 3.2   Applications of 3D printing in healthcare.

durable and can be reproduced. The 3D printed models can improve doctor–patient communication by giving a detailed explanation regarding the diseased organ, pathology, and surgical risks. Recent studies illustrate the significance and requisite of integrating a course on 3D reconstruction and printing for undergraduate medical students in medical schools (Z. Wang et al. 2017).

3.6.2 Surgical Training and Practice

3.6.2.1 Cardiac Surgery

Surgeons commonly use scans from cardiovascular MRI (CMR), echocardiography, angiography, and CT imaging modalities to perform cardiovascular resection and interventional cardiology. Although the imaging modalities provide high-resolution images, still it is hard to anticipate the real anatomical systems in congenital defects due to large morphological variations. Congenital heart disease (CHD) refers to an abnormality when the heart or blood vessels near the heart is underdeveloped, normally before birth. The 3D printed models are accurate in demonstrating the spatial relationships which helps to plan for pre-surgery and surgical simulations, and to guide the surgeons during resection (Greil et al. 2007). These models also help in the localization of coronary arteries and abnormal structures (Mottl-Link et al. 2008), assessment of the abnormalities in great arteries (Vranicar et al. 2008), and understanding of vascular anatomy (Ngan et al. 2006) and pediatric heart transplantation (Sodian et al. 2008b). Coronary artery bypass grafting (CABG) is a risky procedure that involves high mortality rate. Personalized three dimensionally printed model helps to locate the bypass graft and assists in opening the sterum successfully (Sodian et al. 2008a). Cardiac tumors are rare but fatal. The 3D printed cardiovascular model with cardiac fibroma helps surgeons to overcome limited experience in handling the case and plan for the tumor resection (Jacobs et al. 2008). Similarly, these models are used for transcatheter aortic valve replacement (TAVR) (Schmauss et al. 2012), transcatheter percutaneous pulmonary valve implantation (PPVI) (Schievano et al. 2007), left atrial appendage closure (Otton et al. 2015), and trans-apical aortic valve replacement (Abdel-Sayed and von Segesser 2011).

3.6.2.2 Neurosurgery

In 1999, a 3D printed stereolithographic model was developed to assist in the neurosurgical planning of orbital brachytherapy (Poulsen et al. 1999). The planning of skull-based surgeries (Müller et al. 2003), surgery for lesion near motor cortex (Spottiswoode et al. 2013), cerebral aneurysm surgery (Stadie et al. 2008), and simulation of neurosurgical procedures for cerebral tumors (Waran et al. 2014; Waran et al. 2015) were performed using the 3D printed models. These models improve confidence in the candidates as they can repeat the procedures on the model which results in improving the hands-on experience in resection.

3.6.2.3 Craniomaxillofacial Surgery

The surgery performed on the region of upper jaw, face, nose, and eye sockets is called maxillofacial surgery. Back in 1998, 3D printed models were fabricated for presurgical planning of acute maxillofacial trauma (Kermer et al. 1998). These models provide correct defect dimensions and positions to decide the common morphology of the implant. The studies show that 3D printing shortens the surgery time and improves the results for craniofacial surgeries (D'Urso et al. 2000). Orbital reconstruction (Rohner et al. 2013) and surgery on malformed ears (Longfield, Brickman, and Jeyakumar 2015) performed using 3D printed models show that it enhances the learning experience of trainees.

3.6.3 Personalized Implants, Prostheses, Surgical Tools, and Bioprinting

Three-dimensional printing techniques are used to obtain personalized medical implants, prosthesis, and surgical tools from the scan images. Various surgical tools such as forceps, needle drivers, hemostats, army navy retractors, jigs, and scalpel handles are designed and built (George et al. 2017). Complex tools can be designed and produced in a short time and surgeons can specify the modifications. Implants primarily provide a solution to replace the defective or missing parts. Crowns and bridges are the commonly used dental implants. Orthopedic implants include autografts, allografts, and artificial bone scaffolds (Pilipchuk et al. 2015).

Three-dimensionally printed implants can correct complex fractures and dislocations as well as perform deformity correction. While traditional manufacturing of implant production takes days or weeks, 3D printing of personalized implants may take only several hours. Hip prostheses, knee joint prostheses, prosthetic heart valves, mandibular prostheses, hearing aids, screws, prosthetic legs, prosthetic arms, and prosthetic ears and eyes are all fabricated with 3D printing technologies. Organ transplantation currently depends on the availability of donors which leads to the scarcity of organs. Three-dimensional printing provides a prospective solution by creating tissues and organs. Scaffolds, the main components of tissue engineering, possess the properties of natural human tissues such as nutrients absorption, waste disposal, and regeneration. Researchers succeeded in printing tissues of skin, bone, cartilage, heart valve, kidney, and liver.

3.6.4 Pharmaceutical Industry

Three-dimensional printing helps to overcome the challenges involved in traditional pharmaceutical unit operations. It provides flexibility in design and production of personalized medicines. It includes unique dosage forms, personalized drug dosing, and complex drug release profiles. Three-dimensional printing technology is capable to produce loose and porous tablets which reduces swallowing difficulties (Fu et al. 2004). Microneedles for delivering drugs through the skin can be manufactured using 3D printing in a single step fabrication (Pere et al. 2018). Using 3D printing technology, manufacturing of complex drugs in various colors, shapes and sizes is possible. The shape of the drug influences the rate of drug release and drug dissolution. Three-dimensional printing creates drugs with the same dosage in different shapes. Spritam, the first 3D printed drug approved by the FDA, was prepared by powder bed fusion (Jamroz et al. 2017). Three-dimensional printing provides the power to decide the ideal amount of drug administered to a patient based on the age, weight, gender, and metabolism. These personalized medicines can be further adapted to patient's clinical feedback. Polypills are pills that combine many drugs into a single tablet. The whole medication for a patient with multiple chronic disease can be incorporated into a single pill using three-dimensional printing. Moreover, it facilitates on-spot printing for fewer stability drugs and on-demand manufacturing of drugs for natural disasters and military operations. Progress in technology can introduce a chance of on-demand printing of pills in hospitals and pharmacies.

3.6.5 Personal Protective Equipment

In the midst of the COVID-19 pandemic, 3D printing has emerged as a key technology to uphold improved health care. Numerous applications of 3D printing for COVID-19 include medical devices, testing devices, training and visualization aids, personal protective equipment, personal accessories, and emergency dwellings (Choong et al. 2020). Medical devices that can be 3D printed consist of ventilator valves, non-invasive positive end expiratory pressure masks, emergency respiration devices, and mask connectors for continuous positive airways pressure and bilevel positive airways pressure. Testing and training devices include the nasopharyngeal swabs. Medical manikins or bio-models act as training and visualization aids. The examples of 3D printed personal protective equipment are face shields, respirators, and metal respirator filters whereas face masks, mask fitters, mask adjusters, and door openers are the examples of 3D printed personal accessories. Three-dimensional printing fabricated emergency dwellings are used in order to quarantine patients. Three-dimensional printing provides decentralized printing by using designs shared online, which was used in the serious disturbance of supply chains during the pandemic (Tino et al. 2020).

3.7 CHALLENGES AND FUTURE PERSPECTIVES IN MEDICAL 3D RECONSTRUCTION AND PRINTING

The key challenge in 3D reconstruction is that the result depends on the prior step of segmentation. There are manual, semi-automatic, and automatic segmentation process. Although manual segmentation by experts is time consuming, it can provide accurate segmentation results which gives good visualization by 3D reconstruction. The major challenges of 3D printing associated with materials, printer, and issues from a management perspective are discussed in this section. Selection of suitable material for 3D printing is a challenge. The materials must be determined according to the application of the model. The choice of biocompatible or bioresorbable materials is limited. The choice of the material depends on the 3D printing technique used, printing resolution, and printer speed. Another challenge is the selection of appropriate binder for fabricating 3D scaffolds. All binders are not suitable for the sintering process. Good quality 3D printed parts are produced using organic binders, but the binders affect the plastic portions of the 3D printers in the long run. The quality and thickness of the scaffolds depend on the distribution of shape and size of the particles. The mechanical properties of materials play an important role as it directly affects the cellular growth in fabricated bone tissues. In order to interface the scaffolds with the biological system, the materials should have good mechanical properties. Another challenge is the color and texture similarity or dissimilarity of the 3D printed biomedical products with the organs. Multi-extruder 3D printers are also not able to produce realistic results in terms of color and texture. The challenges related to printers involve low dimensional accuracy, as in fused deposition modeling, which depends on the software, screw movements, and the firmware control. Powder agglomeration is another difficulty faced in 3D printing, in which bigger pore agglomeration leads to poor densification. The size of the nozzle is the challenge for achieving a nanoscale design for biomedical products. Cost associated with the materials, investment, utility, and technical servicing is another challenge associated with 3D printing. The lack of guidelines demands a trial and error method to obtain the product, which is also challenging. Finally, there is a risk of cyber-attack, as 3D printing technology uses an internet connection, so data confidentiality and integrity are essential. Further advancements in technologies are required for improving the resolution without surrendering the structure of scaffolds. There is a need to remove the powder particles stuck in small channels. One possible strategy is to create powder particles in spherical form for easy removal. Future research should concentrate on the nanoarchitecture for the direct integration of molecules into scaffolds.

3.8   CONCLUSION

Current developments in mechanical systems as well as in the software field have immensely boosted the resolution, precision, and speed of the 3D printing technology. It has been widely used in medical education, the surgical field, pharmaceutical industry, personal protective equipment, personalized implants, prosthesis, and surgical tools. Some of the aspects that have to be considered for 3D printing applications are the type of software and printer, production time, mechanical characteristics and haptic feedback of the material, costs involved. There is an insufficiency in the precision and effectiveness of the 3D printing of metals, particularly in obtaining a good surface finish. There exists an imbalance between the speed and printing accuracy also. Upon finding solutions to obtain high accuracy, good surface finish, and quick manufacturing, 3D printing can be extensively used in the medical field. There exist only a few well-established materials like titanium alloys, stainless steel, and aluminum alloys, which leads to a lack of raw materials for 3D printing. Research studies need to be carried out to face this limiting factor. The 3D printing techniques such as laser-based, ink-based, extrusion-based methods involve different kinds of factors which determines the properties of printed parts. Therefore, these factors must be optimized relative to the characteristics required, particularly where cells and biomolecules are involved. Although 3D printing in the medical field faces constraints, the continuous expansion and advancement of the biomedical materials industry and 3D printing technology can provide unparalleled growth and opportunities. In the coming years, integration of 3D reconstruction and printing with AI and big data can bring about significant change in the biomedical field.

REFERENCES

Abdel-Sayed, Philippe, and Ludwig Karl von Segesser. 2011. "Rapid Prototyping for Training Purposes in Cardiovascular Surgery." In Md Enamul Hoque, Ed. *Advanced Applications of Rapid Prototyping Technology in Modern Engineering*. 61–74, Books on Demand.

Abdelazeem, Rania M, Doaa Youssef, Jala El-Azab, Salah Hassab-Elnaby, and Mostafa Agour. 2020. "Three-Dimensional Visualization of Brain Tumor Progression Based Accurate Segmentation via Comparative Holographic Projection." *Plos One* 15 (7): e0236835.

Anastasiou, Athanasios, Charalambos Tsirmpas, Alexandros Rompas, Kostas Giokas, and Dimitris Koutsouris. 2013. "3D Printing: Basic Concepts Mathematics and Technologies." In *13th IEEE International Conference on BioInformatics and BioEngineering*, 1–4.

Arakeri, Megha P, G Ram Mohana Reddy. 2013. "An Effective and Efficient Approach to 3D Reconstruction and Quantification of Brain Tumor on Magnetic Resonance Images." *International Journal of Signal Processing, Image Processing and Pattern Recognition* 6 (3): 111.

Bahraminasab, Marjan. 2020. "Challenges on Optimization of 3D-Printed Bone Scaffolds." *BioMedical Engineering OnLine* 19 (1): 1–33.

Balla, Vamsi Krishna, Shashwat Banerjee, Susmita Bose, and Amit Bandyopadhyay. 2010. "Direct Laser Processing of a Tantalum Coating on Titanium for Bone Replacement Structures." *Acta Biomaterialia* 6 (6): 2329–34.

Bencharit, Sompop, Warren C Byrd, Sandra Altarawneh, Bashir Hosseini, Austin Leong, Glenn Reside, Thiago Morelli, and Steven Offenbacher. 2014. "Development and Applications of Porous Tantalum Trabecular Metal-Enhanced Titanium Dental Implants." *Clinical Implant Dentistry and Related Research* 16 (6): 817–26.

Binder, Johannes S, Michael Scholz, Stephan Ellmann, Michael Uder, Robert Grützmann, Georg F Weber, and Christian Krautz. 2021. "Cinematic Rendering in Anatomy: A Crossover Study Comparing a Novel 3D Reconstruction Technique to Conventional Computed Tomography." *Anatomical Sciences Education* 14 (1): 22–31.

Chen, Hao, Yuchen He, and Weidong Jia. 2020. "Precise Hepatectomy in the Intelligent Digital Era." *International Journal of Biological Sciences* 16 (3): 365.

Chen, Shi, Zhouxian Pan, Yanyan Wu, Zhaoqi Gu, Man Li, Ze Liang, Huijuan Zhu, et al. 2017. "The Role of Three-Dimensional Printed Models of Skull in Anatomy Education: A Randomized Controlled Trail." *Scientific Reports* 7 (1): 1–11.

Choong, Yu Ying Clarrisa, Hong Wei Tan, Deven C Patel, Wan Ting Natalie Choong, Chun-Hsien Chen, Hong Yee Low, Ming Jen Tan, Chandrakant D Patel, and Chee Kai Chua. 2020. "The Global Rise of 3D Printing during the COVID-19 Pandemic." *Nature Reviews Materials* 5 (9): 637–39.

D'Urso, Paul S, David J Effeney, W John Earwaker, Timothy M Barker, Michael J Redmond, Robert G Thompson, and Francis H Tomlinson. 2000. "Custom Cranioplasty Using Stereolithography and Acrylic." *British Journal of Plastic Surgery* 53 (3): 200–204.

Demir, Ali Gökhan, Lorenzo Monguzzi, and Barbara Previtali. 2017. "Selective Laser Melting of Pure Zn with High Density for Biodegradable Implant Manufacturing." *Additive Manufacturing* 15: 20–28.

Do, Anh-Vu, Behnoush Khorsand, Sean M Geary, and Aliasger K Salem. 2015. "3D Printing of Scaffolds for Tissue Regeneration Applications." *Advanced Healthcare Materials* 4 (12): 1742–62.

Duan, Fuqing, Donghua Huang, Yun Tian, Ke Lu, Zhongke Wu, and Mingquan Zhou. 2015. "3d Face Reconstruction from Skull by Regression Modeling in Shape Parameter Spaces." *Neurocomputing* 151: 674–82.

Dudina, Dina V, Boris B Bokhonov, and Eugene A Olevsky. 2019. "Fabrication of Porous Materials by Spark Plasma Sintering: A Review." *Materials* 12 (3): 541.

Dworzak, Jalda, Hans Lamecker, Jens von Berg, Tobias Klinder, Cristian Lorenz, Dagmar Kainmüller, Heiko Seim, Hans-Christian Hege, and Stefan Zachow. 2010. "3D Reconstruction of the Human Rib Cage from 2D Projection Images Using a Statistical Shape Model." *International Journal of Computer Assisted Radiology and Surgery* 5 (2): 111–24.

Engelhardt, Sandy, Raffaele De Simone, Peter M Full, Matthias Karck, and Ivo Wolf. 2018. "Improving Surgical Training Phantoms by Hyperrealism: Deep Unpaired Image-to-Image Translation from Real Surgeries." In *International Conference on Medical Image Computing and Computer-Assisted Intervention*, 747–55.

Erbel, Raimund, Carlo Di Mario, Jozef Bartunek, Johann Bonnier, Bernard de Bruyne, Franz R Eberli, Paul Erne, et al. 2007. "Temporary Scaffolding of Coronary Arteries with Bioabsorbable Magnesium Stents: A Prospective, Non-Randomised Multicentre Trial." *The Lancet* 369 (9576): 1869–75.

Farahani, Rouhollah D, Martine Dubé, and Daniel Therriault. 2016. "Three-Dimensional Printing of Multifunctional Nanocomposites: Manufacturing Techniques and Applications." *Advanced Materials* 28 (28): 5794–821.

Fok, Kai-Yin, Chi-Tsun Cheng, K Tse Chi, and Nuwan Ganganath. 2016. "A Relaxation Scheme for TSP-Based 3D Printing Path Optimizer." In *2016 International Conference on Cyber-Enabled Distributed Computing and Knowledge Discovery (CyberC)*, 382–85.

Frazier, William E. 2014. "Metal Additive Manufacturing: A Review." *Journal of Materials Engineering and Performance* 23 (6): 1917–28.

Fu, Yourong, Shicheng Yang, Seong Hoon Jeong, Susumu Kimura, and Kinam Park. 2004. "Orally Fast Disintegrating Tablets: Developments, Technologies, Taste-Masking and Clinical Studies." *Critical Reviews™ in Therapeutic Drug Carrier Systems* 21 (6): 433–475.

Gadia, Akshay, Kunal Shah, and Abhay Nene. 2018. "Emergence of Three-Dimensional Printing Technology and Its Utility in Spine Surgery." *Asian Spine Journal* 12 (2): 365.

Garcia, Justine, ZhiLin Yang, Rosaire Mongrain, Richard L Leask, and Kevin Lachapelle. 2018. "3D Printing Materials and Their Use in Medical Education: A Review of Current Technology and Trends for the Future." *BMJ Simulation and Technology Enhanced Learning* 4 (1): 27–40.

George, Mitchell, Kevin R Aroom, Harvey G Hawes, Brijesh S Gill, and Joseph Love. 2017. "3D Printed Surgical Instruments: The Design and Fabrication Process." *World Journal of Surgery* 41 (1): 314–19.

Gneiger, Stefan, Johannes A Österreicher, Aurel R Arnoldt, Alois Birgmann, and Martin Fehlbier. 2020. "Development of a High Strength Magnesium Alloy for Wire Arc Additive Manufacturing." *Metals* 10 (6): 778.

Gnonnou, Christo, and Nadia Smaoui. 2014. "Segmentation and 3D Reconstruction of MRI Images for Breast Cancer Detection." In *Image Processing, Applications and Systems Conference (IPAS), 2014 First International*, 1–6.

González Izard, Santiago, Ramiro Sánchez Torres, Oscar Alonso Plaza, Juan Antonio Juanes Mendez, and Francisco José Garcia-Peñalvo. 2020. "Nextmed: Automatic Imaging Segmentation, 3D Reconstruction, and 3D Model Visualization Platform Using Augmented and Virtual Reality." *Sensors* 20 (10): 2962.

Goyal, Sukriti, Nikhil Sharma, Bharat Bhushan, Achyut Shankar, and Martin Sagayam. 2021. "IoT Enabled Technology in Secured Healthcare: Applications, Challenges and Future Directions." In: Hassanien A.E., Khamparia A., Gupta D., Shankar K., Slowik A. (Eds.) *Cognitive Internet of Medical Things for Smart Healthcare*, 25–48. Springer, Cham.

Greil, Gerald F, Ivo Wolf, Axel Kuettner, Michael Fenchel, Stephan Miller, Petros Martirosian, Fritz Schick, Matthias Oppitz, Hans-Peter Meinzer, and Ludger Sieverding. 2007. "Stereolithographic Reproduction of Complex Cardiac Morphology Based on High Spatial Resolution Imaging." *Clinical Research in Cardiology* 96 (3): 176–85.

Guo, Lei, Ying Li, Dongbo Miao, Lei Zhao, Weili Yan, and Xueqin Shen. 2011. "3-D Reconstruction of Encephalic Tissue in MR Images Using Immune Sphere-Shaped SVMs." *IEEE Transactions on Magnetics* 47 (5): 870–73.

Hailer, Nils. 2018. "20 Years of Porous Tantalum in Primary and Revision Hip Arthroplasty—Time for a Critical Appraisal." *Acta Orthopaedica* 89 (3): 254.

Haleem, Abid, Mohd Javaid, and Raju Vaishya. 2020. "3D Printing Applications for the Treatment of Cancer." *Clinical Epidemiology and Global Health* 8 (4): 1072–76.

Han, Seungkyu, Matthew Zielewski, David Martinez Holguin, Monica Michel Parra, and Namsoo Kim. 2018. "Optimization of AZ91D Process and Corrosion Resistance Using Wire Arc Additive Manufacturing." *Applied Sciences* 8 (8): 1306.

Hsieh, Tsung-yen, Brian Cervenka, Raj Dedhia, Edward Bradley Strong, and Toby Steele. 2018. "Assessment of a Patient-Specific, 3-Dimensionally Printed Endoscopic Sinus and Skull Base Surgical Model." *JAMA Otolaryngology–Head & Neck Surgery* 144 (7): 574–79.

Ige, Oladeji O, Lasisi E Umoru, and Sunday Aribo. 2012. "Natural Products: A Minefield of Biomaterials." *International Scholarly Research Notices* 2012.

Imanishi, Jungo, and Peter F M Choong. 2015. "Three-Dimensional Printed Calcaneal Prosthesis Following Total Calcanectomy." *International Journal of Surgery Case Reports* 10: 83–87.

Inserra, Alessandro, Luca Borro, Marco Spada, Simone Frediani, and Aurelio Secinaro. 2020. "Advanced 3D 'Modeling' and 'Printing' for the Surgical Planning of a Successful Case of Thoraco-Omphalopagus Conjoined Twins Separation." *Frontiers in Physiology* 11.

Jacobs, Stephan, Ronny Grunert, Friedrich W Mohr, and Volkmar Falk. 2008. "3D-Imaging of Cardiac Structures Using 3D Heart Models for Planning in Heart Surgery: A Preliminary Study." *Interactive Cardiovascular and Thoracic Surgery* 7 (1): 6–9.

Jamroz, Witold, Mateusz Kurek, Ewelina Łyszczarz, Witold Brniak, and Renata Jachowicz. 2017. "Printing Techniques: Recent Developments in Pharmaceutical Technology." *Acta Poloniae Pharmaceutica* 74 (3): 753–763.

Jindal, Mansi, Jatin Gupta, and Bharat Bhushan. 2019. "Machine Learning Methods for IoT and Their Future Applications." In *2019 International Conference on Computing, Communication, and Intelligent Systems (ICCCIS)*, 430–34.

Karayegen, Gökay, and Mehmet Feyzi Aksahin. 2021. "Brain Tumor Prediction on MR Images with Semantic Segmentation by Using Deep Learning Network and 3D Imaging of Tumor Region." *Biomedical Signal Processing and Control* 66: 102458.

Kermer, Christian, Andreas Lindner, Ingrid Friede, Arne Wagner, and Werner Millesi. 1998. "Preoperative Stereolithographic Model Planning for Primary Reconstruction in Craniomaxillofacial Trauma Surgery." *Journal of Cranio-Maxillofacial Surgery* 26 (3): 136–39.

Khamparia, Aditya, Prakash Kumar Singh, Poonam Rani, Debabrata Samanta, Ashish Khanna, and Bharat Bhushan. 2020. "An Internet of Health Things-Driven Deep Learning Framework for Detection and Classification of Skin Cancer Using Transfer Learning." *Transactions on Emerging Telecommunications Technologies*, 32: e3963.

Kigka, Vassiliki I, George Rigas, Antonis Sakellarios, Panagiotis Siogkas, Ioannis O Andrikos, Themis P Exarchos, Dimitra Loggitsi, et al. 2018. "3D Reconstruction of Coronary Arteries and Atherosclerotic Plaques Based on Computed Tomography Angiography Images." *Biomedical Signal Processing and Control* 40: 286–94.

Kumar, Santosh, Bharat Bhusan, Debabrata Singh, and Dilip kumar Choubey. 2020. "Classification of Diabetes Using Deep Learning." In *2020 International Conference on Communication and Signal Processing (ICCSP)*, 651–55.

Lamadé, Wolfram, Gerald Glombitza, Lars Fischer, Peter Chiu, Carlos E Cárdenas Sr, M Thorn, Hans-Peter Meinzer, et al. 2000. "The Impact of 3-Dimensional Reconstructions on Operation Planning in Liver Surgery." *Archives of Surgery* 135 (11): 1256–61.

Laronda, Monica M, Alexandra L Rutz, Shuo Xiao, Kelly A Whelan, Francesca E Duncan, Eric W Roth, Teresa K Woodruff, and Ramille N Shah. 2017. "A Bioprosthetic Ovary Created Using 3D Printed Microporous Scaffolds Restores Ovarian Function in Sterilized Mice." *Nature Communications* 8 (1): 1–10.

Lecron, Fabian, Jonathan Boisvert, Saïd Mahmoudi, Hubert Labelle, and Mohammed Benjelloun. 2013. "Three-Dimensional Spine Model Reconstruction Using One-Class SVM Regularization." *IEEE Transactions on Biomedical Engineering* 60 (11): 3256–64.

Li, Y, H Jahr, K Lietaert, P Pavanram, A Yilmaz, L I Fockaert, M A Leeflang, et al. 2018. "Additively Manufactured Biodegradable Porous Iron." *Acta Biomaterialia* 77: 380–93.

Li, Zhenzhu, Zefu Li, Ruiyu Xu, Meng Li, Jianmin Li, Yongliang Liu, Dehua Sui, Wensheng Zhang, and Zheng Chen. 2015. "Three-Dimensional Printing Models Improve Understanding of Spinal Fracture—A Randomized Controlled Study in China." *Scientific Reports* 5 (1): 1–9.

Longfield, Evan A, Todd M Brickman, and Anita Jeyakumar. 2015. "3D Printed Pediatric Temporal Bone: A Novel Training Model." *Otology & Neurotology* 36 (5): 793–95.

Luffy, Sarah A, Da-Tren Chou, Jenora Waterman, Peter D Wearden, Prashant N Kumta, and Thomas W Gilbert. 2014. "Evaluation of Magnesium-Yttrium Alloy as an Extraluminal Tracheal Stent." *Journal of Biomedical Materials Research Part A* 102 (3): 611–20.

Maidin, Shajahan Bin, Ian Campbell, and Eujin Pei. 2012. "Development of a Design Feature Database to Support Design for Additive Manufacturing." *Assembly Automation* 32 (3): 235–244.

Matthew, Di Prima, James Coburn, David Hwang, Jennifer Kelly, Akm Khairuzzaman, and Laura Ricles. 2016. "Additively Manufactured Medical Products–the FDA Perspective." *3D Printing in Medicine* 2 (1): 1–6.

Matthews, Felix, Peter Messmer, Vladislav Raikov, Guido A Wanner, Augustinus L Jacob, Pietro Regazzoni, and Adrian Egli. 2009. "Patient-Specific Three-Dimensional Composite Bone Models for Teaching and Operation Planning." *Journal of Digital Imaging* 22 (5): 473–82.

More, Sujeet, Jimmy Singla, Sahil Verma, Uttam Ghosh, Joel J P C Rodrigues, A S M Sanwar Hosen, In-Ho Ra, et al. 2020. "Security Assured CNN-Based Model for Reconstruction of Medical Images on the Internet of Healthcare Things." *IEEE Access* 8: 126333–46.

Mottl-Link, Sibylle, Michael Hübler, Titus Kühne, Urte Rietdorf, Julia J Krueger, Bernhard Schnackenburg, Raffaele De Simone, et al. 2008. "Physical Models Aiding in Complex Congenital Heart Surgery." *The Annals of Thoracic Surgery* 86 (1): 273–77.

Müller, Adolf, Kartik G Krishnan, Eberhard Uhl, and Gerson Mast. 2003. "The Application of Rapid Prototyping Techniques in Cranial Reconstruction and Preoperative Planning in Neurosurgery." *Journal of Craniofacial Surgery* 14 (6): 899–914.

Murr, Lawrence E, Sara M Gaytan, Edwin Martinez, Frank Medina, and Ryan B Wicker. 2012. "Next Generation Orthopaedic Implants by Additive Manufacturing Using Electron Beam Melting." *International Journal of Biomaterials* 2012.

Ng, Wei Long, Alvin Chan, Yew Soon Ong, and Chee Kai Chua. 2020. "Deep Learning for Fabrication and Maturation of 3D Bioprinted Tissues and Organs." *Virtual and Physical Prototyping* 15 (3): 340–58.

Ngan, Elizabeth M, Ivan M Rebeyka, David B Ross, Mohamed Hirji, Johan F Wolfaardt, Rosemary Seelaus, Andrew Grosvenor, and Michelle L Noga. 2006. "The Rapid Prototyping of Anatomic Models in Pulmonary Atresia." *The Journal of Thoracic and Cardiovascular Surgery* 132 (2): 264–69.

Niinomi, Mitsuo, Takayuki Narushima, and Masaaki Nakai. "Advances in metallic biomaterials: Tissues, Materials and Biological Reactions." Heidelberg, DE: Springer (2015).

van Noort, Richard. 2012. "The Future of Dental Devices Is Digital." *Dental Materials* 28 (1): 3–12.

Nugroho, Pratomo Adhi, Dwi Kurnia Basuki, and Riyanto Sigit. 2016. "3D Heart Image Reconstruction and Visualization with Marching Cubes Algorithm." In *2016 International Conference on Knowledge Creation and Intelligent Computing (KCIC)*, 35–41.

Otton, James M, Roberto Spina, Romina Sulas, Rajesh N Subbiah, Neil Jacobs, David W M Muller, and Brendan Gunalingam. 2015. "Left Atrial Appendage Closure Guided by Personalized 3D-Printed Cardiac Reconstruction." *JACC: Cardiovascular Interventions* 8 (7): 1004–6.

Panigrahi, Niranjan, Ishan Ayus, and Om Prakash Jena. 2021. "An Expert System-Based Clinical Decision Support System for Hepatitis-B Prediction & Diagnosis." In Sachi Nandan Mohanty, G. Nalinipriya, Om Prakash Jena, Achyuth Sarkar, Eds. *Machine Learning for Healthcare Applications*, 57–75. Wiley Online Library.

Paramesha, K, H L Gururaj, and Om Prakash Jena. 2021. "Applications of Machine Learning in Biomedical Text Processing and Food Industry." In Sachi Nandan Mohanty, G. Nalinipriya, Om Prakash Jena, Achyuth Sarkar, Eds. *Machine Learning for Healthcare Applications*, 151–67. Wiley Online Library.

Patel, Manan Sunil, Johnathon R McCormick, Alexander Ghasem, Samuel R Huntley, and Joseph P Gjolaj. 2020. "Tantalum: The next Biomaterial in Spine Surgery?" *Journal of Spine Surgery* 6 (1): 72.

Patra, Sudhansu Shekhar, Om Praksah Jena, Gaurav Kumar, Sreyashi Pramanik, Chinmaya Misra, and Kamakhya Narain Singh. 2021. "Random Forest Algorithm in Imbalance Genomics Classification." In Rabinarayan Satpathy, Tanupriya Choudhury, Suneeta Satpathy, Sachi Nandan Mohanty, Xiaobo Zhang, Eds. *Data Analytics in Bioinformatics: A Machine Learning Perspective*, 173–90. Wiley Online Library..

Pattanayak, Deepak K, A Fukuda, T Matsushita, M Takemoto, S Fujibayashi, K Sasaki, N Nishida, T Nakamura, and T Kokubo. 2011. "Bioactive Ti Metal Analogous to Human Cancellous Bone: Fabrication by Selective Laser Melting and Chemical Treatments." *Acta Biomaterialia* 7 (3): 1398–1406.

Pattnayak, Parthasarathi, and Om Prakash Jena. 2021. "Innovation on Machine Learning in Healthcare Services–An Introduction." In Sachi Nandan Mohanty, G. Nalinipriya, Om Prakash Jena, Achyuth Sarkar, Eds. *Machine Learning for Healthcare Applications*, 1–15. Wiley Online Library..

Pennarossa, Georgia, Sharon Arcuri, Teresina De Iorio, Fulvio Gandolfi, and Tiziana A L Brevini. 2021. "Current Advances in 3D Tissue and Organ Reconstruction." *International Journal of Molecular Sciences* 22 (2): 830.

Pere, Cristiane Patricia Pissinato, Sophia N Economidou, Gurprit Lall, Clémentine Ziraud, Joshua S Boateng, Bruce D Alexander, Dimitrios A Lamprou, and Dennis Douroumis. 2018. "3D Printed Microneedles for Insulin Skin Delivery." *International Journal of Pharmaceutics* 544 (2): 425–32.

Peuster, Matthias, Carola Hesse, Tirza Schloo, Christoph Fink, Philipp Beerbaum, and Christian von Schnakenburg. 2006. "Long-Term Biocompatibility of a Corrodible Peripheral Iron Stent in the Porcine Descending Aorta." *Biomaterials* 27 (28): 4955–62.

Pilipchuk, Sophia P, Alexandra B Plonka, Alberto Monje, Andrei D Taut, Alejandro Lanis, Benjamin Kang, and William V Giannobile. 2015. "Tissue Engineering for Bone Regeneration and Osseointegration in the Oral Cavity." *Dental Materials* 31 (4): 317–38.

Pillai, Sangeeth, Akshaya Upadhyay, Parisa Khayambashi, Imran Farooq, Hisham Sabri, Maryam Tarar, Kyungjun T Lee, et al. 2021. "Dental 3D-Printing: Transferring Art from the Laboratories to the Clinics." *Polymers* 13 (1): 157.

Pillai, Soumya S, and Rajesh Kannan Megalingam. 2020. "Detection and 3D Modeling of Brain Tumor Using Machine Learning and Conformal Geometric Algebra." In *2020 International Conference on Communication and Signal Processing (ICCSP)*, 257–61.

Poulsen, Michael, Cathy Lindsay, Tim Sullivan, and Paul D'Urso. 1999. "Stereolithographic Modelling as an Aid to Orbital Brachytherapy." *International Journal of Radiation Oncology* Biology* Physics* 44 (3): 731–35.

Pradhan, Nitesh, Vijaypal Singh Dhaka, Geeta Rani, and Himanshu Chaudhary. 2020. "Transforming View of Medical Images Using Deep Learning." *Neural Computing and Applications*, 1–12.

Punyaratabandhu, Thipachart, Boonrat Lohwongwatana, Chedtha Puncreobutr, Arkaphat Kosiyatrakul, Puwadon Veerapan, and Suriya Luenam. 2017. "A Patient-Matched Entire First Metacarpal Prosthesis in Treatment of Giant Cell Tumor of Bone." *Case Reports in Orthopedics* 2017.

Rohner, Dennis, Raquel Guijarro-Martinez, Peter Bucher, and Beat Hammer. 2013. "Importance of Patient-Specific Intraoperative Guides in Complex Maxillofacial Reconstruction." *Journal of Cranio-Maxillofacial Surgery* 41 (5): 382–90.

Saini, Monika, Yashpal Singh, Pooja Arora, Vipin Arora, and Krati Jain. 2015. "Implant Biomaterials: A Comprehensive Review." *World Journal of Clinical Cases: WJCC* 3 (1): 52.

Salmi, Mika. 2016. "Possibilities of Preoperative Medical Models Made by 3D Printing or Additive Manufacturing." *Journal of Medical Engineering* 2016: 1–6.

Schievano, Silvia, Francesco Migliavacca, Louise Coats, Sachin Khambadkone, Mario Carminati, Neil Wilson, John E Deanfield, Philipp Bonhoeffer, and Andrew M Taylor. 2007. "Percutaneous Pulmonary Valve Implantation Based on Rapid Prototyping of Right Ventricular Outflow Tract and Pulmonary Trunk from MR Data." *Radiology* 242 (2): 490–97.

Schinhammer, Michael, Anja C Hänzi, Jörg F Löffler, and Peter J Uggowitzer. 2010. "Design Strategy for Biodegradable Fe-Based Alloys for Medical Applications." *Acta Biomaterialia* 6 (5): 1705–13.

Schmauss, Daniel, Christoph Schmitz, Amir Koshrow Bigdeli, Stefan Weber, Nicholas Gerber, Andres Beiras-Fernandez, Florian Schwarz, Christoph Becker, Christian Kupatt, and Ralf Sodian. 2012. "Three-Dimensional Printing of Models for Preoperative Planning and Simulation of Transcatheter Valve Replacement." *The Annals of Thoracic Surgery* 93 (2): e31–e33.

Sharma, Nikhil, Ila Kaushik, Bharat Bhushan, Siddharth Gautam, and Aditya Khamparia. 2020. "Applicability of WSN and Biometric Models in the Field of Healthcare." In: K. Martin Sagayam, Bharat Bhushan, A. Diana Andrushia, Victor Hugo C. de Albuquerque (Eds.) *Deep Learning Strategies for Security Enhancement in Wireless Sensor Networks*, 304–29. IGI Global.

Shi, Jianping, Huixin Liang, Jie Jiang, Wenlai Tang, and Jiquan Yang. 2019. "Design and Performance Evaluation of Porous Titanium Alloy Structures for Bone Implantation." *Mathematical Problems in Engineering* 2019.

Sodian, Ralf, Daniel Schmauss, Mathias Markert, Stefan Weber, Konstantin Nikolaou, Sandra Haeberle, Ferdinand Vogt, et al. 2008a. "Three-Dimensional Printing Creates Models for Surgical Planning of Aortic Valve Replacement after Previous Coronary Bypass Grafting." *The Annals of Thoracic Surgery* 85 (6): 2105–8.

Sodian, Ralf, Stefan Weber, Mathias Markert, Markus Loeff, Tim Lueth, Florian C Weis, Sabine Daebritz, Edward Malec, Christoph Schmitz, and Bruno Reichart. 2008b. "Pediatric Cardiac Transplantation: Three-Dimensional Printing of Anatomic Models for Surgical Planning of Heart Transplantation in Patients with Univentricular Heart." *The Journal of Thoracic and Cardiovascular Surgery* 136 (4): 1098–99.

Spetzger, Uwe, Alexander S Koenig, and others. 2017. "Individualized Three-Dimensional Printed Cage for Spinal Cervical Fusion." *Digital Medicine* 3 (1): 1.

Spottiswoode, B S, D J den Heever, Y Chang, S Engelhardt, S Du Plessis, F Nicolls, H B Hartzenberg, and A Gretschel. 2013. "Preoperative Three-Dimensional Model Creation of Magnetic Resonance Brain Images as a Tool to Assist Neurosurgical Planning." *Stereotactic and Functional Neurosurgery* 91 (3): 162–69.

Stadie, Axel Thomas, Ralf Alfons Kockro, Robert Reisch, Andrei Tropine, Stephan Boor, Peter Stoeter, and Axel Perneczky. 2008. "Virtual Reality System for Planning Minimally Invasive Neurosurgery." *Journal of Neurosurgery* 108 (2): 382–94.

Tam, Chun Hei Adrian, Yiu Che Chan, Yuk Law, and Stephen Wing Keung Cheng. 2018. "The Role of Three-Dimensional Printing in Contemporary Vascular and Endovascular Surgery: A Systematic Review." *Annals of Vascular Surgery* 53: 243–54.

Tawbe, Khalil, François Cotton, and Laurent Vuillon. 2008. "Evolution of Brain Tumor and Stability of Geometric Invariants." *International Journal of Telemedicine and Applications* 2008.

Thijs, Lore, Maria Luz Montero Sistiaga, Ruben Wauthle, Qingge Xie, Jean-Pierre Kruth, and Jan Van Humbeeck. 2013. "Strong Morphological and Crystallographic Texture and Resulting Yield Strength Anisotropy in Selective Laser Melted Tantalum." *Acta Materialia* 61 (12): 4657–68.

Tino, Rance, Ryan Moore, Sam Antoline, Prashanth Ravi, Nicole Wake, Ciprian N Ionita, Jonathan M Morris, et al. 2020. "COVID-19 and the Role of 3D Printing in Medicine." *3D Print Med* 6, 11(2020).

Vranicar, Mark, William Gregory, William I Douglas, Peter Di Sessa, and Thomas G Di Sessa. 2008. "The Use of Stereolithographic Hand Held Models for Evaluation of Congenital Anomalies of the Great Arteries." *Studies in Health Technology and Informatics* 132: 538.

Wang, Aosen, Chi Zhou, Zhanpeng Jin, and Wenyao Xu. 2017. "Towards Scalable and Efficient GPU-Enabled Slicing Acceleration in Continuous 3D Printing." In 2017 22nd Asia and South Pacific Design Automation Conference (ASP-DAC), 623–28.

Wang, Di, Yimeng Wang, Jianhua Wang, Changhui Song, Yongqiang Yang, Zimian Zhang, Hui Lin, Yongqiang Zhen, and Suixiang Liao. 2016. "Design and Fabrication of a Precision Template for Spine Surgery Using Selective Laser Melting (SLM)." *Materials* 9 (7): 608.

Wang, Fuyou, Hao Chen, Pengfei Yang, Aikeremujiang Muheremu, Peng He, Haquan Fan, and Liu Yang. 2020. "Three-Dimensional Printed Porous Tantalum Prosthesis for Treating Inflammation after Total Knee Arthroplasty in One-Stage Surgery–a Case Report." *Journal of International Medical Research* 48 (3): 0300060519891280.

Wang, Ling, Jianfeng Kang, Changning Sun, Dichen Li, Yi Cao, and Zhongmin Jin. 2017. "Mapping Porous Microstructures to Yield Desired Mechanical Properties for Application in 3D Printed Bone Scaffolds and Orthopaedic Implants." *Materials & Design* 133: 62–68.

Wang, Zhongmin, Yuhao Liu, Hongxing Luo, Chuanyu Gao, Jing Zhang, and Yuya Dai. 2017. "Is a Three-Dimensional Printing Model Better than a Traditional Cardiac Model for Medical Education? A Pilot Randomized Controlled Study." *Acta Cardiologica Sinica* 33 (6): 664.

Waran, Vicknes, Vairavan Narayanan, Ravindran Karuppiah, Devaraj Pancharatnam, Hari Chandran, Rajagopalan Raman, Zainal Ariff Abdul Rahman, Sarah L F Owen, and Tipu Z Aziz. 2014. "Injecting Realism in Surgical Training—Initial Simulation Experience with Custom 3D Models." *Journal of Surgical Education* 71 (2): 193–97.

Waran, Vicknes, Vairavan Narayanan, Ravindran Karuppiah, Hari Chandran Thambynayagam, Kalai Arasu Muthusamy, Zainal Ariff Abdul Rahman, and Ramez Wadie Kirollos. 2015. "Neurosurgical Endoscopic Training via a Realistic 3-Dimensional Model with Pathology." *Simulation in Healthcare* 10 (1): 43–48.

Wei, Feng, Zhehuang Li, Zhongjun Liu, Xiaoguang Liu, Liang Jiang, Miao Yu, Nanfang Xu, et al. 2020. "Upper Cervical Spine Reconstruction Using Customized 3D-Printed Vertebral Body in 9 Patients with Primary Tumors Involving C2." *Annals of Translational Medicine* 8 (6).

Yao, Xiling, Seung Ki Moon, and Guijun Bi. 2017. "A Hybrid Machine Learning Approach for Additive Manufacturing Design Feature Recommendation." *Rapid Prototyping Journal* 23 (6): 983–997.

Yap, Chor Yen, Chee Kai Chua, Zhi Li Dong, Zhong Hong Liu, Dan Qing Zhang, Loong Ee Loh, and Swee Leong Sing. 2015. "Review of Selective Laser Melting: Materials and Applications." *Applied Physics Reviews* 2 (4): 41101.

Yazdimamaghani, Mostafa, Mehdi Razavi, Daryoosh Vashaee, Keyvan Moharamzadeh, Aldo R Boccaccini, and Lobat Tayebi. 2017. "Porous Magnesium-Based Scaffolds for Tissue Engineering." *Materials Science and Engineering: C* 71: 1253–66.

Yi, Xuehan, Chenyu Ding, Hao Xu, Tingfeng Huang, Dezhi Kang, and Desheng Wang. 2019. "Three-Dimensional Printed Models in Anatomy Education of the Ventricular System: A Randomized Controlled Study." *World Neurosurgery* 125: e891–e901.

Yin, Ziying, Xin Lu, Salomon Cohen Cohen, Yi Sui, Armando Manduca, Jamie J Van Gompel, Richard L Ehman, and John Huston. 2021. "A New Method for Quantification and 3D Visualization of Brain Tumor Adhesion Using Slip Interface Imaging in Patients with Meningiomas." *European Radiology* 31: 1–11.

Yoo, Dong-Jin. 2011. "Three-Dimensional Surface Reconstruction of Human Bone Using a B-Spline Based Interpolation Approach." *Computer-Aided Design* 43 (8): 934–47.

Zhang, Binkai, Xiang Wang, Xiao Liang, and Jinjin Zheng. 2017. "3D Reconstruction of Human Bones Based on Dictionary Learning." *Medical Engineering & Physics* 49: 163–70.

Zhang, Jing, Ling-Rui Gong, Keping Yu, Xin Qi, Zheng Wen, Qiaozhi Hua, and others. 2020. "3D Reconstruction for Super-Resolution CT Images in the Internet of Health Things Using Deep Learning." *IEEE Access* 8: 121513–25.

Zhang, Shiying, Yang Zheng, Liming Zhang, Yanze Bi, Jianye Li, Jiao Liu, Youbin Yu, Heqing Guo, and Yan Li. 2016. "In Vitro and in Vivo Corrosion and Histocompatibility of Pure Mg and a Mg-6Zn Alloy as Urinary Implants in Rat Model." *Materials Science and Engineering: C* 68: 414–22.

Zuniga, Jorge, Dimitrios Katsavelis, Jean Peck, John Stollberg, Marc Petrykowski, Adam Carson, and Cristina Fernandez. 2015. "Cyborg Beast: A Low-Cost 3d-Printed Prosthetic Hand for Children with Upper-Limb Differences." *BMC Research Notes* 8 (1): 1–9.

4 Medical Text and Image Processing
Applications, Methods, Issues, and Challenges

Behzad Soleimani Neysiani
and Hassan Homayoun

CONTENTS

4.1 INTRODUCTION

Today, almost all industries save their data in computers and electronic devices, making electronic medical records (EMR) a critical resource for medical analysis and decision making. A Google Scholar search using Publish or Perish (Harzing 1997) tool shows more than 2000 articles about image and text processing since 1974, in which 1953 articles seem to be more related. The distribution of articles by year of publication is shown in Figure 4.1 based on a logarithmic scale to depict lower and higher values simultaneously. The year distribution indicates a progressive study in this field, but its complexity indicates the necessity of this field in research and practical markets.

DOI: 10.1201/9781003226147-4

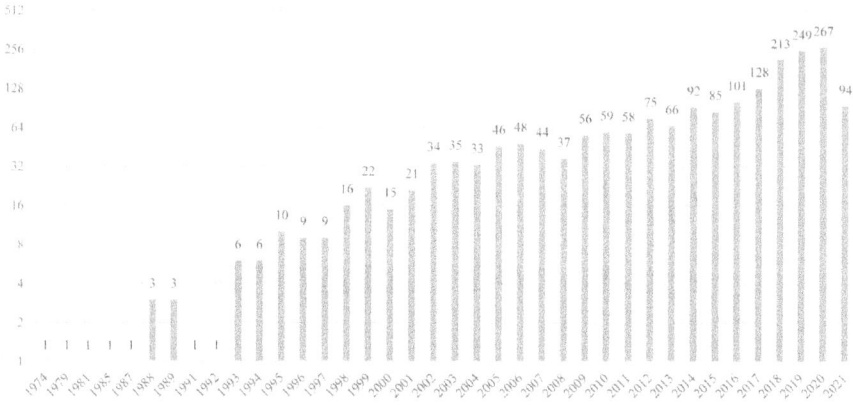

FIGURE 4.1 Yearly distribution of published articles on medical text and image processing based on Google Scholar results (logarithmic scale).

Famous publishers like Elsevier, Springer, Wiley, and IEEE publish a quarter of selected articles, as shown in Figure 4.2. Moreover, there are more than fifty-five books in this field, indicating good progress and maturity. Even though there are many articles in this field, the challenges and issues are vast and need more efforts such as in (AI Multiple 2020) (1) patient care and effective treatment, (2) medical diagnostic, (3) management, and (4) research and development. Every domain has many problems, and their objectives and visions are far from their current states and achievements in most problems. In other words, there is a vast opportunity for research and development on this topic.

A static search based on article titles demonstrates there were more than 200 various review articles in the selected articles, excluding books. These review articles

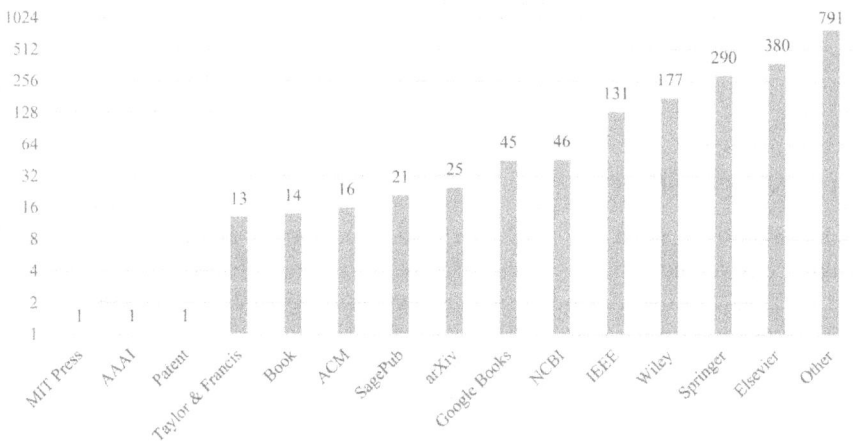

FIGURE 4.2 Distribution of articles on medical text and image processing by publisher based on Google Scholar results (logarithmic scale).

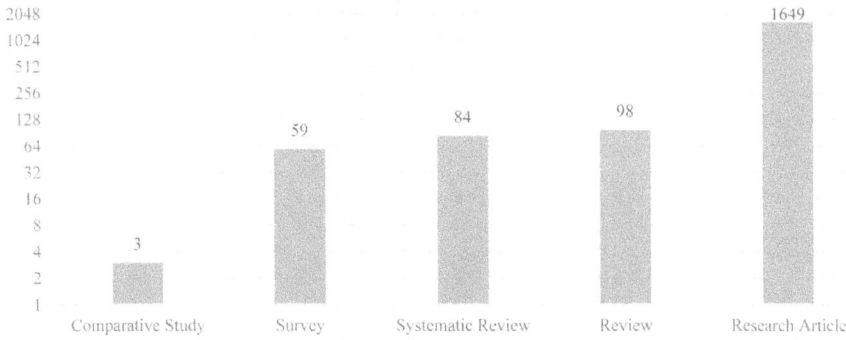

FIGURE 4.3 Distribution of various review articles and research articles on medical text and image processing based on Google Scholar results (logarithmic scale).

can be helpful for beginners to learn about this field from scratch aside from a good background and even can be taught in academies. These review articles can specialize in comparative studies, survey articles, systematic review and simple review. The distribution of various review articles and other research articles is shown in Figure 4.3.

There are many data types in the medical field, but, generally, data can be categorized as structural and non-structural (Manogaran et al. 2017). The structured data are usually nominal or numerical and can be easily compared and used in mathematical or relational operations, essential basic operations for statistical analysis, or machine learning (ML) algorithms (Pattnayak and Jena 2021). Texts and images are unstructured data samples that cannot be processed using the usual mathematical or relational operations, and they need to be converted to structural data, in a process called feature extraction (Soleimani Neysiani, Babamir, and Aritsugi 2020).

There are many researches about both data types and their distribution can be seen in Figure 4.4, which indicates some articles studied both texts and images and

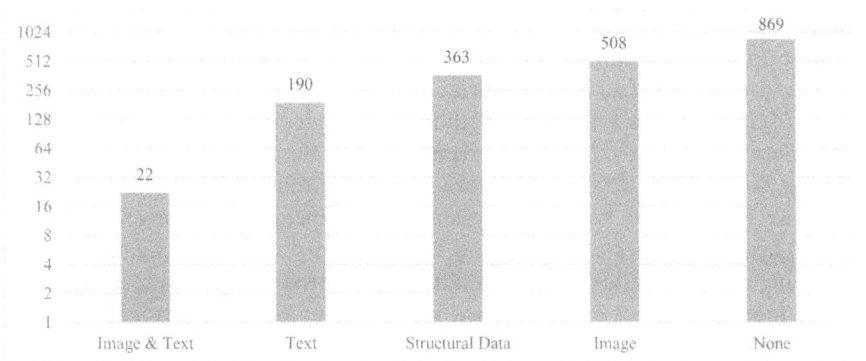

FIGURE 4.4 Distribution of articles on medical text and image processing by data type based on Google Scholar results (logarithmic scale).

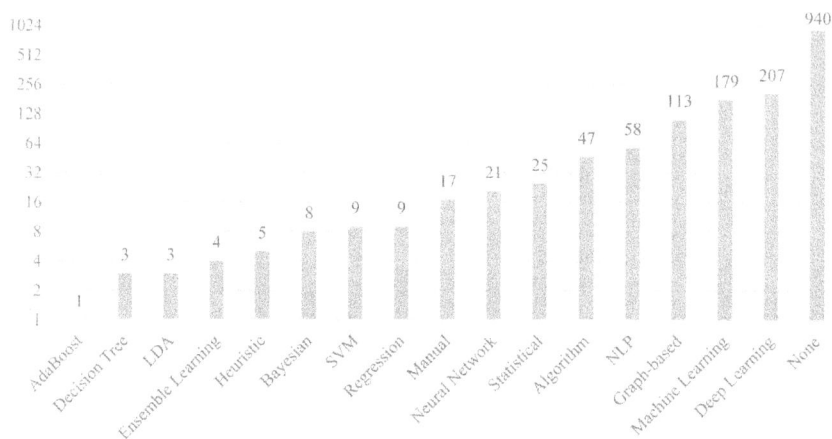

FIGURE 4.5 Distribution of ML algorithms about medical text and image processing based on Google Scholar results (logarithmic scale).

others used just one type, especially those for which our keywords can recognize their data type. Interestingly, images are the most common data type used in studies, then structural data, and, finally, texts. It depends on their dataset and their importance, too. There are fewer available textual data in the medical field, which could be explained by the fact that privacy-preservation for medical images is more accessible than for texts. It should be mentioned that there exists more than 80% of unstructured data in hospital databases (Perera et al. 2013).

ML (Pattnayak and Jena 2021) algorithms primarily use data processing techniques to learn and predict events, categorize data, and find knowledge behind the data. More than 830 articles use various ML algorithms and artificial intelligence techniques for medical data processing based on Figure 4.5, in which deep learning is the most used algorithm. Graph-based algorithms are usually used for network data as another kind of unstructured medical data primarily used in the genetic domain. Natural language processing (NLP) is used to process texts appropriate for prescriptions or social media comments. There are some proposed algorithms for data processing that are categorized in the "Algorithm" method. Besides, statistical analysis is a traditional method for data description and analysis. The neural network refers to traditional artificial neural network methods before deep learning, like a multi-layered feed-forward perceptron model, a primarily used technique, especially in healthcare systems like Diabetes prediction (Kumar et al. 2020). These techniques can be used as keywords for further investigation of data processing methods in this field. It should be considered that 940 articles' data processing methods cannot be determined based on our keywords, excluding books and non-research-based articles.

The articles' topic distribution is shown in Figure 4.6, which indicates that the genetic, mental, and drug domains are the topics most widely studied. Many fields like radiography and breast usually deal with image data, and other diseases usually

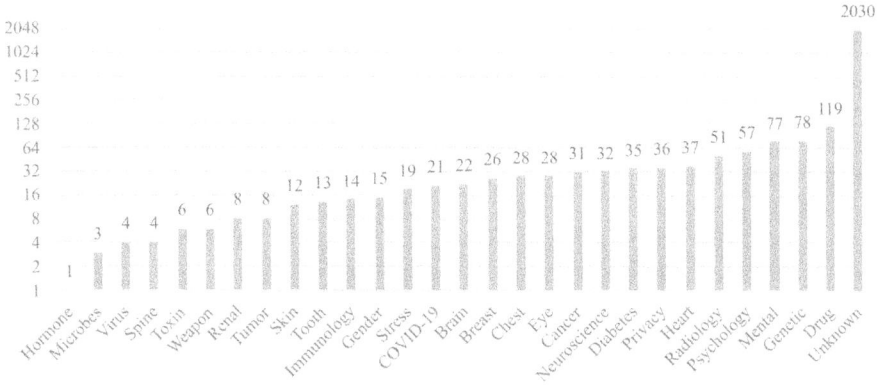

FIGURE 4.6 Distribution of articles on medical text and image processing by topics based on Google Scholar results (logarithmic scale).

use structural data. Viruses, microbes, cancers, tumors, or mental health like stress and psychology have many physical treatment efforts. Drug discovery is another exciting problem based on animal or human experiments or finding their genetic science relations. The privacy consideration is an essential issue for medical records because if patients know their records will be used for other analysis and their case potentially published globally, they will be afraid to visit doctors, discuss about their symptoms, and, finally, voluntarily make noise in their treatments by wrong or imperfect data providing. Thus privacy-preserving is another challenge for medical data processing.

In the following sections, both text and image processing will be discussed to determine their applications, methods, issues, and data processing challenges. It should be considered that unstructured data processing is a complex and time-consuming operation, so many other engineering fields like distributed computing, including cloud, grid, and blockchain, are regarded to deal with big medical data (Biswas et al. 2014). Moreover, unstructured data processing follows the steps outlined in Figure 4.7 (Sun et al. 2018). In the first step, the unstructured data should be gathered from paper or electronic records and then integrated to build a database. Then unstructured data should be pre-processed to clean its noise and prepare it correctly for the primary processing. Central processing usually consists of information extraction and selection and data analyzing. Information selection reduces

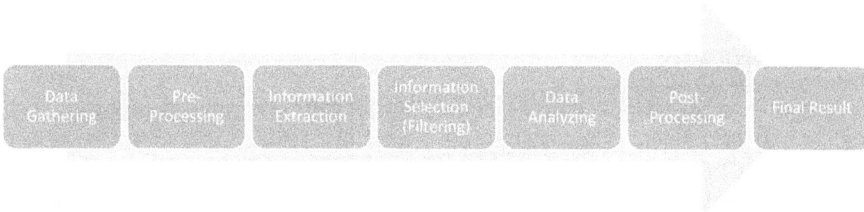

FIGURE 4.7 Unstructured data processing procedure. (See Sun et al. 2018.)

the amount of extracted information by eliminating useless or redundant data that is just time-consuming without significantly affecting the data processing results (Sun et al. 2018). Data analysis depends on the medical objective but usually is an artificial intelligence technology like data mining, which generally uses a machine learning algorithm to extract knowledge from data. Classification, prediction, and clustering are some examples of data analysis. Post-processing usually evaluates and saves extracted knowledge as a new model for further usage, like expert systems (Panigrahi, Ayus, and Jena 2021). The final result will be extracted knowledge and its validation performance as a metric for end-users.

Many other hot topics should be considered, such as the Internet of Things (IoT) (Jindal, Gupta, and Bhushan 2019; Doostali et al. 2020; Goyal et al. 2021) and wireless sensor networks (Nikhil et al. 2020) to collect medical data, and cloud computing (Soltani, Barekatain, and Soleimani Neysiani 2016; Soltani, Soleimani Neysiani, and Barekatain 2017) as an infrastructure for data processing in data science applications like medical healthcare (Soltani, Barekatain, and Soleimani Neysiani 2021). Besides, there are many data science techniques, including data mining, text mining, artificial intelligence, pattern recognition, statistics, and related sciences to process medical data. For example, association rule mining (Hoseini, Shahraki, and Soleimani Neysiani 2015) can find frequent patterns in transactional data; evolutionary algorithms can optimize many tasks like association rule mining (Varzaneh et al. 2018; Soleimani Neysiani et al. 2019) or neural networks (Soleimani Neysiani, Soltani, and Ghezelbash 2015) in a shorter runtime; dimension reduction improves runtime and validation performance (Soleimani Neysiani et al. 2020), dimension expansion (Soleimani Neysiani and Babamir 2019g; Oshnoudi et al. 2021) and new feature generation (Soleimani Neysiani and Babamir 2016) can improve validation performance; ML techniques can improve information retrieval performance (Soleimani Neysiani and Babamir 2020) even though their parameters need to be optimized (Bahadorpour, Soleimani Neysiani, and Shahraki 2017); and feature importance detection and selection can improve runtime and validation performance (Soleimani Neysiani and Shiralizadeh Dezfoli 2020) and eliminate additional useless features in medical use case like pre-diagnosis heart coronary artery disease (Ghasemi, Soleimani Neysiani, and Nematbakhsh 2020).

4.2   MEDICAL TEXT PROCESSING AND ANALYSIS

There are many forms of text data in medical science like medical claims, call center logs, prescriptions, laboratory results, patient records, and notes, all usually written by physicians and nurses about patients and their diseases and symptoms.

4.2.1   APPLICATIONS

Information retrieval (IR) refers to searching documents and finding the most relevant and similar documents (Popowich 2005); a general operation in medical notes and documents is known as information extraction, too (Uramoto et al. 2004). IR techniques usually deal with term frequencies, NLP, and text mining techniques. Disease representation is an IR application to find those records, including diseases or not based on disease symptoms, for further classification (Dreisbach et al. 2019). Fraud detection based on healthcare bills for medical insurance claims is another text mining application involving NLP and IR techniques (Popowich 2005). Question and answering is another application of text processing using NLP and IR techniques, which usually rank the IR results based on the results of the question asked (Iroju and Olaleke 2015).

Medical personnels need to command the computers and devices using speech recognition, especially during critical operations, for searching questions and finding their answers (Q&A), and documenting events. The speech recognition procedure usually converts voice to text and processes texts to extract information (Goss et al. 2019). Moreover, document translation is necessary for international medical agencies to receive international reports (Zhu, Tu, and Huang 2021).

Categorizing and phenotyping clinical text data is another frequent operation, especially with regard to legacy patients' records or big medical data like genetic information which is placed into hierarchical or distinct sets. Clustering is the main technique used for this purpose (Raja et al. 2008). The clustering will find similar documents and keep them in distinct sets, such as a high inter-similarity and low intra-similarity between sets (Trivedi et al. 2018).

Text summarization is essential due to the large volume of text for almost every text-processing application like IR or Q&A to optimize user reading time and finding the most related documents at a glance (Moradi and Ghadiri 2018).

Semantic web improves search engine accuracy to find the more related results using anthologies about objects and terms relationships. It is a symbolic processing act like IR, but this approach extracts related concepts of texts and finds the relationship between extracted concepts to generate its output. The Unified Medical Language System (UMLS) is introduced as a standard knowledge representation for medical purposes. Symbolic processing usually uses finite states and grammars for parsing the input query and produces its output (Meystre and Haug 2005; Iroju and Olaleke 2015).

Medical text reports need de-identification before public publishing for researchers and other studies. De-identification is a privacy-preserving operation to delete the names of patients, doctors, nurses, and hospitals. It needs NLP and IR techniques to find and eliminate sensitive information in EMR as the data integrity retained, for example, substitute patients names with random unique identity numbers (Neamatullah et al. 2008).

Nowadays, the web and social media applications are useful repositories for such purposes as sharing people's viewpoints about diseases, their symptoms, their heuristic treatments, and their opinions about treatments, doctors, and hospitals. Therefore, their comments can be processed to extract their opinion about new events and subjects (Demner-Fushman and Elhadad 2016).

There are already many built tools for processing medical text data which can be categorized based on their application as the following:

1. **Information extraction:** Medical Language Extraction and Encoding (MedLEE)[1] (Friedman et al. 1996), clinical Text Analysis and Knowledge Extraction System (cTAKES)[2] (Savova et al. 2010), Medical Literature Analysis and Retrieval System Online (Medline) (Greenhalgh 1997).

---

[1] https://www.medlee.ca/
[2] https://ctakes.apache.org/

2. **Prediction:** Vaccine Safety Datalink Project (VSD) for vaccination reactions (Hazlehurst et al. 2005).
3. **Symbolic Processing:** Metamap (Aronson 2001).
4. **Question and Answering:** Gene TUC (Sætre 2006).

Machine learning techniques serve almost all application problems to can be automated (Paramesha, Gururaj, and Jena 2021).

4.2.2 METHODS

NLP made texts ready to be used for processing. NLP steps are shown in Figure 4.8, which indicate various processes, including (Iroju and Olaleke 2015):

1. **Phonological analysis:** Speech recognition needs carefully chosen characters primarily based on the sentence, which usually follows three rules, including (1) phonetic rules about word production sounds, (2) phonemic rules about the various pronunciations of spoken words, and (3) prosodic rules considering fluctuation in stress and intonation across a sentence.
2. **Morphological analysis:** Checking a word's form in a language and their relation, including those terms with the same and different form of their primary term as inflectional and derivational analysis, respectively.
3. **Lexical analysis:** This process, also known as tokenization, extracts meaningful terms, called tokens, from sentences like nouns, verbs, and adjectives.
4. **Syntactic analysis:** A parser will check the correctness of sentences and find their language construction, especially the role of each term in the sentence, like subjects, verbs, objectives, and adjectives.
5. **Semantic analysis:** The logical meaning of words will be checked using semantic networks that model word-level interactions in this phase, e.g., checking that an apple cannot eat a mouse, but vice versa is correct.

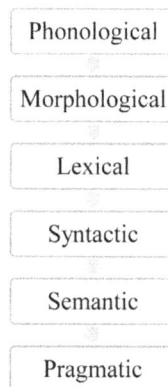

Phonological

Morphological

Lexical

Syntactic

Semantic

Pragmatic

FIGURE 4.8 NLP analysis steps. (See Iroju and Olaleke, 2015.)

6. **Pragmatic analysis:** Every term may have more than one meaning depending on the context, e.g., apple is a fruit and an international brand for electronic devices like cellphones or laptops. Thus, every term's meaning should be considered based on the context of its sentence and even paragraph or entire document.

NLP techniques are usually used in the pre-processing phase of text processing. The usual pre-processing operations for text consider the following steps:

1. **Tokenizing:** It separates meaningful terms, as was mentioned in lexical analysis of NLP steps.
2. **Stemming or lemmatization:** It is a morphological analysis that finds the pure form, especially for verbs or plural nouns with different forms.
3. **Removing stop words:** These are useless words and elements like punctuation, conjunctions, sometimes copula verbs, and frequent terms in a context in which their presence and frequency are not essential. Stop words are just wasting our time and sometimes lead us to misunderstand and misinterpret the results.
4. **Typo detection and correction:** Human reports usually contain many typos (Soleimani Neysiani and Babamir 2018), which can be determined rapidly (Soleimani Neysiani and Babamir 2019a) using NLP tools. Many typos, like interconnected terms (Soleimani Neysiani and Babamir 2019f), can be corrected efficiently (Soleimani Neysiani and Babamir 2019d) to improve text mining and IR validation performance (Soleimani Neysiani and Babamir 2019c).

The IR technique usually uses two famous techniques called term frequency (TF) and inverse document frequency (IDF) which are the number a term is repeated in the selected text and entire documents of the database, respectively. Many other heuristic techniques like minimum, average, and maximum TF/IDF improve IR technique validation performance (Soleimani Neysiani, Babamir, and Aritsugi 2020). TF (equation 4.1) can be calculated for each t term with a specific *length* in a document, including k textual fields like f as $d[f]$ with w_f weight field importance and *average_length$_f$* for all terms in $d[f]$ and b_f is a constant to prevent division by zero.

$$TF_D(t,d) = \sum_{f=1}^{K} \frac{w_f \times occurrences(d[f],t)}{1 - b_f + \dfrac{b_f \times length}{average\_length_f}} \tag{4.1}$$

IDF (equation 4.2) is a logarithm in Euler number base for dividing N documents by the number of d documents, including t in their f textual field as $d[f]$.

$$IDF(t,D) = \log \frac{N}{\left|\{d \in D : t \in d[f]\}\right|} \tag{4.2}$$

BM25F (equation 4.3) is a weighted average of TF and IDF for two documents that can calculate text similarities (Soleimani Neysiani and Babamir 2019b).

$$BM25F_{ext}(d,q) = \sum_{t \in d[f] \cap q[f]} IDF(t, Total\ Text\ Fields\ of\ Bug\ Reports)$$

$$\times \frac{TF_D(t,d[f])}{K_1 + TF_D(t,d[f])}$$

(4.3)

Feature extraction is the most crucial procedure for predictive application. There are many feature extraction methods like using TF/IDF for the most critical terms in texts. The longest common subsequence (LCS) finds the largest similar substring between two texts, a widespread operation in genetic analysis and text mining applications (Soleimani Neysiani and Babamir 2019e). Another recent and innovative approach is word embedding, which uses a deep neural network to represent a term using a vector representation like word2vec (Chiu and Baker 2020).

4.2.3 Issues and Challenges

Texts usually have misspelling and typos as a typical challenge that needs processing and cleaning in the pre-processing phase (Iroju and Olaleke 2015). Every medical domain needs its ontology as an essential resource for semantic search, which needs a database to view these anthologies, extend, and modified them. Another critical challenge in text processing is uncertainty, which needs a fuzzy theorem to manage uncertain symbols like high or low temperature, which demands context and people. Privacy preservation is a historical concern that made textual dataset publishing difficult (Agrawal and Jain 2020).

4.3 MEDICAL IMAGE PROCESSING AND ANALYSIS

Medical imaging is the visual reconstruction task of various body organs and compartments usually covered by skin and bony structures. This visual reconstruction appears in various forms of medical digital images depending on the imaging techniques and technologies. There are various imaging technologies including, X-ray, computed tomography (CT), magnetic resonance (MR), positron-emitting tomography (PET), and ultrasonic imaging. Each imaging technique is sensitive to a specific type of structure and tissue. Therefore, different tissue types appear distinctly in medical images. Physicians use this distinction in medical digital images in different analyses to diagnose and track disease progression.

Image analysis can either be manual by a physician or automatic by using a computer program. Manual analysis is usually time-consuming, laborious, and error-prone, therefore, automatic analysis is preferred. In other words, different computer-aided detection (CADe) and computer-aided diagnosis (CADx) systems are equipped with modules that are capable of analyzing medical images. These modules use intelligent algorithms such as classification, regression, detection, and segmentation to perform analytical tasks. Classification algorithms aim to categorize tumors, pathologies, or tissues as different sub-types; regression algorithms attempt to map images to a numerical score which represents various risks or degrees of a specific disease; detection algorithms attempt to localize pathologies and tissues of interest; and segmentation algorithms are in charge of accurate delineation of various abnormalities. As early diagnosis of diseases improves prognosis, image-based CAD systems are beneficial in screening programs. In other words, early diagnosis reduces the death rate of different diseases.

Deep-based neural networks like convolutional neural networks (CNNs) and multi-view massive training deep neural network (MMTDNN) have more than 90% validation performance for abnormal tissue detection, as highlighted – bold values – in Table 4.1. If lesion and normal areas are considered as positive and negative points, respectively; the algorithm may predict these areas as true or false. So, there exist four states based on the actual points and predict states, including true positive (TP), true negative (TN), false positive (FP), and false negative (FN). These values are usually tabulated in a matrix called the confusion matrix. The validation metrics usually defined based on these values as equations 4.4–4.8 (Khastavaneh and Ebrahimpour-Komleh 2020a).

Accuracy (equation 4.4) is the fraction of true prediction, either positive or negative, based on total points.

$$Accuracy = \frac{TP + TN}{TP + TN + FP + FN} \tag{4.4}$$

TABLE 4.1

Comparison of MMTDNN results for Segmentation and Detection of Abnormal Tissues in Medical Images with Other Methods

Method	Accuracy	Sensitivity	Specificity	Dice Similarity Coefficient	Jaccard Index
Fully CNN using Jaccard Distance (Yuan, Chao, and Lo 2017)	0.963	**0.926**	0.971	0.922	0.861
Very Deep Residual Networks (Yu et al. 2017)	0.949	0.911	0.957	0.897	0.829
Multi-stage fully CNN (Bi et al. 2017)	0.955	0.922	0.965	0.912	0.846
Massive Training ANN (MTANN) (Khastavaneh and Ebrahimpour-Komleh 2017)	0.861	0.790	0.847	0.713	0.580
MMTDNN (Khastavaneh and Ebrahimpour-Komleh 2020a)	**0.973**	0.912	**0.986**	**0.931**	**0.876**

Source: Khastavaneh and Ebrahimpour-Komleh (2020a).

Sensitivity (equation 4.5), or recall, is the fraction of true positive prediction based on total positive points, indicating that the ML algorithm can truly recall how many abnormal points.

$$\text{Sensitivity} = \text{Recall} = \frac{\text{TP}}{\text{TP} + \text{FN}} \qquad (4.5)$$

Specificity (equation 4.6) is like sensitivity, but for negative points, it is the fraction of true negative prediction based on total negative points, indicating that the ML algorithm can truly recall how many normal points.

$$\text{Specificity} = \frac{\text{TN}}{\text{TN} + \text{FP}} \qquad (4.6)$$

Dice similarity coefficient (equation 4.7) and Jaccard index (equation 4.8) indicate true positive prediction based on total actual and predicted positive points because a positive point is an abnormal point, and its prediction is crucial; therefore, many metrics try to reflect its efficiency.

$$\text{Dice similarity coefficient} = \frac{2 \times \text{TP}}{2 \times \text{TP} + \text{FN} + \text{FP}} \qquad (4.7)$$

$$\text{Jaccard index} = \frac{\text{TP}}{\text{TP} + \text{FN} + \text{FP}} \qquad (4.8)$$

Another branch of algorithms focuses on enhancing medical images to differentiate better normal tissues, pathologies, and abnormalities from each other. As a reality, medical images are usually full of noise and artifacts. Enhancement applications aim to remove these noise and artifacts. Medical images which are noise-free and artifact-free better represent organs and abnormalities. Therefore, clear medical images are ideal for both physicians and CAD systems to make accurate clinical decisions. These enhancement algorithms improve the performance of medical images for further analysis either by a physician or a CAD system. Enhancement algorithms are applied to different modalities such as MR and ultrasonic images.

Different images are acquired from different time points to investigate or assess some situations in organs or tissues. These images may be in different modalities. In these cases, these modalities must be aligned together. For such purposes, registration algorithms are employed. Therefore, registration algorithms benefit applications that work with different modalities (Klein et al. 2010).

Different classification, regression, detection, and segmentation applications use ML, and their core components are introduced in the following sections. Moreover, the primary methods and algorithms of regression, classification, detection and segmentation are elaborated. Finally, issues and challenges of these applications and algorithms will be highlighted.

4.3.1 APPLICATIONS

Based on three primary types of algorithms, three main application areas of automated analysis and processing of medical images are available. These applications are very diverse, with various degrees of importance in clinics. Some of these applications play an essential role in the diagnosis and follow-up of the disease. Sometimes, this role has a substantial degree of importance so continuing treatment without it is impossible. In other words, these broad ranges of applications offer optimal treatment to different diseases and assist physicians with a second opinion. Besides optimal treatment, automated medical image analysis is critical and essential to conduct medical research, such as drug development and large screening programs. In these cases, large populations need to be considered for various purposes, such as measuring the risk of diseases and delineating abnormalities. According to the main algorithm, these applications are categorized into three categories: regression/classification-based, localization or detection-based, and segmentation-based.

4.3.1.1   Regression and Classification Applications

The image under analysis is mapped to a continuous number representing the risk or degree of disease in regression-based applications. Classification-based applications attempt to categorize medical images, or a part of them, in different categories or sub-types. This classification aims to diagnose the disease or reveal the stage of the disease. In other words, a typical image is automatically analyzed to check whether there is any sign of a disease in that image to classify the patient whose image it is as healthy or unhealthy.

Classification-based applications work with different image modalities. Some applications focus on the lung's x-ray images to check if there is any sign of infection in those images, for example, classification of thoracic diseases (Wang and Xia 2018), classification of COVID-19 (Pham 2021), and classification of tuberculosis disease (Sathitratanacheewin, Sunanta, and Pongpirul 2020).

Many classification-based applications attempt to categorize tumors as benign or malignant in different modalities. These applications include skin cancer classification (Yu et al. 2017), breast cancer classification (Araujo et al. 2017; Motlagh et al. 2018; Shi et al. 2018), and lung nodule classification (Hua et al. 2015).

4.3.1.2   Detection Applications

In contrast to the classification applications that only assess a typical medical image to see if exciting organ, pathology, or tissue exists in that image, detection applications show that organ, pathology or tissue's location. This localization assists physicians while looking for specific abnormalities in images. Detection-based applications include brain tumor localization, lung nodule localization as early signs of lung cancer (Setio et al. 2016), detection of breast masses as early signs of breast cancer (Cruz-Roa et al. 2014; Samala et al. 2016).

4.3.1.3   Segmentation Applications

Segmentation applications aim to assign a label to the pixels of digital medical images so that pixels with the same label share the same visual characteristics or computed properties. Segmentation applications usually focus on delineating tumors and pathologies; diagnosing colon, prostate, liver, and breast cancers; studying anatomical structures; measuring tissue volume; detecting long nodules; and many other applications. As a result, segmentation-based applications of medical imaging can be widely used in clinics for diagnostic and treatment monitoring by physicians.

As segmentation and analysis of abnormal tissues in medical images are vital, accurate segmentation of these abnormal tissues is of interest for many CAD systems (Homayoun and Ebrahimpour-Komleh 2021). Quantitative measurement of these abnormalities is crucial for monitoring disease progression and optimal treatment.

One proper segmentation application will measure lesion load, including count and volume, in patients with multiple sclerosis (MS) (Khastavaneh and Haron 2014). Lesion load determines the drug dosage a patient should take. Accurate segmentation of MS lesions must be performed to compute the lesion load (Cabezas et al. 2014). Skin lesions are very prevalent in some areas of the world. Segmentation of these lesions is the first step for automatic and accurate determination of lesion type. Therefore, many applications focus on the accurate segmentation of skin lesions (Khastavaneh and Ebrahimpour-Komleh 2020a). Breast cancer is one of the leading causes of death among women worldwide. Therefore, mass breast segmentation is significant for the optimal treatment of the disease.

Many people are suffering from diabetes mellitus. Moreover, diabetes causes some lesions in the retina of diabetic people. Accurate computation of retinal lesion loads is significant for optimal treatment (Khastavaneh and Ebrahimpour-Komleh 2019). Lung nodules, if not treated on time, will develop and change to lung cancer. Therefore, accurate segmentation and detection of these lung CTs' nodules is an exciting application (Kido, Hirano, and Mabu 2020).

Besides the segmentation of abnormalities, some applications focus on the segmentation of normal tissues and organs. Extracting brain tissue from MR images is vital in measuring brain atrophy (Khastavaneh and Ebrahimpour-Komleh 2015a; Khastavaneh and Ebrahimpour-Komleh 2015b). Some applications focus on the parcellation of the brain into its central regions and sub-regions (Akkus et al. 2017). These parcellation applications assist physicians and researchers who study brain compartments (Anbeek et al. 2005).

4.3.2 Methods

This section aims to discuss the primary methods for analyzing and processing of medical images. Nowadays, various simple image processing methods for analyzing medical images and many state-of-the-art based on ML and deep learning are proposed. As shown in Figure 4.9, a typical ML-oriented pipeline for medical image analysis potentially includes seven stages: image acquisition, pre-processing, candidate extraction, feature generation, feature selection, main analysis, and post-processing. A digital image of a specific organ of interest is obtained using one of the previously mentioned medical imaging technologies in the image acquisition stage. The pre-processing, as the next stage, depends on the analysis type and also imaging technique. For example, noise elimination, bias field correction, and histogram normalization are common tasks in the pre-processing stage. The candidate extraction stage produces initial expected results using fast clustering and thresholding

Image Acquisition

Pre-proccessing

Candidate Extraction

Feature Generation

Feature Selection

Main Analysis

Post-proccessing

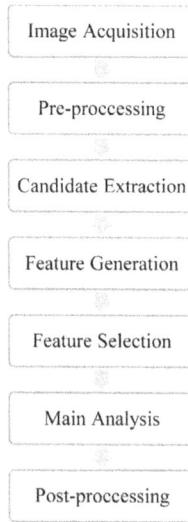

FIGURE 4.9   Block diagram of a typical image analysis method.

algorithms. The description and abstraction of candidate or image regions will be built into the feature generation stage. The feature selection stage selects the best quantifiers that describe candidate regions' surface intensity or sub-images. This selection prevents the curse of dimensionality as a destructive phenomenon. Depending on the method's expected outcome, the main analysis stage applies one of the regression, classification, detection, or segmentation algorithms to perform expected tasks. As the final stage of the pipeline, post-processing attempts to refine the final results by removing false positives or false negatives.

The main analysis stage of the pipeline aims to model the data and perform the main decision-making. Depending on the task, regression, classification, detection, or segmentation algorithms are applied to the data. There are two main directions for building an automated image analysis system, shallow modeling or deep modeling. In shallow modeling, feature generation and feature selection stages are mandatory before the modeling. Moreover, the quality of the leading modeling phase highly depends on the feature generation stage. Quality feature generation is based on trial and error, and depends on the experience of the expert. Many shallow methods such as support vector machines, neural networks, and decision trees contribute to medical applications; decision trees are among the most prevalent algorithms for classification and regression applications, and their main power is their explainability capability. Medical communities are interested to know the causes of the disease or essential factors of the diseases. Therefore, decision trees are widely used in different tasks, including the segmentation of MS lesions (Geremia et al. 2011). These shallow models cannot analyze medical images at the clinic level because they cannot tackle complexities in the medical images. In other words, organs, tissues, and abnormalities in medical images are potentially too complex to be represented accurately by simple shallow models.

In contrast to shallow modeling, deep modeling performs the task of modeling and feature generation simultaneously. Deep modeling is considered a subset of the big concept of representation learning. These methods attempt to generate a new representation of the raw data to perform more superior ML tasks (Khastavaneh and Ebrahimpour-Komleh 2020b). Deep learning methods are deep artificial neural networks. These deep networks amplify informative features from raw input data and suppress irrelevant information. There are many deep neural network architectures for different kinds of data. A CNN is a remarkable deep architecture capable of working with images. The main power of CNNs is their ability to learn and extract features relevant to the task at hand. Multiple CNNs have been proposed for various medical image processing and analysis tasks, including regression, classification, detection, and segmentation. Figure 4.10 demonstrates the difference between shallow modeling or feature-based CAD and deep modeling or image-based CAD. There is a gap between feature extraction and modeling in shallow or feature-based modeling, which causes some problems in the model's generalizability. In contrast, deep modeling utilizes end-to-end learning that can be fed directly with images and remove the gap between the feature extraction and modeling stages.

CNNs are widely used to classify skin lesions as cancerous or non-cancerous (Hosny, Kassem, and Fouad 2020; Khamparia et al. 2020) and classify images if they contain signs of COVID-19 (Yasar and Ceylan 2021). CNNs are widely employed in the task of segmentation, especially the segmentation of abnormal tissues. Conventional CNNs are very powerful in extracting context information from

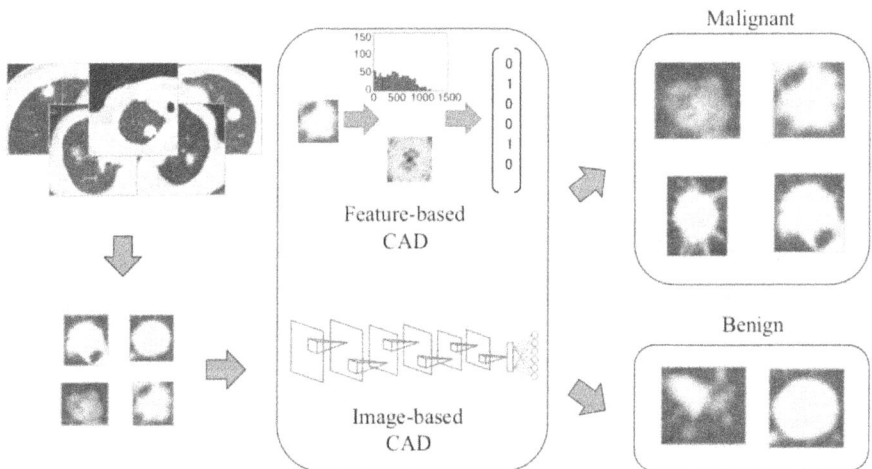

FIGURE 4.10 Image-based CAD/deep modeling versus feature-based CAD/shallow modeling. (See Kido, Hirano, and Mabu 2020.)

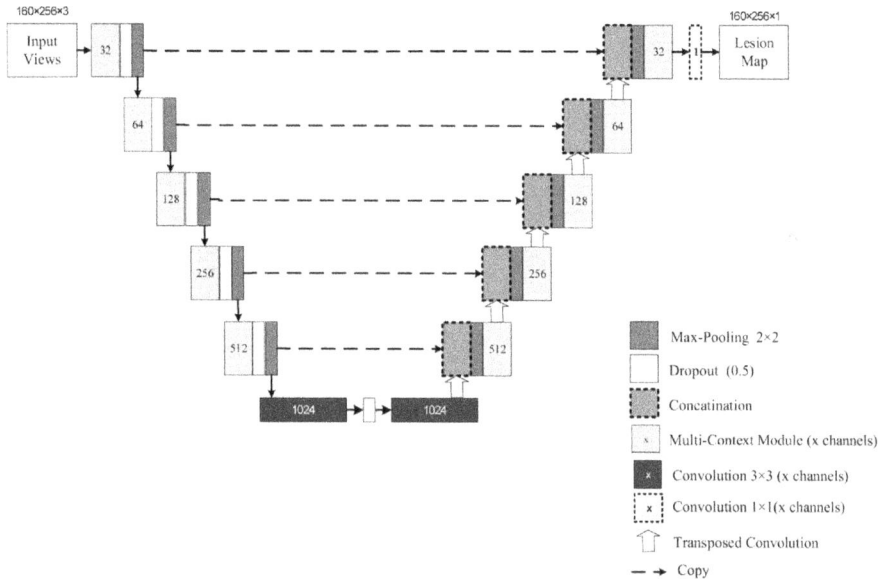

FIGURE 4.11   Block diagram of a typical U-shaped network.

images, but not suitable for capturing localization information. A U-shaped network has been proposed to have a CNN to capture both context and localization information (Noh, Hong, and Han 2015). A typical U-shaped network is an encoder-decoder network with two contraction and expansion paths, as shown in Figure 4.11 The contraction path attempts to extract context information, while the expansion path attempts to generate a segmentation mask. In U-shaped networks, some shortcut connections from the contraction path to the expansion path take care of localization information.

U-shaped networks have been employed for different segmentation tasks, including segmentation of lesions in brain MR images (Duong et al. 2019), segmentation of breast microcalcifications (Hossain 2019) and abnormalities (Almajalid et al. 2018), segmentation of skin lesions (Tang et al. 2019; Goyal et al. 2020), and many other organs and abnormalities.

4.3.3   ISSUES AND CHALLENGES

Automated medical image analysis is considered a challenging and sophisticated task in computer vision. This complexity is related to the inherent characteristics of body tissues and the shortcomings of imaging devices and imaging technologies. Some of these complexities include fuzzy borders of organs and inhomogeneity. Some abnormalities and organs' borders are fuzzy, preventing accurate description of their shapes for better analysis. Also, inhomogeneity means the surface of a specific anatomical structure or pathology is not identical throughout that structure or pathology. These inhomogeneous changes in the gray level of tissues affect the correct interpretation of the tissue properties. Noise, artifacts, and imaging conditions are another reality that always exists in medical images. All of these complexities justify the need for more sophisticated methods and techniques for tackling these challenging conditions.

Another issue for developing state-of-the-art medical image analysis applications and methods is the lack of enough data. In the condition of rare data, ML models cannot fit the data and become generalized. A rare data problem becomes severe if the ML model is deep. The number of free parameters of deep models is vast. Therefore, high amounts of data are needed to set these parameters.

Imbalanced data (Patra et al. 2021), clinical acceptance, and validation problems are other developing medical image analysis applications. Fortunately, many clinics accept the rule of artificial intelligence and ML in diagnosis and medical decision-making.

4.4   CONCLUSION

In this study, representative applications and methods of medical image and text processing are introduced. These applications and methods that serve physicians as a second opinion are used for different purposes, including diagnostic, follow-up, prevention, and medical research. Image analysis applications categorize different tissues as healthily or abnormal, detect tissues and organs of interest in different medical modalities, and accurately delineate organs or pathologies. Text analysis applications are used to detect drug side effects, automated interpretation of medical reports, information extraction, and text summarization.

As medical text and images are inherently unstructured data, typical feature-based ML methods cannot correctly process and analyze these data types. As a result, more sophisticated ML methods and techniques are needed. Deep neural networks are very advanced to act as end-to-end learners for analyzing unstructured data. Deep networks apply multiple layer-wise transformations to the input data to reach the final decision. In other words, unstructured data are abstracted in different layers to facilitate final inference.

Moreover, deep networks can tackle complexities existing in medical data by suppressing irrelevant information such as noise and artifacts, and amplifying relevant information. Therefore, the applications based on deep methods are considered state of the art. Moreover, much literature reported that the methods based on the deep learning family are very successful in medical image and text analysis.

A word cloud is drawn in Figure 4.12 based on titles and abstracts of selected articles in this chapter about images and text medical data processing, in which the boldest words indicate the more frequent and essential terms. This word cloud can be used as a guideline for future work in this field, which relieves this chapter. The word cloud demonstrates that image data are primarily used data against text and structural data. Besides, it refers to many processing methods like deep learning. The MRI technique is one of the boldest techniques in this figure, indicating its importance among research articles.

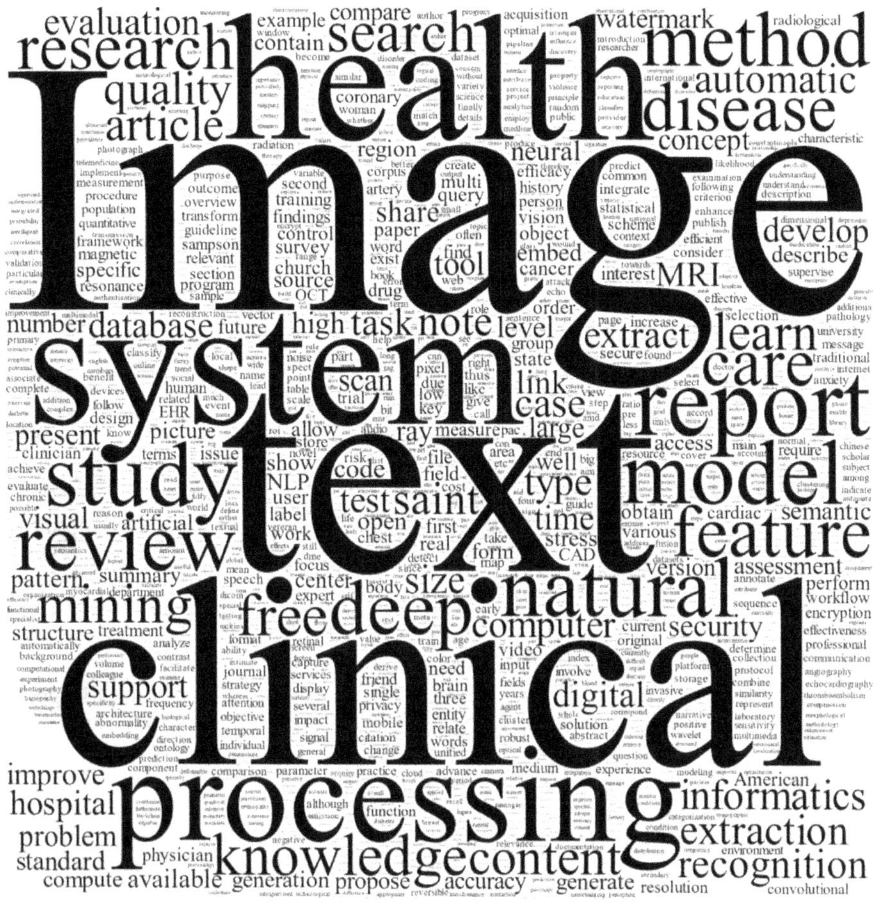

FIGURE 4.12 Word cloud for medical data processing.

REFERENCES

Agrawal, Shweta, and Sanjiv Kumar Jain. 2020. "Medical text and image processing: Applications, issues and challenges." In *Machine Learning with Health Care Perspective*, 237–62. Springer, Cham.

Akkus, Zeynettin, Alfiia Galimzianova, Assaf Hoogi, Daniel L. Rubin, and Bradley J. Erickson. 2017. "Deep learning for brain MRI segmentation: State of the art and future directions." *Journal of Digital Imaging* 30 (4): 449–59. https://doi.org/10.1007/s10278-017-9983-4

Almajalid, Rania, Juan Shan, Yaodong Du, and Ming Zhang. 2018. "Development of a deep-learning-based method for breast ultrasound image segmentation." 2018 17th IEEE International Conference on Machine Learning and Applications (ICMLA). 17-20 Dec, Orlando, FL, USA, https://doi.org/10.1109/ICMLA.2018.00179

Anbeek, Petronella, Koen L. Vincken, Glenda S. van Bochove, Matthias J.P. van Osch, Jeroen van der Grond. 2005. "Probabilistic segmentation of brain tissue in MR imaging." *NeuroImage* 27 (4): 795–804. https://doi.org/10.1016/j.neuroimage.2005.05.046

Araujo, T., G. Aresta, E. Castro, J. Rouco, P. Aguiar, C. Eloy, A. Polonia, and A. Campilho. 2017. "Classification of breast cancer histology images using convolutional neural networks." *PLoS One* 12 (6): 1–14. http://journals.plos.org/plosone/article/file?id=10.1371/journal.pone.0177544\& type=printable

Aronson, Alan R. 2001. "Effective mapping of biomedical text to the UMLS Metathesaurus: the MetaMap program." Proceedings of the AMIA Symposium: 17–21. https://pubmed.ncbi.nlm.nih.gov/11825149

Bahadorpour, Mojdeh, Behzad Soleimani Neysiani, and Mohammad Nadimi Shahraki. 2017. "Determining optimal number of neighbors in item-based kNN collaborative filtering algorithm for learning preferences of new users." *Journal of Telecommunication, Electronic and Computer Engineering (JTEC)* 9 (3): 163–7.

Bi, Lei, Jinman Kim, Euijoon Ahn, Ashnil Kumar, Michael Fulham, and Dagan Feng. 2017. "Dermoscopic image segmentation via multistage fully convolutional networks." *IEEE Transactions on Biomedical Engineering* 64 (9): 2065–74. https://doi.org/10.1109/TBME.2017.2712771

Biswas, Sumon, Tanjina Akhter, MS Kaiser, and SA Mamun. 2014. "Cloud based healthcare application architecture and electronic medical record mining: an integrated approach to improve healthcare system." 2014 17th International Conference on Computer and Information Technology (ICCIT). 22-23 Dec, Dhaka, Bangladesh, https://doi.org/10.1109/ICCITechn.2014.7073139

Cabezas, Mariano, Arnau Oliver, Eloy Roura, Jordi Freixenet, Joan C. Vilanova, and Torrent Rami. 2014. "Automatic multiple sclerosis lesion detection in brain MRI by FLAIR thresholding." *Computer Methods and Programs in Biomedicine* 115 (3): 147–161. https://doi.org/10.1016/j.cmpb.2014.04.006

Chiu, Billy, and Simon Baker. 2020. "Word embeddings for biomedical natural language processing: A survey." *Language and Linguistics Compass* 14 (12): e12402. https://doi.org/10.1111/lnc3.12402

Cruz-Roa, Angel, Ajay Basavanhally, Fabio Gonzlez, Hannah Gilmore, Michael Feldman, Shridar Ganesan, Natalie Shih, John Tomaszewski, and Anant Madabhushi. 2014. "Automatic detection of invasive ductal carcinoma in whole slide images with convolutional neural networks." 9041 (216): 904103. https://doi.org/10.1117/12.2043872

Demner-Fushman, Dina, and Noemie Elhadad. 2016. "Aspiring to unintended consequences of natural language processing: a review of recent developments in clinical and consumer-generated text processing." *Yearbook of medical informatics* (1): 224.

Doostali, Saeed, Seyed Morteza Babamir, Mohammad Shiralizadeh Dezfoli, and Behzad Soleimani Neysiani. 2020. "IoT-based model in smart urban traffic control: Graph theory and genetic algorithm." 2020 11th International Conference on Information and Knowledge Technology (IKT), 22-23 Dec, Tehran, Iran, https://doi.org/10.1109/IKT51791.2020.9345623

Dreisbach, Caitlin, Theresa A Koleck, Philip E Bourne, and Suzanne Bakken. 2019. "A systematic review of natural language processing and text mining of symptoms from electronic patient-authored text data." *International Journal of Medical Informatics* 125: 37–46.

Duong, M. T., J. D. Rudie, J. Wang, L. Xie, S. Mohan, J. C. Gee, and A. M. Rauschecker. 2019. "Convolutional Neural Network for Automated FLAIR Lesion Segmentation on Clinical Brain MR Imaging." *American Journal of Neuroradiology* 40 (8): 1282–90. https://doi.org/10.3174/ajnr.A6138

Friedman, Carol, Lyudmila Shagina, Socrates A. Socratous, and Xiao Zeng. 1996. "A WEB-based version of MedLEE: A medical language extraction and encoding system." Proceedings of the AMIA Annual Fall Symposium: 938. https://www.ncbi.nlm.nih.gov/pmc/articles/PMC2233000/

Geremia, Ezequiel, Olivier Clatz, Bjoern H. Menze, Ender Konukoglu, Antonio Criminisi, and Nicholas Ayache. 2011. "Spatial decision forests for MS lesion segmentation in multi-channel magnetic resonance images." *NeuroImage* 57 (2): 378–390. https://doi. org/10.1016/j.neuroimage.2011.03.080

Ghasemi, Foad, Behzad Soleimani Neysiani, and Naser Nematbakhsh. 2020. "Feature Selection in Pre-Diagnosis Heart Coronary Artery Disease Detection: A heuristic approach for feature selection based on Information Gain Ratio and Gini Index." 2020 6th International Conference on Web Research (ICWR), 22-23 April, Tehran, Iran, https://doi.org/10.1109/ICWR49608.2020.9122285

Goss, Foster R, Suzanne V Blackley, Carlos A Ortega, Leigh T Kowalski, Adam B Landman, Chen-Tan Lin, Marie Meteer, Samantha Bakes, Stephen C Gradwohl, and David W Bates. 2019. "A clinician survey of using speech recognition for clinical documentation in the electronic health record." *International Journal of Medical Informatics* 130: 103938. https://doi.org/10.1016/j.ijmedinf.2019.07.017

Goyal, Manu, Amanda Oakley, Priyanka Bansal, Darren Dancey, and Moi Hoon Yap. 2020. "Skin Lesion Segmentation in Dermoscopic Images with Ensemble Deep Learning Methods." *IEEE Access* 8: 4171–81. https://doi.org/10.1109/ACCESS.2019.2960504

Goyal, Sukriti, Nikhil Sharma, Bharat Bhushan, Achyut Shankar, and Martin Sagayam. 2021. "IoT Enabled Technology in Secured Healthcare: Applications, Challenges and Future Directions." In *Cognitive Internet of Medical Things for Smart Healthcare: Services and Applications*, edited by Aboul Hassanien, Aditya Khamparia, Deepak Gupta, K. Shankar and Adam Slowik, 25–48. Cham: Springer International Publishing.

Greenhalgh, Trisha. 1997. "How to read a paper: the Medline database." *BMJ* 315 (7101): 180–3.

Harzing, Anne-Wil. 1997. *Publish or Perish.* Tarma Software Research Pty Limited, Melbourne, Australia.

Hazlehurst, Brian, John Mullooly, Allison Naleway, and Brad Crane. 2005. "Detecting possible vaccination reactions in clinical notes." AMIA Annual Symposium proceedings 2005: 306–10. https://www.ncbi.nlm.nih.gov/pmc/articles/PMC1560600/

Homayoun, Hassan and Ebrahimpour-komleh, Hossein. 2021. "Automated segmentation of abnormal tissues in medical images." *Journal of Biomedical Physics and Engineering* 11 (4). pp. 415-424. https://doi.org/10.31661/jbpe.v0i0.958

Hoseini, Masome Sadat, Mohammad Nadimi Shahraki, and Behzad Soleimani Neysiani. 2015. "A new algorithm for mining frequent patterns in can tree." 2015 2nd International Conference on Knowledge-Based Engineering and Innovation (KBEI), 5-6 Nov, Tehran, Iran, https://doi.org/10.1109/KBEI.2015.7436153

Hosny, Khalid M., Mohamed A. Kassem, and Mohamed M. Fouad. 2020. "Classification of skin lesions into seven classes using transfer learning with AlexNet." *Journal of Digital Imaging* 33 (5): 1325–34. https://doi.org/10.1007/s10278-020-00371-9

Hossain, Md Shamim. 2019. "Microcalcification segmentation using modified u-net segmentation network from mammogram images." *Journal of King Saud University – Computer and Information Sciences.* https://doi.org/10.1016/j.jksuci.2019.10.014

Hua, Kai-Lung, Che-Hao Hsu, Shintami Chusnul Hidayati, Wen-Huang Cheng, and Yu-Jen Chen. 2015. "Computer-aided classification of lung nodules on computed tomography images via deep learning technique." *OncoTargets and Therapy* 8: 2015–22. https://doi. org/10.2147/OTT.S80733

Iroju, Olaronke G, and Janet O Olaleke. 2015. "A systematic review of natural language processing in healthcare." *International Journal of Information Technology and Computer Science* 7 (8): 44–50.

Jindal, M, J Gupta, and B Bhushan. 2019. "Machine learning methods for IoT and their future applications." 2019 International Conference on Computing, Communication, and Intelligent Systems (ICCCIS), October 18–19, 2019.

Khamparia, Aditya, Prakash Kumar Singh, Poonam Rani, Debabrata Samanta, Ashish Khanna, and Bharat Bhushan. 2020. "An internet of health things-driven deep learning framework for detection and classification of skin cancer using transfer learning." *Transactions on Emerging Telecommunications Technologies.* https://doi.org/10.1002/ett.3963

Khastavaneh, Hassan and Ebrahimpour-Komleh, Hossein. 2015a. "Brain extraction using iso-data clustering algorithm aided by histogram analysis." 2015. International Conference on Knowledge-Based Engineering and Innovation (KBEI), pp. 847-852, https://doi.org/10.1109/KBEI.2015.7436154

_____. 2015b. "Brain extraction: A region based histogram analysis strategy," *Signal Processing and Intelligent Systems Conference (SPIS)*, pp. 20-24, 16-17 Dec, Tehran, Iran, https://doi.org/10.1109/SPIS.2015.7422305.

_____. 2017. "Neural network-based learning kernel for automatic segmentation of multiple sclerosis lesions on magnetic resonance images." *Journal of Biomedical Physics & Engineering* 7 (2): 155–62. https://pubmed.ncbi.nlm.nih.gov/28580337.

_____. 2019. "Segmentation of Diabetic Retinopathy Lesions in Retinal Fundus Images Using Multi-View Convolutional Neural Networks", *Iran Journal of Radiology* 16 (Special Issue). https://doi.org/10.5812/iranjradiol.99148.

_____. 2020a. "MMTDNN: Multi-view massive training deep neural network for segmentation and detection of abnormal tissues in medical images." *Frontiers in Biomedical Technologies* 7 (1): 22–32. https://doi.org/10.18502/fbt.v7i1.2722.

_____. 2020b. "Representation Learning Techniques: An Overview." *In: Bohlouli M., Sadeghi Bigham B., Narimani Z., Vasighi M., Ansari E. (eds) Data Science: From Research to Application. CiDaS 2019. Lecture Notes on Data Engineering and Communications Technologies*, vol 45. Pp. 89-104. Springer, Cham. https://doi.org/10.1007/978-3-030-37309-2_8.

Khastavaneh, Hassan and Haron, Hassan. 2014. "A Conceptual Model for Segmentation of Multiple Scleroses Lesions in Magnetic Resonance Images Using Massive Training Artificial Neural Network," *International Conference on Intelligent Systems, Modelling and Simulation*, pp. 273-278, 27-19 Jan, Langkawi, Malaysia, https://doi.org/10.1109/ISMS.2014.53.

Kido, Shoji, Yasushi Hirano, and Shingo Mabu. 2020. "Deep learning for pulmonary image analysis: Classification, detection, and segmentation." *Advances in Experimental Medicine and Biology* 1213: 47–58. https://doi.org/10.1007/978-3-030-33128-3_3

Klein, Stefan, Marius Staring, Keelin Murphy, Max A Viergever, and Josien P W Pluim. 2010. "Elastix: A toolbox for intensity-based medical image registration." *IEEE Transactions on Medical Imaging* 29 (1): 196–205. https://doi.org/10.1109/TMI.2009.2035616

Kumar, S, B Bhusan, D Singh, and D K Choubey. 2020. "Classification of Diabetes using Deep Learning." International Conference on Communication and Signal Processing (ICCSP), 28–30 July 2020, Chennai, India, https://doi.org/10.1109/ICCSP48568.2020.9182293

Manogaran, Gunasekaran, Chandu Thota, Daphne Lopez, V Vijayakumar, Kaja M Abbas, and Revathi Sundarsekar. 2017. "Big data knowledge system in healthcare." In Chintan Bhatt, Nilanjan Dey, Amira S. Ashour, *Internet of Things and Big Data Technologies for Next Generation Healthcare*, 133–157. Springer International Publishing, Cham, https://doi.org/10.1007/978-3-319-49736-5_7.

Meystre, Stéphane M, and Peter J Haug. 2005. "Comparing natural language processing tools to extract medical problems from narrative text." *AMIA Annual Symposium Proceedings* 2005: 525–29. https://pubmed.ncbi.nlm.nih.gov/16779095

Moradi, Milad, and Nasser Ghadiri. 2018. "Different approaches for identifying important concepts in probabilistic biomedical text summarization." *Artificial Intelligence in Medicine* 84: 101–16. https://doi.org/10.1016/j.artmed.2017.11.004

Jannesari, Mahboobeh, Mehdi Habibzadeh, Hamidreza Aboulkheyr, Pegah Khosravi, Olivier Elemento, Mehdi Totonchi and Iman Hajirasouliha. 2018. *"Breast Cancer Histopathological Image Classification: A Deep Learning Approach."* IEEE International Conference on Bioinformatics and Biomedicine (BIBM), 2405–2412, 3-6 Dec, Madrid, Spain, https://doi.org/10.1109/BIBM.2018.8621307.

Multiple, AI. 2020. "15 AI applications/usecases/examples in healthcare in 2020." Accessed 12/13/2020. https://research.aimultiple.com/healthcare-ai/

Neamatullah, Ishna, Margaret M Douglass, H Lehman Li-wei, Andrew Reisner, Mauricio Villarroel, William J Long, Peter Szolovits, George B Moody, Roger G Mark, and Gari D Clifford. 2008. "Automated de-identification of free-text medical records." *BMC Medical Informatics and Decision Making* 8 (1): 1–17.

Sharma, Nikhil, Ila Kaushik, Bharat Bhushan, Siddharth Gautam, and Aditya Khamparia. 2020. "Applicability of WSN and Biometric Models in the Field of Healthcare." In *Deep Learning Strategies for Security Enhancement in Wireless Sensor Networks*, edited by K. Martin Sagayam, Bharat Bhushan, A Diana Andrushia and C de Albuquerque Victor Hugo, 304–329. Hershey, PA,: IGI Global.

Noh, Hyeonwoo, Seunghoon Hong, and Bohyung Han. 2015. *"Learning Deconvolution Network for Semantic Segmentation."* IEEE International Conference on Computer Vision: 1520–8. 7-13 Dec, Santiago, Chile, https://doi.org/10.1109/ICCV.2015.178

Oshnoudi, Arash., Behzad Soleimani Neysiani, Zahra Aminoroaya, and Naser Nematbakhsh. 2021. "Improving Recommender Systems Performances Using User Dimension Expansion by Movies' Genres and Voting-Based Ensemble Machine Learning Technique." 2021 7th International Conference on Web Research (ICWR), May, 19–20 2021, Tehran, Iran, https://doi.org/10.1109/ICWR51868.2021.9443146

Panigrahi, Niranjan, Ishan Ayus, and Om Prakash Jena. 2021. "An Expert System-Based Clinical Decision Support System for Hepatitis-B Prediction & Diagnosis." In: Sachi Nandan Mohanty,G. Nalinipriya,Om Prakash Jena,Achyuth Sarkar, *Machine Learning for Healthcare Applications*, 57–75. Wiley Online Library, Scrivener Publishing LLC, Beverly, MA, https://doi.org/10.1002/9781119792611.ch4

Paramesha, K., H.L. Gururaj, and Om Prakash Jena. 2021. "Applications of Machine Learning in Biomedical Text Processing and Food Industry." In *Machine Learning for Healthcare Applications*, 151–67. Wiley Online Library, Scrivener Publishing LLC, Beverly, Massachusetts, https://doi.org/10.1002/9781119792611.ch10

Patra, Sudhansu Shekhar, Om Praksah Jena, Gaurav Kumar, Sreyashi Pramanik, Chinmaya Misra, and Kamakhya Narain Singh. 2021. "Random forest algorithm in imbalance genomics classification." In *Data Analytics in Bioinformatics*, 173–90.

Pattnayak, Parthasarathi, and Om Prakash Jena. 2021. "Innovation on Machine Learning in Healthcare Services–An Introduction." In *Machine Learning for Healthcare Applications*, 1–15.

Perera, Sujan, Amit Sheth, Krishnaprasad Thirunarayan, Suhas Nair, and Neil Shah. 2013. "Challenges in understanding clinical notes: Why NLP engines fall short and where background knowledge can help." *Proceedings of the 2013 international workshop on Data management & analytics for healthcare.*

Pham, Tuan D. 2021. "Classification of COVID-19 chest X-rays with deep learning: new models or fine tuning?" *Health Information Science and Systems* 9 (1). https://doi.org/10.1007/s13755-020-00135-3

Popowich, Fred. 2005. "Using text mining and natural language processing for health care claims processing." *ACM SIGKDD Explorations Newsletter* 7 (1): 59–66.

Raja, Uzma, Tara Mitchell, Timothy Day, and J Michael Hardin. 2008. "Text mining in healthcare. Applications and opportunities." *J Healthc Inf Manag* 22 (3): 52–6.

Sætre, Rune. 2006. "GeneTUC: Natural Language Understanding in Medical Text." Doctoral Thesis, Norwegian University of Science and Technology (NTNU), Trondheim, Norway, https://ntnuopen.ntnu.no/ntnu-xmlui/handle/11250/249975

Samala, Ravi K., Heang-Ping Chan, Lubomir Hadjiiski, Mark A. Helvie, Jun Wei, and Kenny Cha. 2016. "Mass detection in digital breast tomosynthesis: Deep convolutional neural network with transfer learning from mammography." *Medical Physics* 43 (12): 6654–6. https://doi.org/10.1118/1.4967345

Sathitratanacheewin, Seelwan, Panasun Sunanta, and Krit Pongpirul. 2020. "Deep learning for automated classification of tuberculosis-related chest X-Ray: dataset distribution shift limits diagnostic performance generalizability." *Heliyon* 6 (8): e04614. https://doi.org/10.1016/j.heliyon.2020.e04614

Savova, Guergana K, James J Masanz, Philip V Ogren, Jiaping Zheng, Sunghwan Sohn, Karin C Kipper-Schuler, and Christopher G Chute. 2010. "Mayo clinical Text Analysis and Knowledge Extraction System (cTAKES): Architecture, component evaluation and applications." *Journal of the American Medical Informatics Association* 17 (5): 507–13. https://doi.org/10.1136/jamia.2009.001560

Setio, Arnaud Arindra Adiyoso, Francesco Ciompi, Geert Litjens, Paul Gerke, and Colin Jacobs. 2016. "Pulmonary nodule detection in CT images: False positive reduction using multi-view convolutional networks." *IEEE Transactions on Medical Imaging* 35 (5): 1160–9. https://doi.org/10.1109/TMI.2016.2536809

Shi, Peng, Jing Zhong, Andrik Rampun, and Hui Wang. 2018. "A hierarchical pipeline for breast boundary segmentation and calcification detection in mammograms." *Computers in Biology and Medicine* 96 (February): 178–188. https://doi.org/10.1016/j.compbiomed.2018.03.011

Soleimani Neysiani, Behzad, and Seyed Morteza Babamir. 2016. "Methods of feature extraction for detecting the duplicate bug reports in software triage systems." International Conference on Information Technology, Communications and Telecommunications (IRICT), 2 March. Tehran, Iran, http://www.sid.ir/En/Seminar/ViewPaper.aspx?ID=7677

_____. 2018. "Automatic Typos Detection in Bug Reports." IEEE 12th International Conference Application of Information and Communication Technologies, 8 July, Almaty, Kazakhstan.

_____. 2019a. "Automatic Interconnected Lexical Typo Correction in Bug Reports of Software Triage Systems." International Conference on Contemporary Issues in Data Science, 8 March, Zanjan, Iran.

_____. 2019b. "Duplicate detection models for bug reports of software triage systems: A survey." *Current Trends in Computer Sciences & Applications* 1 (5): 128–34. https://doi.org/10.32474/CTCSA.2019.01.000123

_____. 2019c. "Effect of typos correction on the validation performance of duplicate bug reports detection." 10th International Conference on Information and Knowledge Technology (IKT), Tehran, Iran, 2020-Jan-2.

_____. 2019d. "Fast language-independent correction of interconnected typos to finding longest terms: Using Trie for typo detection and correction." 24th International Conference on Information Technology (IVUS), Lithuania. http://ceur-ws.org/Vol-2470/

_____. 2019e. "Improving Performance of Automatic Duplicate Bug Reports Detection Using Longest Common Sequence." IEEE 5th International Conference on Knowledge-Based Engineering and Innovation (KBEI), 28 Feb-1 March, Tehran, Iran, https://doi.org/10.1109/KBEI.2019.8735038

_____. 2019f. "New labeled dataset of interconnected lexical typos for automatic correction in the bug reports." *SN Applied Sciences* 1 (11): 1385.

_____. 2019g. "New methodology for contextual features usage in duplicate bug reports detection: Dimension expansion based on Manhattan distance similarity of topics." IEEE 5th International Conference on Web Research (ICWR), Tehran, Iran, 28 Feb-1 March, https://doi.org/10.1109/ICWR.2019.8765296

_____. 2020. "Automatic duplicate bug report detection using information retrieval-based versus machine learning-based approaches." IEEE 6th International Conference on Web Research (ICWR), 22-23 April, Tehran, Iran, https://doi.org/10.1109/ICWR49608.2020.9122288

Soleimani Neysiani, Behzad, Seyed Morteza Babamir, and Masayoshi Aritsugi. 2020. "Efficient feature extraction model for validation performance improvement of duplicate bug report detection in software bug triage systems." *Information and Software Technology* 126: 106344–106363. https://doi.org/10.1016/j.infsof.2020.106344

Soleimani Neysiani, Behzad, Saeed Doostali, Seyed Morteza Babamir, and Zahra Aminoroaya. 2020. "Fast duplicate bug reports detector training using sampling for dimension reduction: Using Instance-based learning for contiuous query in real-world." 2020 11th International Conference on Information and Knowledge Technology (IKT), 22-23 Dec, Tehran, Iran, https://doi.org/10.1109/IKT51791.2020.9345611

Soleimani Neysiani, Behzad, and Mohammad Shiralizadeh Dezfoli. 2020. "Identifying affecting factors on prediction of students' educational statuses: A case study of educational data mining in Ashrafi Esfahani University of Isfahan of Iran." 10th International Conference on Information and Knowledge Technology (IKT). 2 Jan, Tehran, Iran.

Soleimani Neysiani, Behzad, Nasim Soltani, and Shima Ghezelbash. 2015. "A framework for improving find best marketing targets using a hybrid genetic algorithm and neural networks." 2015 2nd International Conference on Knowledge-Based Engineering and Innovation (KBEI), 5-6 Nov, Tehran, Iran, https://doi.org/10.1109/KBEI.2015.7436136

Soleimani Neysiani, Behzad, Nasim Soltani, Reza Mofidi, and Mohammad Hossein Nadimi-Shahraki. 2019. "Improve performance of association rule-based collaborative filtering recommendation systems using genetic algorithm." *International Journal of Information Technology and Computer Science* 11 (2): 48–55.

Soltani, Nasim, Behrang Barekatain, and Behzad Soleimani Neysiani. 2021. "MTC: Minimizing Time and Cost of Cloud Task Scheduling based on Customers and Providers Needs using Genetic Algorithm." *International Journal of Intelligent Systems and Applications (IJISA)* 13 (2): 38–51. https://doi.org/10.5815/ijisa.2021.02.03.

Soltani, Nasim, Behrang Barekatain, and Behzad Soleimani Neysiani. 2016. "Job scheduling based on single and multi objective meta-heuristic algorithms in cloud computing: A survey." *International Conference on Information Technology, Communications and Telecommunications (irICT)*, 2 March, Tehran, Iran, https://www.sid.ir/en/Seminar/ViewPaper.aspx?ID=7678.

Soltani, Nasim, Behzad Soleimani Neysiani, and Behrang Barekatain. 2017. "Heuristic algorithms for task scheduling in cloud computing: a survey." *International Journal of Computer Network and Information Security* 11 (8): 16.

Sun, Wencheng, Zhiping Cai, Yangyang Li, Fang Liu, Shengqun Fang, and Guoyan Wang. 2018. "Data processing and text mining technologies on electronic medical records: A review." *Journal of Healthcare Engineering* 2018, 4302425, Hindawi, https://doi.org/10.1155/2018/4302425.

Tang, Peng, Qiaokang Liang, Xintong Yan, Shao Xiang, Wei Sun, Dan Zhang, and Gianmarc Coppola. 2019. "Efficient skin lesion segmentation using separable-Unet with stochastic weight averaging." *Computer Methods and Programs in Biomedicine* 178: 289–301. https://doi.org/10.1016/j.cmpb.2019.07.005

Trivedi, Gaurav, Phuong Pham, Wendy W Chapman, Rebecca Hwa, Janyce Wiebe, and Harry Hochheiser. 2018. "NLPReViz: an interactive tool for natural language processing on clinical text." *Journal of the American Medical Informatics Association* 25 (1): 81–7. https://doi.org/10.1093/jamia/ocx070

Uramoto, Naohiko, Hirofumi Matsuzawa, Tohru Nagano, Akiko Murakami, Hironori Takeuchi, and Koichi Takeda. 2004. "A text-mining system for knowledge discovery from biomedical documents." *IBM Systems Journal* 43 (3): 516–33.

Varzaneh, Hossein Hatami, Behzad Soleimani Neysiani, Hassan Ziafat, and Nasim Soltani. 2018. "Recommendation systems based on association rule mining for a target object by evolutionary algorithms." *Emerging Science Journal* 2 (2): 100–107.

Wang, Hongyu, and Yong Xia. 2018. "ChestNet: A deep neural network for classification of thoracic diseases on chest radiography." 1–8. https://arxiv.org/abs/1807.03058v1.

Yasar, Huseyin, and Murat Ceylan. 2021. "A novel comparative study for detection of Covid-19 on CT lung images using texture analysis, machine learning, and deep learning methods." *Multimedia Tools and Applications* 80 (4): 5423–47. https://doi.org/10.1007/s11042-020-09894-3

Yu, Lequan, Hao Chen, Qi Dou, Jing Qin, and Pheng-Ann Heng. 2017. "Automated Melanoma Recognition in Dermoscopy Images via Very Deep Residual Networks." *IEEE Transactions on Medical Imaging* 36 (4): 994–1004. https://doi.org/10.1109/TMI.2016.2642839

Yuan, Yading, Ming Chao, and Yeh-Chi Lo. 2017. "Automatic Skin Lesion Segmentation Using Deep Fully Convolutional Networks With Jaccard Distance." *IEEE Transactions on Medical Imaging* 36 (9): 1876–86. https://doi.org/10.1109/TMI.2017.2695227

Zhu, Runjie, Xinhui Tu, and Jimmy Xiangji Huang. 2021. "Utilizing BERT for biomedical and clinical text mining." In *Data Analytics in Biomedical Engineering and Healthcare*, 73–103. Elsevier, London, United Kingdom.

5 Usage of ML Techniques for ASD Detection
A Comparative Analysis of Various Classifiers

Ashima Sindhu Mohanty, Priyadarsan Parida, and Krishna Chandra Patra

CONTENTS

5.1 INTRODUCTION

Autism spectrum disorder (ASD) is a neurodevelopment state characterized by the presence of repetitive behaviors and impairments in socio-communicative skills (Mohanty, Patra, and Parida 2021). When the individual is 6 to 18 months old, the beginning indications of ASD are noticed. Following the initial symptoms, the individual further suffers from social as well as communication disability as a result of unusual motor development during the first 18 to 36 months of life (Backer 2015). Some of the abnormal behaviors associated with the individual include uncertain giggling, problems in making eye contact, no response to sound as well as physical pain, no interest in cuddling with parents, repeating words and sentences, no proper attachment towards object, and less considerate to sudden light or noise.

Identifying behavioral alterations due to ASD in children is much simpler than in adolescent and adult cases, the reason being overlapping of some ASD signs with other mental health disorders with the increase in individual's age. This research highlights the classification of ASD class as "ASD" or "no ASD" in the following individuals: toddler (up to 36 months), child (4–11 years), adolescent (12–16 years) as well as adult (17 years and over).

The "Qualitative Checklist for Autism in Toddlers (Q-CHAT-10)" (Robins et al. 2001) and "Autism Spectrum Quotient (AQ-10)" (Baron-Cohen et al. 2006; Auyeung et al. 2008) based on ten screening questions form the basis of investigation in the proposed approach. The screening questionnaires also exist in the ASD data sets upon which investigation is done (Autism Research Centre – University of Cambridge 1998).

The data sets used in this study are developed by Fadi Fayez Thabtah. The researcher developed a mobile-based ASDTest app which is a screening application and formulated toddler, child, adolescent, and adult ASD data sets, which are utilized in this research. The toddler data set has 18 attributes with an output ASD class whereas there are 21 attributes with an output ASD class in the case of child, adolescent as well as adult data sets.

Successful classification of ASD classes on child, adolescent and adult cases were found but the toddler case was left out. In the toddler dataset, major number of toddler instances is of no ASD class which unbalances the respective data set. This study emphasizes ASD classification on all categories of individuals including toddler by using a minimum number of features from the data sets. Utilizing ML, classifier models are built (Patra et al. 2021) to classify ASD classes. The classifier model is trained by training data and then the trained models get tested by the test data. On-going analysis on classification of ASD highlights feature selection and dimension reduction, evolution of latest ML approaches for classification of ASD class, enhancement of evaluation parameters, and reducing the diagnosis time for ASD.

Healthcare is not only confined to neurological disorders which can be technically handled by artificial intelligence (Pattnayak and Jena 2021). But in addition to neurology, there are numerous healthcare areas like skin cancer (which can be detected from skin images by the application of deep learning along with the framework of Internet of Health and Things (Khamparia et al. 2020)) and prediction of Hepatitis-B (Panigrahi, Ayus, and Jena 2021). The implementation of Internet of Things (IoT) in the healthcare sector increases productivity as well as examination of data in healthcare unit (Goyal et al. 2021) Furthermore, application of wireless sensor network (WSN) and biometric models in verifying fingerprint operations has enhanced security and helped to preserve privacy in the healthcare sector (Sharma et al. 2020). Presently, urban IoT systems, with the implementation of ML, supports smart cities as well as advanced communication technologies (Jindal, Gupta, and Bhushan 2019) in addition to biomedical text processing (Paramesha, Gururaj, and

Jena 2021). In the domain of medical applications, deep learning is utilized for the classification of diabetes (Kumar et al. 2020).

Medical professionals can be positively benefitted by the method used in this paper in providing awareness to the individuals with ASD symptoms for further evaluation.

In this chapter, Section 5.2 outlines the related research work with classifier models, Section 5.3 outlines the data sets collected for the investigation followed by the description of the proposed methodology in Section 5.4. The results obtained for each category of individual are discussed in Section 5.5 and, finally, the conclusion is outlined in Section 5.6.

5.2 LITERATURE SURVEY

Thabtah (2019) came up with a mobile-based ASDTest app as a screening tool which took into account Q-CHAT as well as AQ-10 screening questions with a time efficient feature. Utilizing the tool, the researcher gathered 1452 instances for all classes of individuals including toddler, child, adolescent, and adult. However, due to the unbalanced nature of the toddler dataset, it was kept out of the investigation, reducing the number of instances to 1100 with 21 features. For feature extraction, wrapping filtering method was implemented. The investigation further classified the ASD classes using Naïve Bayes (NB) (Liu, Zhu, and Yang 2013) and Logistic Regression (LR) (Thabtah, Abdelhamid, and Peebles 2019) by computing different performance parameters. The adult dataset attained higher performance rates with the implementation of the LR model.

Al-diabat (2018) investigated the ASD class upon the category of child using fuzzy data mining models. The source of dataset is the UCI ML repository consisting of 509 instances with 21 features. The fuzzy data mining classification algorithms FURIA, JRIP, RIDOR (Caluza 2019), and PRISM (Cendrowska 1987) were utilized for classifying ASD class. The results of the FURIA classification model was more accurate and sensitive, outperforming the rest of the models. The JRIP algorithm showed the maximum specificity rate.

Vaishali and Sasikala (2018) confined the investigation to the child dataset only. The source of the dataset is the UCI ML repository and consists of 292 instances with 21 attributes. The investigation employed binary firefly feature selection wrapper based on swarm intelligence. Followed by feature selection, the investigator classified the ASD class into "ASD" or "no ASD" category utilizing NB, J48 DT (Salzberg 1994), surface vector machine (SVM) (Keerthi et al. 2001), k-nearest neighb (KNN) (Aha, Kibler, and Albert 1991), and Multilayer Perceptron (MLP) (Pal and Mitra 1992). The resulting accuracy of more than 90 percent validated the performance of classifier models.

To improve the effectiveness of ASD detection, Thabtah (2019) further identified lesser number of influential features (Thabtah, Kamalov, and Rajab 2018). The investigation utilized the same datasets used in Thabtah (2019) where once again the toddler data set was excluded from the investigation due to its unbalanced nature. The experimentation employed variable analysis (VA) as filtration method and compared the result from VA against CHI-SQ (Liu and Setiono 1995), IG (Pratiwi and Adiwijaya 2018), CFS (Wosiak and Zakrzewska 2018) and correlation attribute evaluation analysis (Quinlan 1986). The ML classifiers are repeated incremental pruning to produce error reduction (RIPPER) and C4.5 (DT) (Salzberg 1994) classifying VA features with evaluation of performance parameters. VA selected minimum features in case of all the datasets unlike the former mentioned filtering approaches followed by ML classification with acceptable rate of performance parameters. The adolescent dataset outperformed the rest of the datasets in the investigation.

The author in Thabtah (2019) put forward a rule-based machine learning (RML) (Thabtah and Peebles 2020). The research covered the datasets used in Thabtah (2019) over the same category of individuals having 1100 instances with 21 features thereby dropping the toddler dataset from the investigation. There was the comparison of RML performance with eight ML classifiers: RIDOR, RIPPER, Bagging, Nnge, Boosting, C4.5, CART, and PRISM (Gaines and Compton 1995; Salzberg 1994). The research experienced standard performance of RML compared with other models of evaluation parameters.

The investigators in Akter et al. (2019) identified and detected ASD upon adult, adolescent, child as well as toddler datasets. The source once again being the UCI ML repository having 2009 instances. Three feature transformation (FT) approaches – log, Z-score, and sine – were implemented. Following the feature transformation, nine ML classifier models – Adaboost (Zhang et al. 2019) flexible discriminant analysis (FDA), LDA, penalized discriminant analysis (PDA) (Kassambara 2018), C5.0, mixture discriminant analysis (MDA), boosted generalized linear model (Glmboost) (Hofner et al. 2014), CART, and SVM – were utilized for the purpose of ASD classification followed by evaluation of performance parameters. The result of investigation showed that the SVM and Glmboost classifiers got maximum performance for toddler as well as adolescent datasets respectively and Adaboost classifier showed standard performance for child as well as adult datasets.

Raj and Masood (2020) made use of LR, NB, SVM, and KNN classifiers in addition to artificial neural network (ANN), as well as convolution neural network (CNN) and speculated the probability of ASD in adult, adolescent, and child data sets. The data sets were gathered from UCI ML repository covering 1100 instances with 21 features where the toddler data set was excluded due to its unbalanced nature. CNN yielded maximum performance in case of all data sets. The category of adult data set yielded maximum results. Table 5.1 summarizes the ASD classification approaches as discussed in the literature survey.

5.3   DATA COLLECTION

Kaggle and the UCI ML repository being the authenticated and public access sites for research purpose, the ASD data sets are gathered from those repositories (Thabtah 2017a; 2017b; 2017c; 2018). The mobile-based ASDTest app developed by Thabtah (2019) collected the ASD data from individuals via screening questionnaire. The

TABLE 5.1

ASD Classification Approaches

Research in	Year of Research	Data Collection Source	Category of Individuals	Classifier Models Used	Number of features/ Attributes Extracted	Performance Parameters
(Thabtah 2019)	2018	ASD Screening Test App	Adult, Adolescent, Child	LR, NB	12, 8, 4	Accuracy, Sensitivity, Specificity
(Al-diabat 2018)	2018	UCI Repository	Child	FURIA, PRISM, JRIP, RIDOR	16	Accuracy, Sensitivity, Specificity
(Vaishali and Sasikala 2018)	2018	UCI Repository	Child	NB, J48 (DT), SVM, KNN, MLP	10	Accuracy, TP Rate, ROC area, RMSE
(Thabtah, Kamalov, and Rajab 2018)	2018	ASD Screening Test App	Adult, Adolescent, Child	RIPPER, C4.5 (DT)	6,8,8	Accuracy, Sensitivity, Specificity, PPV rate, NPV rate
(Thabtah and Peebles 2020)	2019	ASD Screening Test App	Adult, Adolescent, Child	RML, RIDOR, RIPPER, Bagging, Nnge, Adaboost, C4.5 (DT), CART, PRISM	19	Error rate, Sensitivity, Specificity, Harmonic Mean (F1), Accuracy
(Akter et al. 2019)	2019	UCI Repository, Kaggle	Adult, Adolescent, Child, Toddler	Adaboost, FDA, LDA, PDA, C5.0, MDA, Glmboost, CART, SVM	No feature extracted	Accuracy, Kappa statistics, AUROC, Sensitivity, Specificity, Log-loss
(Raj and Masood 2020)	2020	UCI Repository	Adult, Adolescent, Child	LR, NB, SVM, KNN, ANN, CNN	No feature extracted	Accuracy, Sensitivity, Specificity

Note: Data gathered by ASDTest app are stored in UCI repository for experimental purposes.

TABLE 5.2
ASD Data Sets

Sl no.	Name of Data Set	Source	Attribute Type	Number of Attributes	Number of Cases	Number of Cases with ASD Class	Number of Cases with no ASD Class
1	"Toddler"	Kaggle (Thabtah 2018)	"Categorical, continous and binary"	18	1054	728	326
2	"Child"	UCI ML repository (Thabtah 2017a)	"Categorical, continous and binary"	21	292	141	151
3	"Adolescent"	UCI ML repository (Thabtah 2017b)	"Categorical, continous and binary"	21	104	63	41
4	"Adult"	UCI ML repository (Thabtah 2017c)	"Categorical, continous and binary"	21	704	189	515

research is conducted on toddler, child, adolescent as well as adult data sets. The details of all data sets are encapsulated in Table 5.2.

All the data sets, excluding the toddler one, are characterized by some missing values in the attributes: "age", "ethnicity" as well as "Who_completed_the_test". The detail of missing value is summarized in Table 5.3.

Table 5.4 illustrates the details of common attribute in all data sets.

TABLE 5.3
Missing Values Present in ASD Data Sets

Data Set	Adult		Adolescent		Child	
Class Name	Total Number of Cases	Number of Cases After Dropping Missing Value	Total Number of Cases	Number of Cases After Dropping Missing Value	Total Number of Cases	Number of Cases After Dropping Missing Value
ASD	189	180	63	62	141	126
No ASD	515	429	41	36	151	123
Total	704	609	104	98	292	249

TABLE 5.4
Common Attributes in all ASD Data Sets

Name of Attribute	Nature of Attribute	Description of Attribute
"Case Number"	"Numeric"	"Number of cases in dataset"
"Question item 1-10 Answer"	"Either 0 or 1"	"The answers to questions in Q-CHAT-10 and AQ-10"
"Age_Months"	"Numeric"	"Ages of toddler (in months), child, adolescent and adult (in years)"
"Score"	"Numeric"	"Screening score from Q-CHAT-10 and AQ-10 questionnaire"
"Sex"	"String"	"Male/Female"
"Ethnicity"	"String"	"Ethnicity List"
"Jaundice"	"Boolean (Yes/No)"	"Born with jaundice or without jaundice"
"Family_mem_ with_ASD"	"Boolean (Yes/No)"	"If any immediate family member had ASD"
"Who_completed_the_test"	"String"	"The individual performing ASD test"
"Used screening app before"	"Boolean (Yes/No)"	"Whether user used screening app beforehand"
"Country of residence"	"String"	"Country list"
"Screening methodology"	"Numeric"	"Type of screening method selected based on age description"
"ASD class"	"Boolean (Yes/No)"	"Whether case has ASD/no ASD"

5.4 METHODOLOGY

In the proposed work, the input ASD data for all categories of individuals collected from Kaggle as well as the UCI ML repository are pre-processed before classifying under ASD class. The missing data in the data sets are dropped before standardization. The first phase of pre-processing is characterized by conversion of the input data sets into numeric data followed by standardization, which is performed to fit the data into ML models within a specific range. During the second phase of pre-processing, the standardized inputs are applied to different dimension reduction models for reducing the number of attributes in the data sets. Then, after the training data trains the ML classifier models, the trained models are tested by test data for classification. The predicted outputs are finally found and compared against the targets to evaluate the parameters such as accuracy, specificity, sensitivity, precision, recall, Dice as well as F-measure. The workflow of the proposed technique is shown in Figure 5.1

5.4.1 PRE-PROCESSING

The raw data collected from the mentioned repositories are pre-processed in the first stage. In this research the steps involved in pre-processing are standardization and dimension reduction.

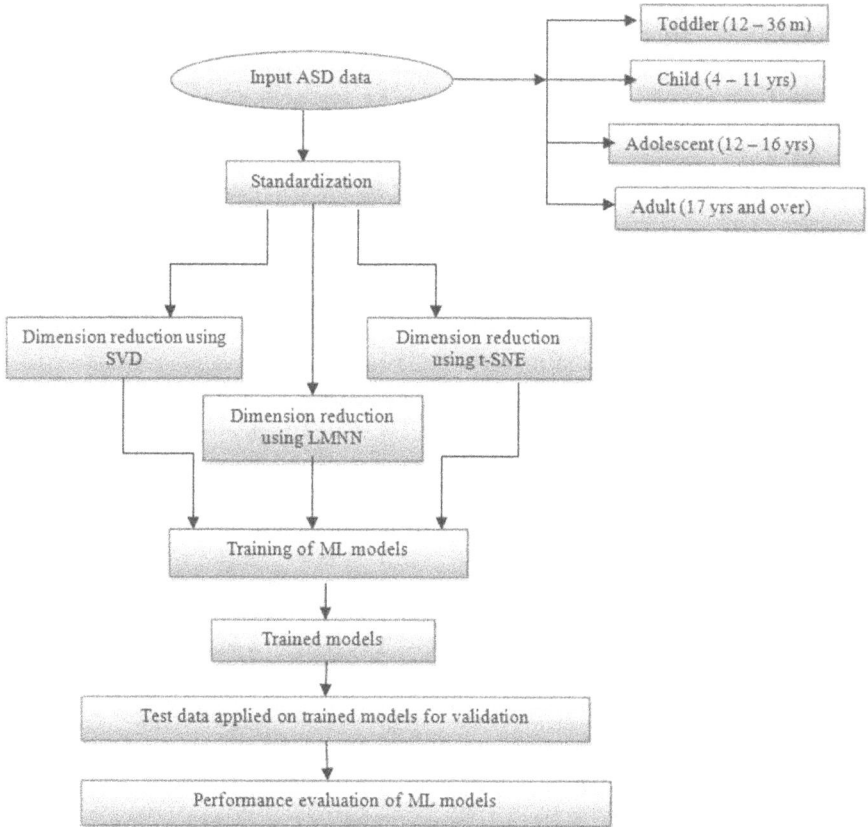

FIGURE 5.1   Architecture of the proposed method indicating processing and classification using ML.

5.4.1.1   Standardization

After analyzing the data sets, it is observed that the attributes present in the datasets are not properly scaled. Hence in order to properly scale the input attributes within a proper range, standardization (Andrade 2020) is implemeted. Mean and standard deviation approach is utilized to carry out the process of standardization for every single attribute in the data set. Mathematically the standardized data is represented by equation 5.1,

$$Sta\_X = \frac{(x - x_{mean})}{(x_{std})} \qquad (5.1)$$

where, x is current value of input X, x_{mean} is mean value of X, and x_{std} is standard deviation of input X.

5.4.1.2   Dimension Reduction Methods

In ML, ensuring to provide the same information, dimension reduction methods convert higher dimension datasets into lower ones for obtaining a better predictive model.

5.4.1.2.1 Singular Value Decomposition Method

When a matrix undergoes singular value decomposition (SVD) (Golub and Kahan 1965), then the matrix is factorized into three matrices. The SVD for a matrix has numerous algebraic properties which mainly focus on linear transformations. The most important application of SVD in ML is dimension reduction.

To analyze SVD deeply, first the eigenvalue decomposition of a matrix is required to be understood. Let us consider a matrix A which is the transformation and it acts on a vector x as multiplication and produce resultant vector as Ax. The denotion aij or $[A]_{ij}$ represents the element of matrix A in row I as well as column j.

Let both A and B be (m×p) as well as (p×n) matrices respectively, then the matrix C is a (m×n) matrix given by, C=AB, as shown in equation 5.2,

$$[C]_{ij} = \sum_{k=1}^{p} a_{ik} b_{kj} \qquad (5.2)$$

Example: In 2-D space, the rotation matrix is defined in equation 5.3,

$$A = \begin{bmatrix} \cos(\theta) & -\sin(\theta) \\ \sin(\theta) & \cos(\theta) \end{bmatrix} \qquad (5.3)$$

This matrix spins a vector about the origin by an angle of θ. One more instance is to stretch matrix B in a 2-D space, as defined in equation 5.4,

$$B = \begin{bmatrix} k & 0 \\ 0 & 1 \end{bmatrix} \qquad (5.4)$$

Along the x-axis, this matrix stretches one vector via k, which is a constant factor, but somehow y-direction remains unaffected. The stretching matrix in y-direction is shown in equation 5.5,

$$B = \begin{bmatrix} k & 0 \\ 0 & 1 \end{bmatrix} \qquad (5.5)$$

5.4.1.2.2 Large-Margin Nearest Neighbor Method

To successfully implement KNN classification, the target neighbors of every input x_i should be nearer in comparison to other differently labeled inputs. For each input, it can be imagined that a perimeter is established by the target neighbors which should not be invaded by different labeled inputs. Imposters are those labeled inputs in the training set that invade the perimeter, should be minimized. However, to enhance the robustness of KNN ML classifier, a stringent goal is adopted for maintaining ample distance between impostors and the perimeter formed by target neighbors. The KNN decision boundries are maintained with marginal safety around them to ensure the robustness of the model against small noise while training the inputs. This robust quality assigns the name of our analysis: large margin nearest neighb

(LMNN) dimension reduction (Sun and Chen 2011). Mathematically, impostors are explicated by a simple inequality. For input a_i with the label b_i and target neighbor a_j, imposer is any output with label $b_l \neq b_i$ such that,

$$\left\|L(a_i - a_l)\right\|^2 \leq \left\|L(a_i - a_j)\right\|^2 + 1 \qquad (5.6)$$

5.4.1.2.3 t-Distributed Stochastic Neighbor Embedding Method

t-Distributed Stochastic Neighbor Embedding (t-SNE) (Melit Devassy and George 2020) is based on conversion of high-dimensional Euclidean separation among data points into conditional probabilities representing the similarities. The similarity of data points a_i to a_j represents the conditional probability $P_{j|i}$. a_i will choose a_j to be its neighbor only if neighbors are picked up in accordance with their probability density under Gaussian at center a_j. For closely placed data points, $P_{j|i}$ is relatively high, but in case of highly gapped data points, $P_{j|i}$ is almost infinitesimal (for reasonable variance values of Gaussian, σ_i). The mathematical expression of conditional probability $P_{j|i}$ is represented by,

$$P_{j|i} = \frac{\exp\left(-\left\|a_i - a_j\right\|^2 / 2\sigma_i^2\right)}{\sum\limits_{k \neq i} \exp\left(-\left\|a_i - a_k\right\|^2 / 2\sigma_i^2\right)} \qquad (5.7)$$

where, σ_i is the variance of the Gaussian that is centered on data point a_i.

In case of low-dimensional data points b_i as well as a_j of high-dimensional data points a_i as well as a_j, computation of a similar conditional probability is possible which is denoted by $q_{j|i}$

$$q_{j|i} = \frac{\exp\left(-\left\|b_i - b_j\right\|^2\right)}{\sum\limits_{k \neq i} \exp\left(-\left\|b_i - b_k\right\|^2\right)} \qquad (5.8)$$

Reasonably, the conditional probabilities $P_{j|i}$ and $q_{j|i}$ should be the same for representing the similarity of data points in distinct dimensional spaces so that difference between $P_{j|i}$ and $q_{j|i}$ is nil for which the plot can be perfectly replicated in different dimensions.

Through this concept, t-SNE minimizes the difference for conditional probability. It also minimizes the sum of differences in case of conditional probabilites.

5.4.2 Machine Learning Models

ML builds classifier models for classifying ASD classes. Training data trains the classifier models and the trained model evaluates the testing data.

5.4.2.1 k-Nearest Neighbors

KNN (Aha, Kibler, and Albert 1991) is one of the oldest classification models used in many areas like pattern recognition, data mining, prediction, and many other areas related to applied science. The closeness of k in data sets is tested which identifies the similar class unclassified data. By determining following distances the nearest neighbor is decided. Assuming k as the total sample, m_i as the ith input, n_i as the output for the respective input then,

Euclidean distance,

$$d(m,n) = \sqrt{\sum_{i=1}^{k} (m_i - n_i)^2} \qquad (5.9)$$

Manhattan distance,

$$d(m,n) = \sum_{i=1}^{k} |m_i - n_i| \qquad (5.10)$$

Minkowski distance,

$$d(m,n) = \left(\sum_{i=1}^{k} (m_i - n_i)^q \right)^{1/q}, q = 1,2,3,..... \qquad (5.11)$$

5.4.2.2 Support Vector Machine

SVM (Keerthi et al. 2001), as one of the fast classification ML methods, deals with regression and classification problems with high accuracy. SVM is also known as the hyperplane method where the data samples are classified in N-dimensional space by a hyperplane. However, the basic objective of SVM is to maximize the separation linking the data samples of both classes. The mathematical formulation is as:

$$\min_{w,b,\xi} \left\{ \frac{1}{2} w^T w + C \sum_{i=1}^{l} \xi_i \right\}, \text{ constraints to}$$

$$n_i \left(w^T \phi(m_i) + b \right) \geq 1 - \xi_i, \xi \geq 0,$$

where, $(m_i, n_i), i = 1,....,1$ represents an instance-label pair, $m_i \in \Re^p, n \in \{1,-1\}^l, \phi$ represents a mapping function, $C > 0$ represents a penalty parameter.

The kernel function is represented as,

$$K(m_i, m_j) \equiv \phi(m_i)^T \phi(m_j) \qquad (5.12)$$

Other form of kernel functions are:
Linear function,

$$K(m_i, m_j) = m_i^T m_j \qquad (5.13)$$

Polynomial function:

$$K(m_i, m_j) = \left(\gamma m_i^T m_j + r \right)^d, \gamma > 0 \qquad (5.14)$$

Radial basis function,

$$K\left(m_i, m_j\right) \tag{5.15}$$

Sigmoid function:

$$K\left(m_i, m_j\right) = \tanh\left(\gamma m_i^T + r\right)$$

5.4.2.3 Naive Bayes

This classification technique is based on Bayes' theorem which is assumption of independence among predictors (Liu, Zhu, and Yang 2013). In another way, an NB classifier assumes that the presence of a single feature in a class which is unrelated to the presence of other features. NB model is easy to prepare and very useful for a large data set. It is very simple to implement and better than other classification methods. By using Bayes' theorem, the posterior probability P(c|y) from P(c), P(y) and P(y|c) can be calculated as,

$$P\left(c \mid y\right) = \frac{P\left(y \mid c\right) P\left(c\right)}{P\left(y\right)} \tag{5.16}$$

where, P(c|y) is posterior probability of class 'c' with the given predictor y, P(c) is prior probability of class 'c', P(y|c) is likelihood which is probability of predictor given class, and P(y) is prior probability of predictor.

5.4.2.4 Decision Tree

Decision tree (DT) (Salzberg 1994) is one of the well-known supervised learning algorithms implemented to solve statistical classification as well as problems related to regression. In this work, the DT designs a training model for predicting target variables (YES or NO).

A DT is constructed top-down from a root node and the data is partitioned into subsets. The subsets contain the instances with similar values.

While building a DT, two sorts of entropy are evaluated utilizing the data sets as follows:

a. Evaluation of entropy with a single attribute:

$$E(T) = \sum_{i=1}^{c} - p_i \log_2 p_i \tag{5.17}$$

where E is the entropy, T is the output class, p_i is probability of ith class, and c is number of output class.

b. Evaluation of entropy with two attributes:

$$E(T, X) = \sum_{c \in X} P(c) E\left(c_1, c_2\right) \tag{5.18}$$

where output class is represented by T, one of the inputs is represented by X, probability of output for a specific input is represented by P(c), and number of counts for class1 with respect to input X_1 as well as class2 with respect to input X_2 are represented by c_1 and c_2 respectively.

c. Repetition of step a) and step b) for every input and then calculation of total sum of (5.17) and total sum of (5.18) to yield information gain mathematically represented by,

$$G(T,X) = E(T) - E(T,X) \tag{5.19}$$

d. Continuation of the same process until entropy reaches 0. At that point, the leaf node is assessed where all data are classified.

5.4.3 PERFORMANCE PARAMETERS

The performance parameters such as accuracy (Acc), sensitivity (Sn), specificity (Sp), Dice coefficient (DC), precision (Pre), and F-measure (F1) evaluated the efficacy of the proposed approach (Mohanty, Parida, and Patra 2021). All the performance parameters are calculated from true positive (TP), true negative (TN), false positive (FP) and false negative (FN) values. The values are achieved from the confusion matrix (Thabtah and Peebles 2020). Mathematically the performance parameters are represented in equations 5.20–5.25.

$$Acc = \frac{(TP + TN)}{(TP + TN) + (FP + FN)} \tag{5.20}$$

$$SN = \frac{(TP)}{(TP + FN)} \tag{5.21}$$

$$SPE = \frac{(TN)}{(TN + FP)} \tag{5.22}$$

$$DC = \frac{2(TP)}{(2TP + FP + FN)} \tag{5.23}$$

$$Pre = \frac{TP}{TP + FP} \tag{5.24}$$

$$F_1 = \frac{(TP)}{TP + \frac{1}{2}(FP + FN)} \tag{5.25}$$

5.5 RESULTS AND DISCUSSION

Investigation into the different category of individual data sets resulted in accepted rate of performance. Table 5.5 illustrates the performance of distinct classifiers upon the different dimension reduction techniques.

TABLE 5.5
Classifier Performance

Dimension Reduction Techniques	Classifiers/ Performance Parameters	Acc	Sn	Sp	DC	Pre	F1	Individuals
SVD	KNN	1	1	1	1	1	1	TODDLER
	SVM	0.988	0.989	0.985	0.991	0.993	0.991	
	NB	0.978	0.979	0.975	0.984	0.989	0.984	
	DTREE	0.997	0.997	0.997	0.998	0.999	0.998	
LMNN	KNN	1	1	1	1	1	1	
	SVM	1	1	1	1	1	1	
	NB	0.961	0.952	0.982	0.971	0.991	0.971	
	DTREE	0.995	0.999	0.988	0.997	0.995	0.997	
t-SNE	KNN	1	1	1	1	1	1	
	SVM	0.691	1.000	0.000	0.817	0.691	0.817	
	NB	0.691	1.000	0.000	0.817	0.691	0.817	
	DTREE	0.968	0.973	0.957	0.977	0.981	0.977	
SVD	KNN	1	1	1	1	1	1	ADULT
	SVM	0.980	0.967	0.986	0.967	0.967	0.967	
	NB	0.938	0.883	0.960	0.893	0.903	0.893	
	DTREE	0.992	0.994	0.991	0.986	0.978	0.986	
LMNN	KNN	1	1	1	1	1	1	
	SVM	1	1	1	1	1	1	
	NB	0.959	0.956	0.960	0.932	0.910	0.932	
	DTREE	0.998	1.000	0.998	0.997	0.994	0.997	
t-SNE	KNN	1	1	1	1	1	1	
	SVM	0.834	0.728	0.879	0.722	0.716	0.722	
	NB	0.806	0.689	0.855	0.678	0.667	0.678	
	DTREE	0.980	0.956	0.991	0.966	0.977	0.966	
SVD	KNN	1	1	1	1	1	1	CHILD
	SVM	0.960	0.952	0.967	0.960	0.968	0.960	
	NB	0.960	0.960	0.959	0.960	0.960	0.960	
	DTREE	0.984	0.984	0.984	0.984	0.984	0.984	
LMNN	KNN	1	1	1	1	1	1	
	SVM	0.952	0.960	0.943	0.953	0.945	0.953	
	NB	0.884	0.881	0.886	0.884	0.888	0.884	
	DTREE	0.976	0.960	0.992	0.976	0.992	0.976	
t-SNE	KNN	1	1	1	1	1	1	
	SVM	0.570	0.595	0.545	0.584	0.573	0.584	
	NB	0.699	0.627	0.772	0.678	0.738	0.678	
	DTREE	0.952	0.921	0.984	0.951	0.983	0.951	
SVD	KNN	1	1	1	1	1	1	ADOLESCENT
	SVM	0.949	0.968	0.917	0.960	0.952	0.960	
	NB	0.888	1.000	0.694	0.919	0.849	0.919	
	DTREE	0.959	0.952	0.972	0.967	0.983	0.967	
LMNN	KNN	1	1	1	1	1	1	
	SVM	0.888	0.968	0.750	0.916	0.870	0.916	
	NB	0.837	0.871	0.778	0.871	0.871	0.871	
	DTREE	0.959	0.968	0.944	0.968	0.968	0.968	
t-SNE	KNN	1	1	1	1	1	1	
	SVM	0.724	0.823	0.556	0.791	0.761	0.791	
	NB	0.714	0.887	0.417	0.797	0.724	0.797	
	DTREE	0.929	0.984	0.833	0.946	0.910	0.946	

For the category of toddler data set, KNN classifier model for SVD attributes resulted in 100 percent performance for no wrongly classified individuals under ASD class. Following the KNN model is the performance of DT classifier model with more than 99 percent performance. For DT model, it is found that one toddler was wrongly classified as ASD and two toddlers were wrongly classified as no ASD. For the LMNN attributes, KNN and SVM classifier models produced 100 percent performance following which DT classifier model produced more than 99 percent performance with four and one toddlers wrongly classified as ASD and no ASD classes, respectively. In the case of t-SNE attributes, KNN classifier model suppressed all other classifier models with 100 percent performance. Following the KNN model is the DT classifier model with more than 95 percent performance. The performance of the DT model slightly dropped due to a minor increase in the number of wrongly classified individuals under ASD class, that is, 14 and 20 toddlers were wrongly classified as ASD and no ASD classes, respectively. Somehow the performance of SVM and NB classifier models for t-SNE attributes is not found so appealing due to the misclassification of 326 toddlers as ASD class. Figure 5.2 shows the performance of applied ML algorithms in terms of performance parameters on the toddler dataset.

In the category of the child data set, KNN classifier model in case of SVD attributes outperformed the rest of the classifier models with 100 percent performance with no wrong classification of individuals under ASD class. Next to the KNN model is the performance of the DT classifier model which is beyond 98 percent with two children wrongly classified as ASD and no ASD classes respectively. For the LMNN attributes, the KNN model resulted in 100 percent performance with not a single instance of wrong classification of individuals under ASD class. Following the KNN

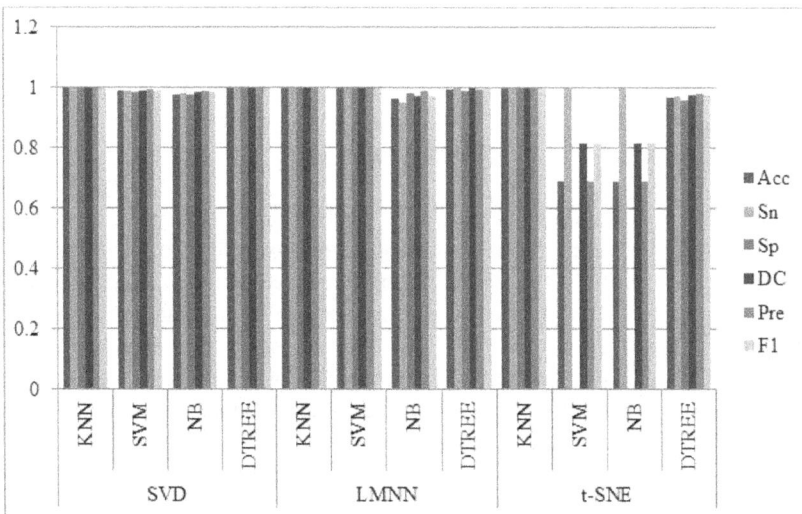

FIGURE 5.2   Performance rate of the ML algorithms on the toddler dataset.

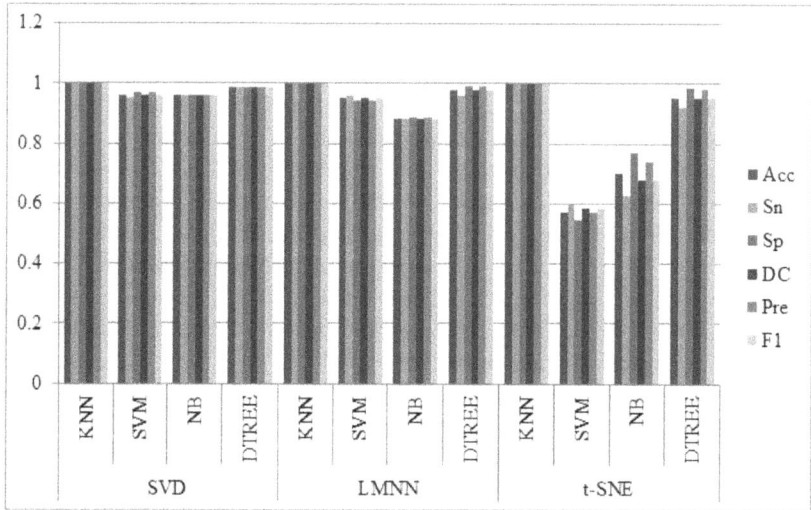

FIGURE 5.3   Performance rate of the ML algorithms on the child dataset.

model, the DT classifier model is the next one for LMNN attributes to produce more than 95 percent performance with a small increase in misclassification of individuals as 1 and 5 child individuals got misclassified as ASD and no ASD classes, respectively. In case of t-SNE attributes, the performance of the KNN model outperformed the rest of the classifier models with 100 percent performance followed by the DT model with more than 90 percent performance, as well as two and ten children were misclassified as ASD and no ASD classes, respectively. Somehow the performance of SVM and NB classifier models for t-SNE attributes was not up to mark with t-SNE attributes because of a greatly increased number of individual misclassifications. In the case of the SVM model, 56 and 51 children were misclassified as ASD and no ASD classes, respectively, and for the NB model, 28 and 47 children faced misclassification as ASD and no ASD classes, respectively. Figure 5.3 shows the performance of applied ML algorithms in terms of performance parameters on the child dataset.

For the category of adolescent data set, the KNN classifier model for SVD attributes resulted in 100 percent performance with no instance of individual misclassification. Next to the KNN model is the performance of the DT classifier model which reached more than 90 percent performance with one and three adolescent individuals misclassified as ASDF and no ASD classes, respectively. In addition, the performance of SVM and NB classifier models was also acceptable. In the case of LMNN attributes, the performance of the KNN classifier model outperformed the rest of the classifier models with 100 percent performance with no instance of individual misclassification. Following the KNN model is the performance of the DT classifier model whose performance is more than 94 percent with two adolescent individuals misclassified as ASD and two as no ASD. Somehow, the performance

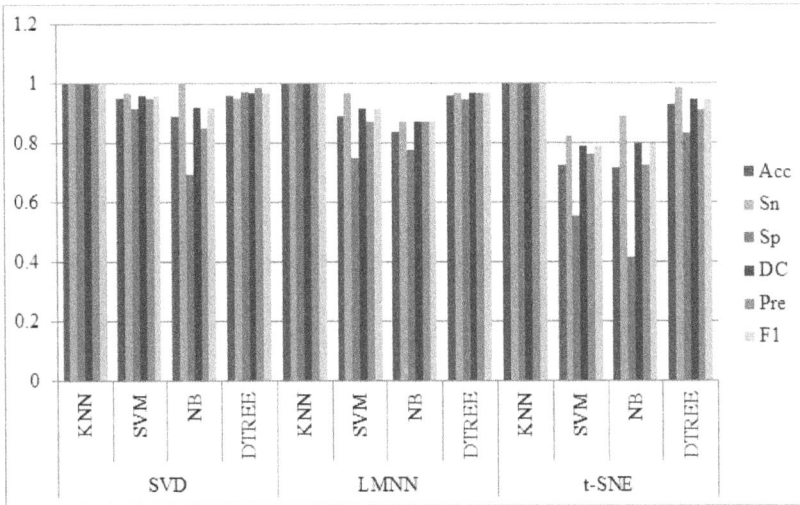

FIGURE 5.4 Performance rate of the ML algorithms on the adolescent dataset.

of SVM and NB is also acceptable up to far extent. Finally, for t-SNE attributes, the KNN classifier model resulted in 100 percent performance with no instance of individual misclassification. Following the KNN model is the DT classifier model with more than 90 percent performance, except for specificity which is found to be 83.33 percent due to the misclassification of six and one adolescent individuals as ASD and no ASD classes, respectively. The performance of SVM and NB is not found to be very appealing due to the greatly increased number of individual misclassification. Figure 5.4 shows the performance of applied ML algorithms in terms of performance parameters on the adolescent dataset.

In the category of adult data set, the best outcome for SVD attributes is shown by the KNN classifier model with 100 percent performance and no instance of individual misclassification. Following the KNN model is the performance of the DT classifier model whose evaluation rate is more than 97 percent, with four and one misclassified individuals as ASD and no ASD classes, respectively. However, a remarkable rate of acceptance is also found in the case of SVM and NB classifier models. For LMNN attributes, the KNN and SVM classifier models resulted in the best performance with 100 percent evaluation rates and no instances of individual misclassification. Next to KNN and SVM models, is the performance of the DT classifier model with more than 99 percent of evaluation rate and one instance misclassified as ASD class. However, the result of the NB classifier model is to a greater degree or extent very acceptable with more than 90 percent performance. Finally, for the t-SNE attributes, the best performance is shown by the KNN classifier model with no misclassified instance. Following the KNN model is the performance of the DT classifier model which is more than 95 percent with four and eight adult individuals being misclassified as ASD and no ASD classes, respectively. But the performance of SVM and NB is not up to the mark for t-SNE

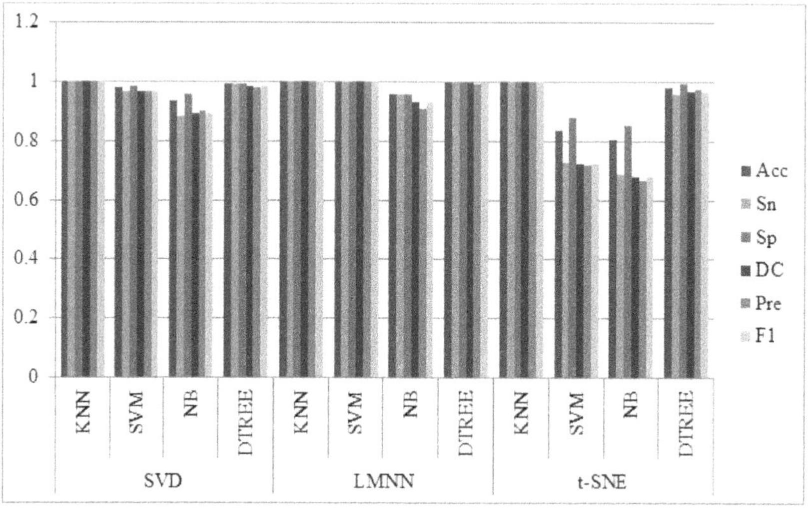

FIGURE 5.5   Performance rate of the ML algorithms on the adult dataset.

attributes. Figure 5.5 shows the performance of applied ML algorithms in terms of performance parameters on the adult dataset.

Table 5.6 below summarizes the comparative analysis of different classification approaches:

TABLE 5.6
Performance Comparison Analysis

Research in	Individual's ASD Dataset	Classifiers Utilized	Acc	Sn	Sp	DC	Pre	F1
(Thabtah 2019)	Adult	LR	0.998	0.999	0.997	-	-	-
(Al-diabat 2018)	Child	FURIA	0.913	0.914		-	-	-
		JRIP			0.928	-	-	-
(Vaishali and Sasikala 2018)	Child	SVM, MLP	0.996	-	-	-	-	-
(Thabtah, Kamalov, and Rajab 2018)	Adolescent	C4.5		0.905	-	-	-	-
	Adult	C4.5	0.890		0.925	-	-	-
(Thabtah and Peebles 2020)	Adult	RML	0.940	0.940	0.970	-	-	0.945
(Akter et al. 2019)	Toddler	SVM	0.987	0.993	-	-	-	-
		Adaboost	-	-	0.995	-	-	-
(Raj and Masood 2020)	Adult	CNN	0.995	0.993	1.000	-	-	-
Proposed method	Child, Adolescent	KNN	1.000	1.000	1.000	1.000	1.000	1.000
	Toddler, Adult	KNN, SVM	1.000	1.000	1.000	1.000	1.000	1.000

5.6 CONCLUSION

ASD greatly hampers the quality of life an individual should lead. Individuals with ASD suffer a lot and their standard of living deteriorates. To improve the quality and standard of life for the people with ASD, advanced detection with treatment is crucial. The proposed procedure focuses on prior detection of ASD. In this work, using dimension reduction techniques – SVD, LMNN, and t-SNE – the number of attributes in all data sets are reduced followed by 80 percent training data to train the various ML classifier models and the remaining 20 percent is used as testing data to carry out testing. Finally, the classifier models detected ASD classes for all categories of individuals – adult, adolescent, child, and toddler. The distinct performance parameters in this work such as accuracy, sensitivity, specificity, dice, precision, recall, and F-measure are evaluated by utilizing various ML classifiers like KNN, SVM, NB, and DT and proved to be clinically acceptable. The performance of KNN and DT classifiers on all dimension reduction techniques proved to be leading whereas that of SVM and NB classifiers somehow lagged in performance due to some misclassification of individuals under ASD classes. Overall, it can be assured that ML classifier models can be applied in detecting ASD. Generally, in most of the related investigations, the toddler data set is dropped due to its unbalanced characteristics. As a result of the unbalanced nature, researchers found the respective data set difficult to investigate. In this research, the toddler data set is investigated in addition to other categories of data sets with successful ASD detection in toddlers.

REFERENCES

Aha, David W., Dennis Kibler, and Marc K. Albert. 1991. "Instance-Based Learning Algorithms." *Machine Learning* 6 (1): 37–66. https://doi.org/10.1007/BF00153759

Akter, Tania, Md. Shahriare Satu, Md. Imran Khan, Mohammad Hanif Ali, Shahadat Uddin, Pietro Lio, Julian M. W. Quinn, and Mohammad Ali Moni. 2019. "Machine Learning-Based Models for Early Stage Detection of Autism Spectrum Disorders." *IEEE Access* 7: 166509–27. https://doi.org/10.1109/ACCESS.2019.2952609

Al-diabat, Mofleh. 2018. "Fuzzy Data Mining for Autism Classification of Children." *International Journal of Advanced Computer Science and Applications* 9 (7). https://doi.org/10.14569/IJACSA.2018.090702

Andrade, Chittaranjan. 2020. "Understanding the Difference Between Standard Deviation and Standard Error of the Mean, and Knowing When to Use Which." *Indian Journal of Psychological Medicine* 42 (4): 409–10. https://doi.org/10.1177/0253717620933419

Autism Research Centre - University of Cambridge. 1998. https://www.autismresearchcentre.com/

Auyeung, Bonnie, Simon Baron-Cohen, Sally Wheelwright, and Carrie Allison. 2008. "The Autism Spectrum Quotient: Children's Version (AQ-Child)." *Journal of Autism and Developmental Disorders* 38 (7): 1230–40. https://doi.org/10.1007/s10803-007-0504-z

Backer, Nouf Backer Al. 2015. "Developmental Regression in Autism Spectrum Disorder." *Sudanese Journal of Paediatrics* 15 (1): 21–6. http://www.ncbi.nlm.nih.gov/pubmed/27493417

Baron-Cohen, Simon, Rosa A Hoekstra, Rebecca Knickmeyer, and Sally Wheelwright. 2006. "The Autism-Spectrum Quotient (AQ)—Adolescent Version." *Journal of Autism and Developmental Disorders* 36 (3): 343–50. https://doi.org/10.1007/s10803-006-0073-6

Caluza, Las Johansen B. 2019. "Fuzzy Unordered Rule Induction Algorithm Application Basic Programming Language Competence: A Rule-Based Model." *Indian Journal of Science and Technology* 12 (12): 1–10. https://doi.org/10.17485/ijst/2019/v12i12/142575

Cendrowska, Jadzia. 1987. "PRISM: An Algorithm for Inducing Modular Rules." *International Journal of Man-Machine Studies* 27 (4): 349–70. https://doi.org/10.1016/S0020-7373(87)80003-2

Gaines, B. R., and P. Compton. 1995. "Induction of Ripple-down Rules Applied to Modeling Large Databases." *Journal of Intelligent Information Systems* 5 (3): 211–28. https://doi.org/10.1007/BF00962234

Golub, G., and W. Kahan. 1965. "Calculating the Singular Values and Pseudo-Inverse of a Matrix." *Journal of the Society for Industrial and Applied Mathematics Series B Numerical Analysis* 2 (2): 205–24. https://doi.org/10.1137/0702016

Goyal, Sukriti, Nikhil Sharma, Bharat Bhushan, Achyut Shankar, and Martin Sagayam. 2021. "IoT Enabled Technology in Secured Healthcare: Applications, Challenges and Future Directions." In Janusz Kacprzyk (Ed.) *Cognitive Internet of Medical Things for Smart Healthcare*. 25–48. https://doi.org/10.1007/978-3-030-55833-8_2

Hofner, Benjamin, Andreas Mayr, Nikolay Robinzonov, and Matthias Schmid. 2014. "Model-Based Boosting in R: A Hands-on Tutorial Using the R Package Mboost." *Computational Statistics* 29 (1–2): 3–35. https://doi.org/10.1007/s00180-012-0382-5

Liu, H. and R. Setiono. 1995 "Chi2: Feature Selection and Discretization of Numeric Attributes." In *Proceedings of 7th IEEE International Conference on Tools with Artificial Intelligence*, 388–91. IEEE Comput. Soc. Press. https://doi.org/10.1109/TAI.1995.479783

Jindal, Mansi, Jatin Gupta, and Bharat Bhushan. 2019. "Machine Learning Methods for IoT and Their Future Applications." In *2019 International Conference on Computing, Communication, and Intelligent Systems (ICCCIS)*, 430–34. IEEE. https://doi.org/10.1109/ICCCIS48478.2019.8974551

Kassambara, A. 2018. "Classification Methods Essentials." Statistical Tools for High-Throughput Data Analysis. http://www.sthda.com/english/articles/36-classification-methods-essentials/146-discriminant-analysis-essentials-in-r/

Keerthi, S. S., S. K. Shevade, C. Bhattacharyya, and K. R. K. Murthy. 2001. "Improvements to Platt's SMO Algorithm for SVM Classifier Design." *Neural Computation* 13 (3): 637–49. https://doi.org/10.1162/089976601300014493

Khamparia, Aditya, Prakash Kumar Singh, Poonam Rani, Debabrata Samanta, Ashish Khanna, and Bharat Bhushan. 2020. "An Internet of Health Things-driven Deep Learning Framework for Detection and Classification of Skin Cancer Using Transfer Learning." *Transactions on Emerging Telecommunications Technologies*, May. https://doi.org/10.1002/ett.3963

Kumar, Santosh, Bharat Bhusan, Debabrata Singh, and Dilip kumar Choubey. 2020. "Classification of Diabetes Using Deep Learning." In *2020 International Conference on Communication and Signal Processing (ICCSP)*, 0651–55. IEEE. https://doi.org/10.1109/ICCSP48568.2020.9182293

Liu, Sanyang, Mingmin Zhu, and Youlong Yang. 2013. "A Bayesian Classifier Learning Algorithm Based on Optimization Model." *Mathematical Problems in Engineering* 2013: 1–9. https://doi.org/10.1155/2013/975953

Melit Devassy, Binu, and Sony George. 2020. "Dimensionality Reduction and Visualisation of Hyperspectral Ink Data Using T-SNE." *Forensic Science International* 311 (June): 110194. https://doi.org/10.1016/j.forsciint.2020.110194

Mohanty, Ashima Sindhu, Priyadarsan Parida, and K. C. Patra. 2021. "Identification of Autism Spectrum Disorder Using Deep Neural Network." *Journal of Physics: Conference Series* 1921 (May): 012006. https://doi.org/10.1088/1742-6596/1921/1/012006

Mohanty, Ashima Sindhu, Krishna Chandra Patra, and Priyadarsan Parida. 2021. "Toddler ASD Classification Using Machine Learning Techniques." *International Journal of Online and Biomedical Engineering (IJOE)* 17 (07): 156. https://doi.org/10.3991/ijoe.v17i07.23497

Pal, S. K., and S. Mitra. 1992. "Multilayer Perceptron, Fuzzy Sets, and Classification." *IEEE Transactions on Neural Networks* 3 (5): 683–97. https://doi.org/10.1109/72.159058

Panigrahi, Niranjan, Ishan Ayus, and Om Prakash Jena. 2021. "An Expert System-Based Clinical Decision Support System for Hepatitis-B Prediction & Diagnosis." In Om Prakash Jena, ed., *Machine Learning for Healthcare Applications*, 57–75. Wiley-Scrivener Publisher. https://doi.org/10.1002/9781119792611.ch4

Paramesha, K., H. L. Gururaj, and Om Prakash Jena. 2021. "Applications of Machine Learning in Biomedical Text Processing and Food Industry." In Om Prakash Jena, ed., *Machine Learning for Healthcare Applications*, 151–67. Wiley-Scrivener Publisher. https://doi.org/10.1002/9781119792611.ch10

Patra, Sudhansu Shekhar, Om Praksah Jena, Gaurav Kumar, Sreyashi Pramanik, Chinmaya Misra, and Kamakhya Narain Singh. 2021. "Random Forest Algorithm in Imbalance Genomics Classification." In Rabinarayan Satpathy, Tanupriya Choudhury, Suneeta Satpathy, Sachi Nandan Mohanty, Xiaobo Zhang, ed., *Data Analytics in Bioinformatics*, 173–90. Wiley-Scrivener Publisher. https://doi.org/10.1002/9781119785620.ch7

Pattnayak, Parthasarathi, and Om Prakash Jena. 2021. "Innovation on Machine Learning in Healthcare Services–An Introduction." In Om Prakash Jena, *Machine Learning for Healthcare Applications*, 1–15. Wiley-Scrivener Publisher. https://doi.org/10.1002/9781119792611.ch1

Pratiwi, Asriyanti Indah, and Adiwijaya. 2018. "On the Feature Selection and Classification Based on Information Gain for Document Sentiment Analysis." *Applied Computational Intelligence and Soft Computing* 2018: 1–5. https://doi.org/10.1155/2018/1407817

Quinlan, J. Ross. 1986. "Induction of Decision Trees." *Machine Learning* 1 (1): 81–106. https://doi.org/10.1007/BF00116251

Raj, Suman, and Sarfaraz Masood. 2020. "Analysis and Detection of Autism Spectrum Disorder Using Machine Learning Techniques." *Procedia Computer Science* 167: 994–1004. https://doi.org/10.1016/j.procs.2020.03.399

Robins, D. L., D. Fein, M. L. Barton, and J. A. Green. 2001. "The Modified Checklist for Autism in Toddlers: An Initial Study Investigating the Early Detection of Autism and Pervasive Developmental Disorders." *Journal of Autism and Developmental Disorders* 31 (2): 131–44. https://doi.org/10.1023/a:1010738829569

Salzberg, Steven L. 1994. "C4.5: Programs for Machine Learning by J. Ross Quinlan. Morgan Kaufmann Publishers, Inc., 1993." *Machine Learning* 16 (3): 235–40. https://doi.org/10.1007/BF00993309

Sharma, Nikhil, Ila Kaushik, Bharat Bhushan, Siddharth Gautam, and Aditya Khamparia. 2020. *"Applicability of WSN and Biometric Models in the Field of Healthcare."* In *Deep Learning Strategies for Security Enhancement in Wireless Sensor Networks*, IGI Global, 304–29. https://doi.org/10.4018/978-1-7998-5068-7.ch016

Sun, Shiliang, and Qiaona Chen. 2011. "Hirarchical Distance Metric Learning for Large Margin Nearest Neighbor Classification." *International Journal of Pattern Recognition and Artificial Intelligence* 25 (07): 1073–87. https://doi.org/10.1142/S021800141100897X

Thabtah, Fadi Fayez. 2017a. "Machine-Learning-Databases/00419." https://archive.ics.uci.edu/ml

Thabtah, Fadi. 2017b. "Machine-Learning-Databases/00420." https://archive.ics.uci.edu/ml

Thabtah, Fadi. 2017c. "Machine-Learning-Databases/00426." https://archive.ics.uci.edu/ml

Thabtah, Fadi. 2018. "Autism-Screening-for-Toddlers/Version/1." https://www.kaggle.com/fabdelja/

Thabtah, Fadi. 2019. "An Accessible and Efficient Autism Screening Method for Behavioural Data and Predictive Analyses." *Health Informatics Journal* 25 (4): 1739–55. https://doi.org/10.1177/1460458218796636

Thabtah, Fadi, Firuz Kamalov, and Khairan Rajab. 2018. "A New Computational Intelligence Approach to Detect Autistic Features for Autism Screening." *International Journal of Medical Informatics* 117 (September): 112–24. https://doi.org/10.1016/j.ijmedinf.2018.06.009

Thabtah, Fadi, Neda Abdelhamid, and David Peebles. 2019. "A Machine Learning Autism Classification Based on Logistic Regression Analysis." *Health Information Science and Systems* 7 (1): 1–11. https://doi.org/10.1007/s13755-019-0073-5

Thabtah, Fadi, and David Peebles. 2020. "A New Machine Learning Model Based on Induction of Rules for Autism Detection." *Health Informatics Journal* 26 (1): 264–86. https://doi.org/10.1177/1460458218824711

Vaishali R., and R. Sasikala. 2018. "A Machine Learning Based Approach to Classify Autism with Optimum Behavior Sets." *International Journal of Engineering and Technology (IJET)* 7 (4): 4216–19. https://doi.org/10.14419/ijet.v7i3.18.14907

Wosiak, Agnieszka, and Danuta Zakrzewska. 2018. "Integrating Correlation-Based Feature Selection and Clustering for Improved Cardiovascular Disease Diagnosis." *Complexity* 2018 (October): 1–11. https://doi.org/10.1155/2018/2520706

Zhang, Yanqiu, Ming Ni, Chengwu Zhang, Shuang Liang, Sheng Fang, Ruijie Li, and Zhouyu Tan. 2019. "Research and Application of AdaBoost Algorithm Based on SVM." In *2019 IEEE 8th Joint International Information Technology and Artificial Intelligence Conference (ITAIC)*, 662–66. IEEE. https://doi.org/10.1109/ITAIC.2019.8785556

6 A Framework for Selection of Machine Learning Algorithms Based on Performance Metrices and Akaike Information Criteria in Healthcare, Telecommunication, and Marketing Sector

A. K. Hamisu and K. Jasleen

CONTENTS

DOI: 10.1201/9781003226147-6

6.1 INTRODUCTION

The growth of the internet has seen a profusion of data and a surge in technology for extracting information from big data for marketing strategy, adding value to products and services, and personalizing the consumer experience. Recently, there has been a remarkable increase in interest in the era of artificial intelligence (AI), ML, and deep learning (DL), as more individuals become aware of the breadth of new applications enabled by ML and DL methodologies. The applications of ML and DL range from home to hospital, domestic to enterprise, agriculture to military, and include all aspects of life. The main focus of this chapter is on applications of ML methodologies in three separate sub-domains: healthcare, marketing, and telecommunications. In the healthcare sector, two significant problems are considered for this research work. One is cardiovascular disease and another one is fetal health. The reason for choosing both these diseases is the rate at which they affect the people. Cardiovascular disease, also known as coronary ailment, is one of the most serious ailments in India and around the world. Heart disease is estimated to be the cause of 28.1% of deaths. It is also the leading cause of death, accounting for more than 17.6 million fatalities in 2016 across the world (Shan et al. 2017). As a result, accurate and early diagnosis and treatment of such diseases necessitates a system that can forecast with pinpoint accuracy and consistency. The second problem that is considered for this work is fetal health classification which includes classification of fetal as healthy or unhealthy. A total of three datasets (two cardiovascular datasets and one fetal health dataset) were used under healthcare sector. In this chapter, a framework for the selection of ML algorithm has been proposed. ML algorithm was selected based on dataset attributes, performance metrics, and AIC score. For experimentation purposes, ML algorithms were divided into eager, lazy, and hybrid learners. For the evaluation of the proposed framework, a total of eight datasets from three sectors (healthcare, telecommunication, and marketing) were selected for experimentation. This paper contributes in context of framework for recommendation of the best ML algorithm/model according to the input attributes. Model recommendation was based on performance evaluation parameters (accuracy, precision, and recall) as well as on model selection parameter (AIC).

The rest of this chapter is organized as follows. Section 6.2 presents related work carried out in proposed direction. Complete methodology followed for implementation of this work is presented in Section 6.3. Detailed results and analysis are presented in Section 6.4 followed by concluding remarks in Section 6.5.

6.2 MACHINE LEARNING APPLICATIONS

ML has potential applications in various domains and sectors. This section provides a brief glimpse of applications of ML in healthcare, telecommunication, marketing, and other sectors.

Goyal et al. (2021) introduced the concept of Internet of Health Things and discusses about potential challenges, advancement and benefits for IoT based healthcare and healthcare aided living. Pattnayak and Jena (2021) discussed and explained the need of ML for healthcare systems. Potential application of ML in healthcare and healthcare aided areas which includes from patient to doctor, from diagnosis to treatment, from surgery to decision support system were well elaborated. Panigrahi et al. (2021) developed an expert system-based clinical decision support system (CDSS) for prediction and diagnosis of hepatitis-B. This system comprises 59 rules and implementation is done using web-based Expert System Shell. Paramesha et al. (2021) discussed ML-based approach for sentiment analysis of narrated drug reviews and engineering in food technology which are indirectly related to the healthcare sector. Mohapatra et al. (2021) experimented with convolutional neural network (CNN) for early detection of skin cancer. They have also performed comparative analysis of MobileNet and ResNet50 CNN architectures for skin cancer classification task. Ramakrishnudu et al. (2021) proposed a system that predicts the overall health status of a person using ML techniques. Various parameters such as person's sleeping pattern, his/her physical activity, and his/her eating habits were used for predicting the overall health of the person. Panicker et al. (2021) proposed lightweight CNN model for classifying tuberculosis bacilli from non-bacilli objects. The performance of the proposed model in terms of accuracy is close to the existing ML models Panicker et al. 2021). Islam et al. discussed the use of DL techniques for autonomous disease diagnosis from symptoms. They proposed a graph convolution network (GCN) as a disease–symptom network to link the disease and symptoms. GCN-based deep neural network determines the most probable diseases associated with the given symptoms with 98% accuracy (Islam et al. 2021). Khamparia et al. (2020) proposed transfer learning based novel DL internet of health and things driven method for skin cancer classification. The proposed method performed well as compared to earlier reported techniques. Güldoğan et al. (2021) proposed a transfer learning-based technique for the detection and classification of breast cancer (benign or malignant) based on the ultrasound images. Performance metrices such as accuracy, sensitivity, and specificity with 95% confidence intervals were 0.974 (0.923–1.0), 0.957 (0.781–0.999), and 1 (0.782–1.0), respectively (Güldoğan et al. 2021). Said et al. (2021) proposed a new transfer learning-based approach for the classification of breast cancer in histopathological images. Block wise fine tuning strategy has been employed to handle CNN RESNET-18 (Said et al. 2021). Yang et al. (2021) explored the potential of DL models in the identification of lung cancer subtypes and cancer mimics from whole slide images. Irene et al. (2021) elaborated the ethics of ML in healthcare through the lens of social justice. Recent developments, challenges, and solutions to address those challenges were discussed in detail. Danton et al. (2020) proposed a systematic approach to identify the ethics in ML-based healthcare applications. Elements such as conceptual model, development, implementation, and evaluation were considered while framing the approach (Danton et al. 2020). Muhammad et al. (2020) discussed the challenges, requirements, and opportunities in the area of fairness in healthcare AI and the various nuances associated with it. Liu et al. (2020) proposed DL approaches for automatic diagnosis of Alzheimer's disease (AD) and its prodromal stage, that is, mild cognitive impairment (MCI). Baskar et al. (2020) proposed a framework for wearable sensors (WS) so that it can be applicable as a part of smart healthcare tracking applications. Andre et al. (2019) discussed the application of computer vision, natural language processing in the context of medical domain. Siddique and Chow (2021) discussed the application of ML/AI in healthcare communication. This work includes chatbots for the COVID-19 health education, cancer therapy, and medical imaging. The challenges, issues, and problems for the implementation of ML- and DL-based applications in healthcare and healthcare-aided sector have been discussed (Riccardo et al. 2018). Mateen et al. (2020) presented a framework for improving the accuracy of ML algorithms in healthcare by incorporating reporting guidelines such as SPIRIT-AI and CONSORT-AI in clinical and health science in ML approaches. Ferdous et al. (2020) presented a review on ML when applied to prediction of different diseases. The contribution of ML in healthcare is discussed with aim to provide the best suitable ML algorithm (Ferdous et al. 2020). Utsav et al. (2019) presented a technique to use ML algorithms for predicting the probability of cardiac arrest based on various attributes. Zoabi et al. (2021) proposed an ML-based technique to predict whether an individual is infected with SARS-CoV-2 or not. The model takes different parameters such as age, gender, and presence of various COVID symptoms. Faizal and Sultan (2020) explored the application of AI and data analytics techniques for mobile health. These techniques can be used for providing valuable insights to users and accordingly resources can be planned for mobile health. AI-based models have been proposed for mobile health. Futoma et al. (2020) emphasized for clinical utility and generalizability of ML algorithms and answers the various questions (when, how, and why) on ML applicability for both clinicians and for patients. Wang et al. (2020) proposed an alternative COVID-19 diagnosis methodology based on COVID-19 radio graphical changes in computerized tomography (CT) images. They experimented with DL methods to extract the hidden features from CT scans and provide the diagnosis for COVID-19 (Wang et al. 2020). Song et al. (2020) proposed DeepPneumonia technique (as DL based COVID detection from CT scans) to identify patients with COVID-19. Punn et al. (2020) proposed ML- and DL-based model to analyze predictive behavior of COVID-19 using a dataset published on the Johns Hopkins dashboard.

Authors proposed a technique to predict the customer churn rate (who are likely to cancel the subscription). Various ML algorithms such as DT, Random Forest, and XGBoost have been experimented (Kavitha et al. 2020). Researchers presented analysis to leverage ML methods in marketing research. Comparison between ML methods with statistical methods was also presented. A unified conceptual framework for ML methods have been proposed in this work (Liye and Baohong 2020). Dev et al. (2016) used ML to predict heart disease.

In Galván et al.'s (2009) study, a lazy learning strategy was proposed for building classification learning models. In this work, authors compared the accuracy of SVM and KNN algorithms on student performance data sets. SVM performed well as compared to KNN with accuracy of 91.07% (Nuranisah et al. 2020). Thanh and Kappas (2017) examined and compared the performance of ML algorithm for land use/cover classification. The classification results showed a high overall accuracy of all the algorithms In this paper, authors experimented with ML algorithms on healthcare datasets (Raj and Sonia 2017). Zhenlong et al. (2017) explored the usefulness of ML algorithms for driver drowsiness detection. The results revealed that SVM performed well. In this paper, authors proposed the application of lazy learning techniques to Bayesian tree induction and presents the resulting lazy Bayesian rule learning algorithm, called Lbr (Zheng and Webb 2000). Solomon et al. (2014) presented evaluation of eager and lazy classification algorithms using UCI Bank Marketing data set. Results revealed that eager learners outperform the lazy learners with accuracy of 98%.

6.3 DESIGN AND IMPLEMENTATION OF FRAMEWORK FOR MODEL SELECTION

Proposed architecture is explained in Figure 6.1. Proposed system consists of various phases: data collection, data pre-processing, feature extraction, model building, and performance evaluation.

6.3.1 PHASE 1: INPUT ANALYSIS PHASE

6.3.1.1 Input Attributes

In this phase, attributes are input into the system. The selection of attributes entirely depends upon the problem for which the most suitable algorithm is to be identified.

6.3.1.2 Attribute Analysis

In this sub-phase, input attributes are analyzed. Various kinds of analysis such as size of input attributes, type of input attributes, and nature of input attributes are

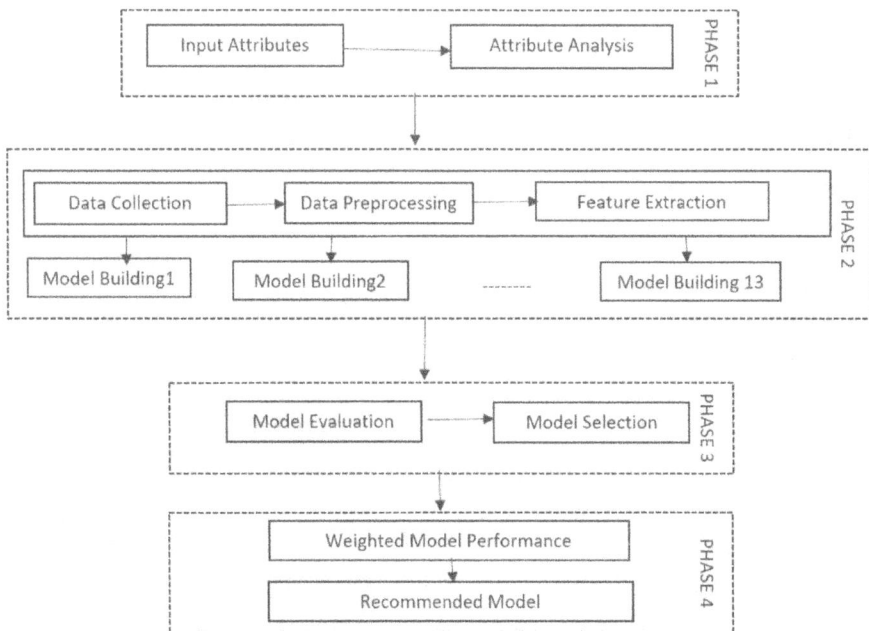

FIGURE 6.1 Architecture of proposed system.

performed for better understanding of data. Visualization technique was used to identify the relationship between input attributes whether it is linear or non-linear, based on which set of ML algorithms were selected. For input attributes where a linear relationship exists among the attributes, algorithms like SVM can be selected for initial evaluation. If the size of input attributes is small, algorithm like Naïve Bayes can be preferable for initial evaluation. As nature of data concerns, it depends upon the output target variable type. In our work, target variable is categorical in nature.

6.3.2   PHASE 2: MODEL BUILDING PHASE

In this phase, various selected ML algorithms were trained and tested for datasets from each of the sectors. The ML algorithm training and testing process is described in the following sub-phases.

6.3.2.1   Data collection

For this research work, three sectors (healthcare, telecommunication, and marketing) were selected. A total of eight datasets were collected in three sectors. Details of dataset by sector are presented in Table 6.1. The description includes the number of records, attributes, and class labels in each dataset.

6.3.2.2   Data Pre-Processing

Raw data need to be pre-processed to organize them into the form which is good for training the ML algorithm (Han and Kamber 2001). In this work, raw data passes through various pre-processing stages such as label encoding and handling missing values with mean of that attribute.

6.3.2.3   Features Extraction

To reduce the computational cost and time for building the model, subsets of features/attributes were selected. Multifactor dimensionality reduction methods were used for reducing the dimensionality of the data. Some attributes were not considered for model building based upon co-linearity matrices (used for finding relationship with indented class label).

TABLE 6.1
Dataset Description

Sector	Dataset	Description
Marketing	(Avocado 2020)	18,249 records; 13 attributes; 2 class labels
	(Bank in Marketing 2020)	11,162 records; 17 attributes; 2 class labels
Telecommunication	(Telecom 2020)	4000 records; 12 attributes; 2 class labels
	(Cell2cell train 2020)	51047 records; 38 attributes; 2 class labels
	(Churn in Telecom 2020)	3333 records; 21 attributes; 2 class labels
Healthcare	(Cardio-Vascular 2020)	70,000 records; 13 attributes; 2 class labels
	(Fetal_Health 2020)	2126 records; 22 attributes; 2 class labels
	(Health_heart 2020)	1025 records; 14 attributes; 2 class labels

6.3.2.4 Model Building

In this research work, 13 machine algorithms were experimented. These ML algorithms were divided into the following categories: eager or lazy depending upon the learning procedure and third category is hybrid (Huang et al. 2014; Dev et al. 2016).

1. **Eager learning:** This category of ML algorithms includes DT, SVM, and Neural Network (NN).

    A DT is built using recursive partitioning-based approach. A tree-like structure is generated using input attributes and leaf nodes of those generated trees represent the class labels. In this research work, C4.5 version of DT was built using the gain ratio of attribute.

$$Gain \ Rtio\left(X_i, D\right) = \frac{Information \ Gain \ (X_i, D)}{Entropy \ (P_{X_i}(D))} \tag{6.1}$$

   Where $Gain \ Ratio\left(X_i, D\right)$ is ratio of attribute X_i with regard to Dataset D (Han and Kamber 2001).

   SVM is statistical ML algorithm which is based on the structural risk minimization principle (Han and Kamber 2001). Linear SVM tries to find maximal marginal hyperplane using the following equation:

$$f(\vec{x}) = \begin{cases} 1 & if \ \vec{w} \cdot \vec{x} + b \geq 1 \\ -1 & if \ \vec{w} \cdot \vec{x} + b \leq -1 \end{cases} \tag{6.2}$$

   Where $\vec{w}$ and b parameters are identified from training data.

   NN is supervised ML algorithm which is based on backprogation where weights in hidden layer and output layer are updated according to error in estimation. For weights updation, the following equation is utilized.

$$w_j^{k+1} = w_j^k + \lambda(y_i - \widehat{y_i^k}) \, x_{ij} \tag{6.3}$$

   Where k is iteration, x_{ij} is input attribute value, w_j^k is weight assigned in k^{th} iteration, and λ learning rate (Han and Kamber 2001).

2. **Lazy learning:** This category includes KNN algorithm and LNB algorithm.

    KNN algorithm is a distance-based ML algorithm which has application in classification as well as regression problems. In this research work, distance is calculated based on Euclidean distance measure. Distance between test point (x) and existing training point (y) is given by,

$$Eucidean \ distance = \sqrt{\sum_{i=1}^{n}\left(x_i - y_i\right)^2} \tag{6.4}$$

   For each dataset, hyper-parameter for KNN, that is, k, is tuned using elbow method.

TABLE 6.2
Category-Wise Machine Learning Algorithms

S. No.	Category	Algorithm
1	Eager	Decision Tree (DT)
		Support Vector Machine (SVM)
		Neural Network (NN)
2	Lazy	K-nearest Neighbhour (KNN)
		Lazy Naïve Bayes (LNB)
3	Hybrid	KNN+LNB
		SVM+DT+NN
		SVM+KNN
		DT+KNN
		NN+KNN
		SVM+LNB
		DT+LNB
		NN+LNB

3. **Hybrid Learning:** This category of ML algorithms was formed by combining different ML algorithms. Algorithms in this category are generated by stacking up the different ML algorithms from the eager and lazy categories. Count in eager, lazy, and hybrid ML categories is 3, 2, and 8 respectively. Table 6.2 provides the details about the categories of ML algorithms.

6.3.3 Phase 3: Model Evaluation Phase

6.3.3.1 Model Analysis Module

In this phase, analysis of each ML model is carried out in terms of performance evaluation parameters and model selection parameters. Accuracy, precision, recall, F-measure, receiver operating characteristic (ROC) curve, and ROC area under curve (AUC) are used as performance metrices for evaluation. For model selection purposes, the AIC score was calculated for each algorithm (Akaike 1973).

6.3.4 Phase 4: Model Recommendation Phase

Based on the attributes passed on in phase 1, this phase identifies the most suitable ML algorithm based on performance metrices and AIC score. Recommendation of ML algorithm is based on the weighted average of performance parameters and AIC score.

6.4 RESULT AND ANALYSIS

The purpose of this research is to find the best performing ML algorithm in each sector (telecommunication, health, and marketing). For this purpose, a total 104 experiments were performed where every dataset (8 in total) is experimented with 13 ML algorithms (as listed in the previous section). Selection of ML algorithm is carried out on the basis of performance parameters as well as AIC score. Implementation of this work has been carried out in Python.

6.4.1 SELECTION OF MODEL BASED ON ACCURACY, PRECISION, RECALL, AND F-MEASURE

Tables 6.3–6.5 show the results of ML algorithms in each sector. For interpretation purposes, the average of each metric (accuracy, precision, recall, and f-measure) is obtained.

From Tables 6.3–6.5, it can be observed that the eager learner category of ML algorithms performed well as compared to lazy and hybrid learner. Overall average

TABLE 6.3
Result Obtained with Marketing Sector

Learning Methods	Average Accuracy	Average Precision	Average Recall	Average F-measure
Eager learner	94	0.92	0.99	0.95
Lazy learner	91	0.86	0.74	0.78
Hybrid learner	92	0.88	0.93	0.93

TABLE 6.4
Result Obtained with Healthcare Sector

Learning Methods	Average Accuracy	Average Precision	Average Recall	Average F-measure
Eager learner	90	0.88	0.83	0.88
Lazy learner	85	0.86	0.88	0.87
Hybrid learner	76	0.78	0.77	0.79

TABLE 6.5
Result Obtained with Telecommunication Sector

Learning Methods	Average Accuracy	Average Precision	Average Recall	Average F-measure
Eager learner	90	0.89	0.99	0.92
Lazy learner	86	0.90	0.84	0.86
Hybrid learner	85	0.78	0.87	0.88

TABLE 6.6

Average Accuracy-Based Comparison of Machine Learning Algorithms

Learning Methods	Marketing Dataset Average Accuracy	Telecommunication Dataset Average Accuracy	Healthcare Dataset Average Accuracy
Eager learner	94	90	90
Lazy learner	91	86	85
Hybrid learner	92	85	76

TABLE 6.7

Average Precision-Based Comparison of Machine Learning Algorithms

Learning Methods	Marketing Dataset Average Precision	Telecommunication Dataset Average Precision	Healthcare Dataset Average Precision
Eager learner	0.92	0.89	0.88
Lazy learner	0.86	0.90	0.86
Hybrid learner	0.88	0.78	0.78

accuracy of eager learners ranges from 90% to 94%. Accuracy- and precision-based comparative analysis is presented in Tables 6.6 and 6.7.

From Figures 6.2 and 6.3, it can be observed that the eager learner category of algorithms performed well for the healthcare sector based on accuracy and precision. For identification of the best ML algorithm in each sector, performance analysis of ML algorithms in the eager learner category is carried out. From Figures 6.2 and 6.3,

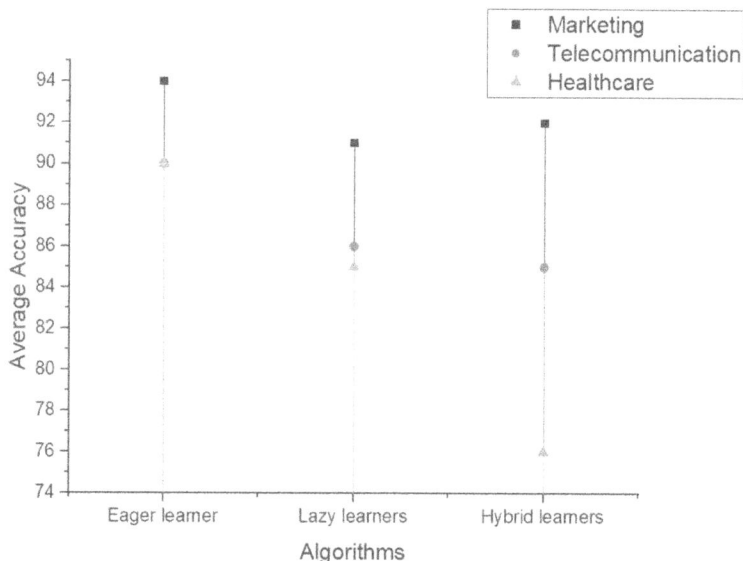

FIGURE 6.2 Comparison of algorithms based on accuracy.

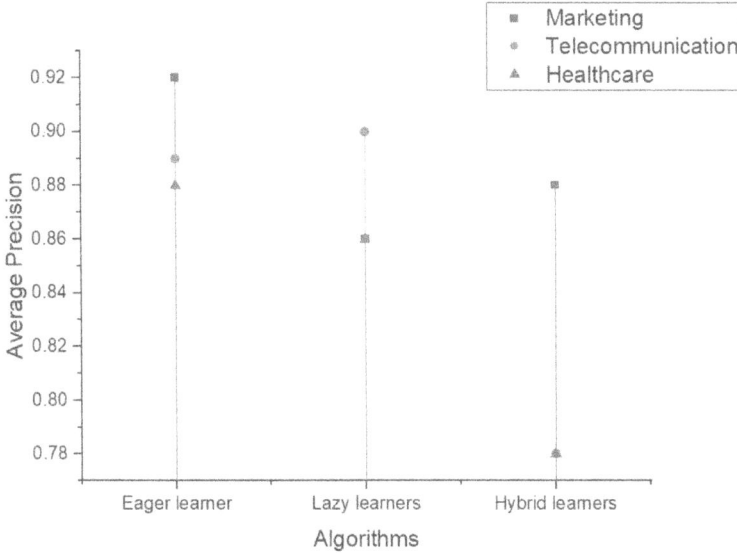

FIGURE 6.3   Comparison of algorithms based on precision.

it can be observed that the eager learner category of algorithms performed well for the healthcare sector based on accuracy and precision. For identification of the best ML algorithm in each sector, performance analysis of ML algorithms in the eager learner category is carried out. In the case of the healthcare dataset, SVM is proven to be the best ML algorithm, whereas in the case of the telecommunication and marketing dataset, DT comes out as the top performing one. NN was the worst performing algorithm in each sector. Furthermore, ROC curve (refer to Figures 6.4–6.6) and ROC-AUC score was analyzed for top performing algorithms. ROC-AUC score comes out to be 1.0 for all top performing ones.

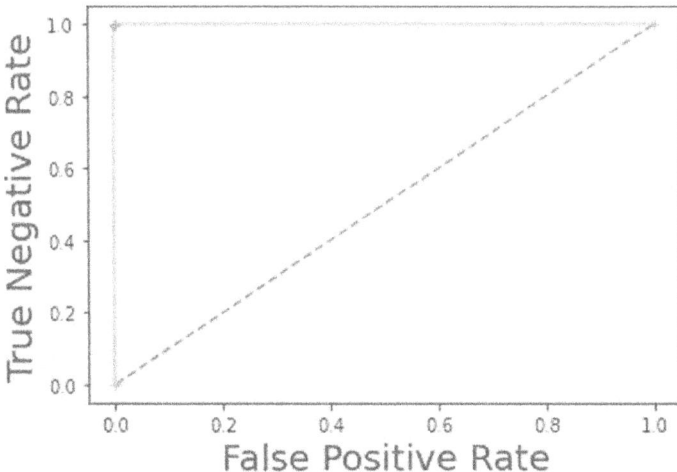

FIGURE 6.4   ROC curve for DT algorithm in the marketing sector.

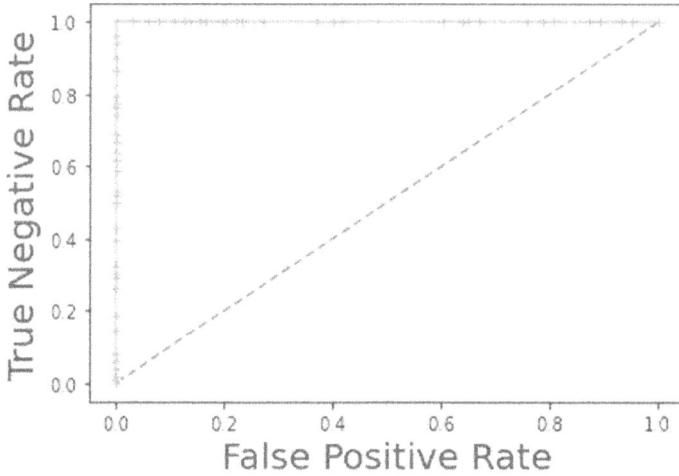

FIGURE 6.5   ROC curve for SVM algorithm in the healthcare sector.

As performance of all the ML algorithms is on the same scale, further analyses is carried out using AIC.

6.4.2   SELECTION OF MODEL BASED ON AKAIKE INFORMATION CRITERIA

In this section, algorithm performance is measured in terms of AIC. The best model is chosen with the help of probability framework of log-likelihood under maximum likelihood estimation. The AIC score can be calculated using:

$$AIC = 2*k - 2\,\log(L) \tag{6.5}$$

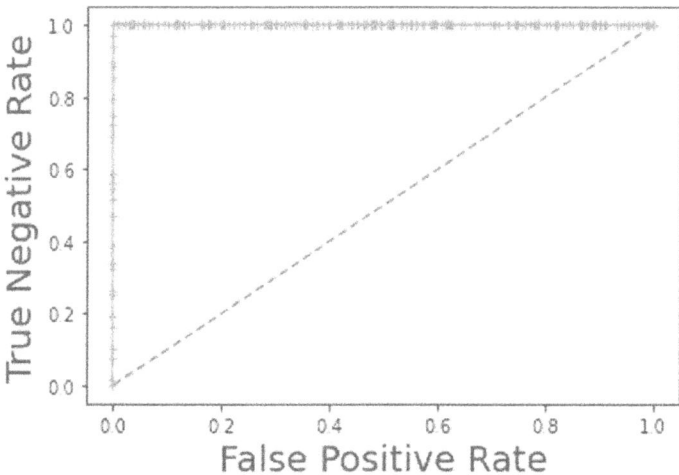

FIGURE 6.6   ROC curve for DT algorithm in the telecommunication sector.

TABLE 6.8

Results Based on Average AIC Score

Learning Methods	Marketing Dataset Average AIC	Telecommunication Dataset Average AIC	Healthcare Dataset Average AIC
Eager learner	15.41	21.92	24.07
Lazy learner	16.35	19.91	21.76
Hybrid learner	17.38	22.19	24.96

where k indicates the number of independent variables used to build the model and L indicates maximum likelihood estimate of model (Akaike 1973). The best model is one which minimizes the information loss and has the minimum score for AIC.

From Table 6.8 it can be observed that in the marketing dataset, the lowest AIC score of 15.41 is reported by the eager learner category of ML algorithms, whereas for the telecommunication and healthcare datasets, the lowest AIC score is reported by the lazy learner category of ML algorithms with a score of 19.91 and 21.76, respectively.

From Figure 6.7 it can be observed that for the marketing sector, the lowest AIC score is reported by eager learners, whereas in the case of telecommunication and healthcare sectors, the lazy learner category reported the lowest AIC. To find the best suitable algorithm for each sector, comparative analysis has been

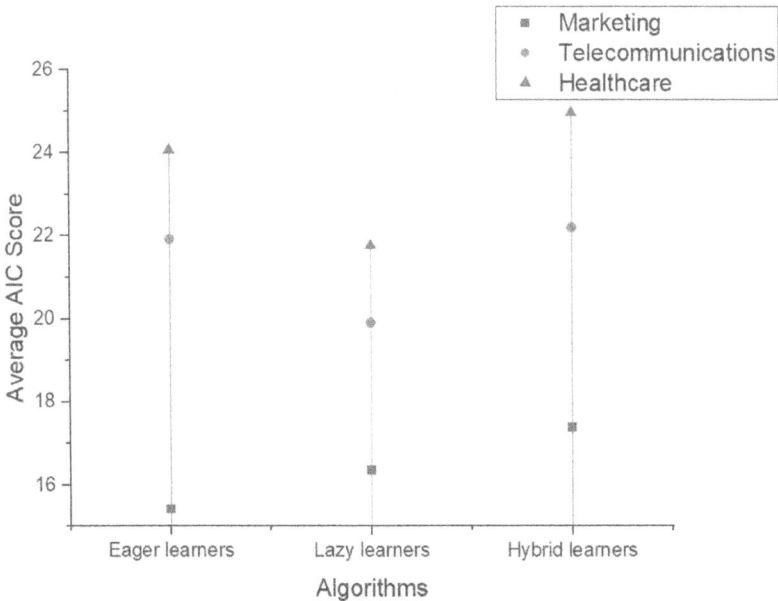

FIGURE 6.7   Comparison of algorithms based on AIC score.

TABLE 6.9

Accuracy- v/s AIC Score-Based Comparative Analysis of Algorithms

	Accuracy-Based Analysis		AIC-Based Analysis	
	Category	Algorithm	Category	Algorithm
Marketing	Eager	DT	Eager	SVM
Telecommunication	Eager	DT	Lazy	KNN
Healthcare	Eager	SVM	Lazy	KNN

carried out. Comparative analysis of algorithms based on accuracy and AIC score is presented in Table 6.9.

Figure 6.7 Three different ML model categories (lazy, eager, hybrid) for three different sectors are compared using AIC for model selection.

From Table 6.9 it can be observed that for the marketing dataset, the eager learner category is the better option as compared to lazy learners. Based on accuracy and AIC score, the most suitable ML algorithms are DT and SVM. On the basis of accuracy, eager learner is the best performing category of ML algorithms. DT and SVM are the most suitable algorithms for the telecommunication as well as healthcare sectors. On the basis of AIC score, lazy learner category of ML algorithms is the best option for the telecommunication and healthcare sectors. Out of all lazy learners, KNN performed well on telecommunication as well as on the healthcare sector.

6.5 CONCLUSION

In this research work, a framework for recommendation of ML algorithm has been formulated. The purpose was to find the most suitable ML algorithm for three different sectors. For experimentation purpose, ML algorithm were divided into three categories: eager, lazy, and hybrid learner. KNN, LNB, SVM, DT, NN, and the hybrid classifier using stacking were used on eight different datasets (from three different sectors: marketing, healthcare, and telecommunication). On the basis of accuracy, results revealed that eager learner ML algorithms are the best performing ones in all three sectors. Among eager learners, SVM is proven to be the top performing in healthcare with precision of 0.98. DT is the best suited for the telecommunication and marketing datasets with precision of 0.99 and 0.94, respectively. Whereas, on the basis of AIC score, SVM is the best suited for the marketing dataset, whereas KNN is the best suited for telecommunication and healthcare dataset.

REFERENCES

Akaike, H 1973. Information theory and an extension of the maximum likelihood principle. In: Petrov, B. N. and Csáki, F. (eds.), *2nd International Symposium on Information Theory, Tsahkadsor, Armenia, USSR, September 2–8, 1971.* Budapest: Akadémiai Kiadó, pp. 267–81.

Andre, E., Alexandre, R., Bharath, R., Volodymyr, K., Mark, D., Katherine, C., Claire, C., Greg, C., Sebastian, T., Jeff, D. 2019. A guide to deep learning in healthcare. *Nature Medicine*, 25: 24–29. https://doi.org/10.1038/s41591-018-0316-z

Avocado dataset accessed from https://www.kaggle.com/neuromusic/avocado-prices in Dec 2020.

Bank in Marketing dataset accessed from https://www.kaggle.com in Dec 2020.

Baskar, S., Mohamed, S. P., Kumar, R., Burhanuddin, M. A., Sampath, R. 2020. A dynamic and interoperable communication framework for controlling the operations of wearable sensors in smart healthcare applications. *Computer Communications*,149: 17–26. https://doi.org/10.1016/j.comcom.2019.10.004

Cardio_Vascular dataset accessed from https://www.kaggle.com in Dec 2020.

Cell2celltrain dataset accessed from https://www.kaggle.com in Dec 2020.

Churn in Telecom dataset accessed from https://www.kaggle.com in Dec 2020.

Danton, S. C., Michael, D. A., Chris, F. 2020. Identifying ethical considerations for machine learning healthcare applications. *The American Journal of Bioethics*, 20(11): 7–17. https://doi.org/10.1080/15265161.2020.1819469

Dev, S. K., Krishnapriya, S., Kalita, D. 2016. Prediction of heart disease using data mining techniques. *Indian Journal of Science and Technology*, 9(39): 1–5.

Faizal, K. Z., Sultan, R. A. 2020. Applications of artificial intelligence and big data analytics in m-health: A healthcare system perspective. *Journal of Healthcare Engineering*, 2020: 1–15. https://doi.org/10.1155/2020/8894694

Ferdous, M., Debnath, J., Chakraborty, N. R. 2020. Machine Learning Algorithms in Healthcare: A Literature Survey. *11th International Conference on Computing, Communication and Networking Technologies (ICCCNT)*, Kharagpur, India, 2020, pp. 1–6, https://doi.org/10.1109/ICCCNT49239.2020.9225642

Fetal_Health dataset accessed from https://www.kaggle.com in Dec 2020.

Futoma, J., Simons, M., Panch, T., Doshi-Velez, F., Celi, L. A. 2020. The myth of generalisability in clinical research and machine learning in health care. *The Lancet. Digital health*, 2(9): e489–e492. https://doi.org/10.1016/S2589-7500(20)30186-2

Galván, I. M., Valls, J. M., Lecomte, N., Isasi, P. 2009. A Lazy Approach for Machine Learning Algorithms. *Artificial Intelligence Applications and Innovations III. AIAI 2009. IFIP International Federation for Information Processing*, vol 296. Boston, MA: Springer. https://doi.org/10.1007/978-1-4419-0221-4_60

Goyal, S., Sharma, N., Bhushan, B., Shankar, A., Sagayam, M. 2021. *IoT Enabled Technology in Secured Healthcare: Applications, Challenges and Future Directions*. In Hassanien A.E., Khamparia A., Gupta D., Shankar K., Slowik A. (eds) *Cognitive Internet of Medical Things for Smart Healthcare. Studies in Systems, Decision and Control*, 311: 25–48. https://doi.org/10.1007/978-3-030-55833-8_2

Güldoğan, E., Ucuzal, H., Küçükakçalı, Z., Çolak, C. 2021. Transfer learning-based classification of breast cancer using ultrasound images. *Middle Black Sea Journal of Health Science*, 7(1): 74–80. https://doi.org/10.19127/mbsjohs.876667

Han, J., Kamber, M. 2001. *Data Mining: Concepts and Techniques*. San Diego, USA: Morgan Kaufmann.

Health_heart dataset accessed from https://www.kaggle.com in Dec 2020.

Huang, G., Song, S., Gupta, J. N. D., Wu, C. 2014. Semi-supervised and unsupervised extreme learning machines. *IEEE Transactions on Cybernetics*, 44(1): 2405–17. https://doi.org/10.1109/TCYB.2014.2307349

Irene, Y. C., Emma, P., Sherri, R., Shalmali, J., Kadija, F., Marzyeh, G. 2021. Ethical machine learning in healthcare. *Annual Review of Biomedical Data Science*, 4(1): 1–24. https://doi.org/10.1146/annurev-biodatasci-092820-114757

Islam, S. R., Sinha, R., Maity, S. P., Ray, A. K. 2021. Deep Learning on Symptoms in Disease Prediction. In: Mohanty, S. N., Nalinipriya, G., Jena, O. P. and Sarkar, A. (eds), *Machine Learning for Healthcare Applications,* Wiley Online Library, pp. 77–87. https://doi.org/10.1002/9781119792611.ch5

Kavitha, V., Hemanth, K. G., Mohan, K. S. V., Harish, M. 2020. Churn prediction of customer in telecom industry using machine learning algorithms. *International Journal of Engineering Research & Technology*, 09(05). http://dx.doi.org/10.17577/IJERTV9IS050022

Khamparia, A., Singh, P. K., Rani, P., Samanta, D., Khanna, A., Bhushan, B. 2020. An internet of health things-driven deep learning framework for detection and classification of skin cancer using transfer learning. *Transactions on Emerging Telecommunication Technologies*: 32, e3963. https://doi.org/10.1002/ett.3963

Liu, M., Lian, C., Shen, D. 2020. Anatomical-Landmark-Based Deep Learning for Alzheimer's Disease Diagnosis with Structural Magnetic Resonance Imaging. In: Chen, Y. W. and Jain, L. (eds), *Deep Learning in Healthcare. Intelligent Systems*. Reference Library, vol 171. Cham: Springer. https://doi.org/10.1007/978-3-030-32606-7_8

Liye, M., Baohong, S. 2020. Machine learning and AI in marketing – Connecting computing power to human insight. *International Journal of Research in Marketing*, 37(3): 481–504. https://doi.org/10.1016/j.ijresmar.2020.04.005

Mateen, B. A., Liley, J., Denniston, A. K. 2020. Improving the quality of machine learning in health applications and clinical research. *Nature Machine Intelligence*, 2: 554–6. https://doi.org/10.1038/s42256-020-00239-1

Mohapatra, S., Abhishek, N., Bardhan, D., Ghosh, A. A., Mohanty, S. 2021. Comparison of MobileNet and ResNet CNN Architectures in the CNN-Based Skin Cancer Classifier Model. In: Mohanty, S. N., Nalinipriya, G., Jena, O. P. and Sarkar, A. (eds), *Machine Learning for Healthcare Applications*, Wiley Online Library, 169–86. https://doi.org/10.1002/9781119792611.ch11

Muhammad, A. A., Arpit, P., Carly, E., Vikas, K., Ankur, T. 2020. Fairness in Machine Learning for Healthcare. In *Proceedings of the 26th ACM SIGKDD International Conference on Knowledge Discovery & Data Mining (KDD '20)*. New York, NY: Association for Computing Machinery, 3529–3530. https://doi.org/10.1145/3394486.3406461

Nuranisah, Syahril E., Poltak, S. 2020. Analysis of algorithm support vector machine learning and k-nearest neighbor in data accuracy. *IOP Conf. Series: Materials Science and Engineering*, 725: 1–7.

Panicker, R. O., Pawan, S., Rajan, J., Sabu, M. 2021. A Lightweight Convolutional Neural Network Model for Tuberculosis Bacilli Detection From Microscopic Sputum Smear Images. In: Mohanty, S. N., Nalinipriya, G., Jena, O. P. and Sarkar, A. (eds), *Machine Learning for Healthcare Applications*, Wiley Online Library, 343–51. https://doi.org/10.1002/9781119792611.ch22

Panigrahi, N., Ayus, I., Jena, O. P. 2021. An Expert System-Based Clinical Decision Support System for Hepatitis-B Prediction & Diagnosis. In: Mohanty, S. N., Nalinipriya, G., Jena, O. P. and Sarkar, A. (eds), *Machine Learning for Healthcare Applications*, Wiley Online Library, 57–75. https://doi.org/10.1002/9781119792611.ch4

Paramesha, K., Gururaj, H., Jena, O. P. 2021. Applications of Machine Learning in Biomedical Text Processing and Food Industry. In: Mohanty, S. N., Nalinipriya, G., Jena, O. P. and Sarkar, A. (eds), *Machine Learning for Healthcare Applications*:, Wiley Online Library, 151–67. https://doi.org/10.1002/9781119792611.ch10

Pattnayak, P., Jena, O. P. 2021. Innovation on Machine Learning in Healthcare Services– An Introduction. In: Mohanty, S. N., Nalinipriya, G., Jena, O. P. and Sarkar, A. (eds), *Machine Learning for Healthcare Applications*, Wiley Online Library, 1–15. https://doi.org/10.1002/9781119792611.ch1

Punn, N. S., Sonbhadra, S. K., Agarwal, S. 2020. COVID-19 epidemic analysis using machine learning and deep learning algorithms. *medRxiv*. https://doi.org/10.1101/2020.04.08.20057679

Raj, K., Sonia. 2017. SVM & KNN based classification of healthcare data sets using weka. *IJCSC*, 8(1): 50–54. https://doi.org/10.031206/IJCSC.2016.012

Ramakrishnudu, T., Prasen, T. S., Chakravarthy, V. T. 2021. A Framework for Health Status Estimation Based on Daily Life Activities Data Using Machine Learning Techniques. In: Mohanty, S. N., Nalinipriya, G., Jena, O. P. and Sarkar, A. (eds), *Machine Learning for Healthcare Applications*, Wiley Online Library, 17–32. https://doi.org/10.1002/9781119792611.ch2

Riccardo, M., Fei, W., Shuang, W., Xiaoqian, J., Joel, T. D. 2018. Deep learning for healthcare: review, opportunities and challenges. *Briefings in Bioinformatics*, 19(6): 1236–46, https://doi.org/10.1093/bib/bbx044

Said, B., Xiabi, L., Zhongshu, Z., Xiaohong, M., Chokri, F. 2021. A new transfer learning based approach to magnification dependent and independent classification of breast cancer in histopathological images. *Biomedical Signal Processing and Control*, 63. https://doi.org/10.1016/j.bspc.2020.102192

Shan, X., Tiangang, Z., Zhen, Z., Daoxian, W., Junfeng, H., Xiaohui, D. 2017. Cardiovascular Risk Prediction Method Based on CFS Subset Evaluation and Random Forest Classification Framework. *2017 IEEE 2nd International Conference on Big Data Analysis (ICBDA)*, 228–32. https://doi.org/10.1109/ICBDA.2017.8078813

Siddique, S, Chow, J. C. L. 2021. Machine learning in healthcare communication. *Encyclopedia*, 1(1): 220–39. https://doi.org/10.3390/encyclopedia1010021

Solomon, G. F., Abebe, D. A., Bhabani, S. D. M. 2014. A comparative study on performance evaluation of eager versus lazy learning methods. *International Journal of Computer Science and Mobile Computing*, 3(3): 562–8.

Song, Y., Shuangjia, Z., Liang, L., et al. 2020. Deep learning Enables Accurate Diagnosis of Novel Coronavirus (COVID-19) with CT images. *IEEE/ACM Transactions on Computational Biology and Bioinformatics* https://doi.org/10.1101/2020.02.23.20026930

Telecom dataset accessed from https://www.kaggle.com/blastchar/telco-customer-churn in Dec 2020.

Thanh, N. P., Kappas, M. 2017. Comparison of Random Forest, k-Nearest Neighbor, and support vector machine classifiers for land cover classification using Sentinel-2 imagery. *Sensors (Basel)*. 18(1). doi: 10.3390/s18010018. PMID: 29271909; PMCID: PMC5796274.

Utsav, C., Vikas, K., Vipul, C., Sumit, T., Amit, K. 2019. Cardiac arrest prediction using machine learning algorithms. *2019 2nd International Conference on Intelligent Computing Instrumentation and Control Technologies (ICICICT)*, 1, 886–90. https://doi.org/10.1109/ICICICT46008.2019.8993296

Wang, S., Kang, B., Ma, J., Zeng, X., Xiao, M., Guo, J., Cai, M., Yang, J., Li, Y., Meng, X., Xu, B. 2020. A deep learning algorithm using CT images to screen for Corona Virus Disease (COVID-19). *European Radiology*. https://doi.org/10.1007/s00330-021-07715-1

Yang, H., Chen, L., Cheng, Z., Yang, M., Wang, J., Lin, C., Wang, Y., Huang, L., Chen, Y., Peng, S., Ke, Z., Li.,W. 2021. Deep learning-based six-type classifier for lung cancer and mimics from histopathological whole slide images: a retrospective study. *BMC Medicine*. 19(80). https://doi.org/10.1186/s12916-021-01953-2

Zheng, Z., Webb, G. I. 2000. Lazy learning of Bayesian rules. *Machine Learning*, 41: 53–84. https://doi.org/10.1023/A:1007613203719

Zhenlong, L., Qingzhou, Z., Xiaohua, Z. 2017. Performance analysis of K-Nearest neighbor, support vector machine, and artificial neural network classifiers for driver drowsiness detection with different road geometries. *International Journal of Distributed Sensor Systems*, 13(9): 1–12. https://doi.org/10.1177/1550147717733391

Zoabi, Y., Deri-Rozov, S., Shomron, N. 2021. Machine learning-based prediction of COVID-19 diagnosis based on symptoms. *npj Digital Medicine*, 4(3): 1–5. https://doi.org/10.1038/s41746-020-00372-6

7 Hybrid Marine Predator Algorithm with Simulated Annealing for Feature Selection

Utkarsh Mahadeo Khaire, R. Dhanalakshmi, and K. Balakrishnan

CONTENTS

DOI: 10.1201/9781003226147-7

7.1 INTRODUCTION

This section presents the rigorous overview of feature selection (FS), the meta-heuristic (MH) algorithm, motivation, contributions, and organization of the research work.

7.1.1 FEATURE SELECTION

The large volume of data and high dimensionality harms classification accuracy and computational cost. In general, an irrelevant, irredundant, or missing value reduces the predictive model's accuracy. Typically, most microarray datasets have over 60,000 features or attributes with fewer samples. This high dimensionality of the microarray dataset hinders the diagnosis, prognosis, and treatment of life-threatening diseases (Patra et al. 2021). Extracting a significant component from a microarray dataset for optimal results has been a bottleneck for many data science researchers. FS is a crucial pre-processing technique for dealing with high-dimensional problems and improving accuracy. The general procedure of selecting significant features is given in Algorithm 7.1. A valid search procedure is used to generate a subset from the microarray dataset in the first step. The second step evaluates the subsets' list and compares the optimal subset with the antecedent subset; the newly updated subset is highly recommended over the older one, implying that it will restore the existing one. The procedure repeats until the end of maximum iterations. Finally, the best subset score is chosen and used in the following classification technique.

Algorithm 7.1: Selecting Feature Subset

> **Step 1:** Starts with subset generation
> **Step 2:** Subset evaluation
> **Step 3:** Stopping condition
> **Step 4:** Validating the feature subset
> - **If** requirement satisfies, test n number of times
> - Select the best feature set
> - **Else** repeat Steps 2 and 3
> **Step 5:** End process

7.1.2 FEATURE SELECTION TECHNIQUES

In general, FS techniques are classified into three parts: filter, wrapper, and embedded. Figure 7.1 depicts the taxonomy of feature selection techniques. The filter method uses statistical measures like information gain (IG) (Lei 2012), Pearson correlation (PC) (Sundarrajan and Arumugam 2016), and relief (Urbanowicz et al. 2018) to evaluate the selected features. In contrast, the wrapper method uses a standard learning algorithm like particle swarm optimization (PSO) (Eberhart and Kennedy 1995), genetic algorithm (GA) (Nag and Pal 2016), and whale optimization algorithm (WOA) (Mirjalili and Lewis 2016). Wrapper methods usually produce the best results because they use the learning algorithm, but they are more computationally demanding than the filter approach. In this case, embedded practices incorporate both filter and wrapper methods to reduce the computational complexity in the model building phase. The well-known embedded methods are LASSO (Muthukrishnan and Rohini 2017) and ridge regression (Paul and Drineas 2016). Embedded methods are less

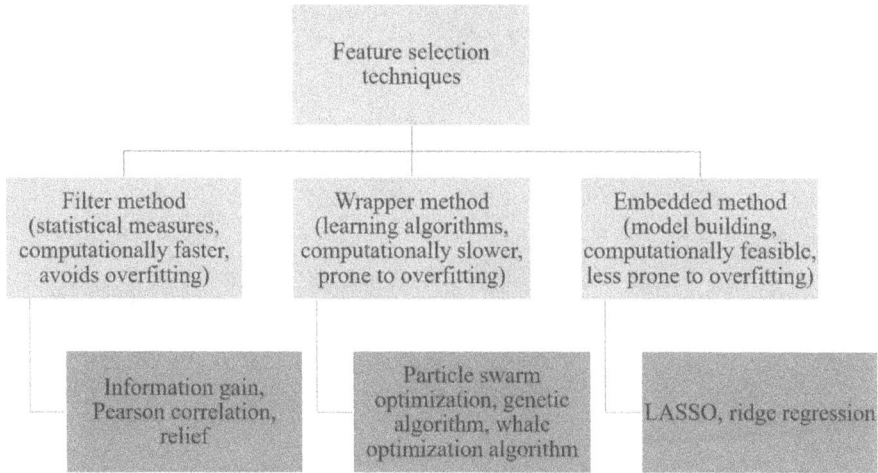

FIGURE 7.1 Taxonomy of feature selection techniques.

prone to overfitting. The diversity of the search space in nature is very high, but it is limited. When compared to random search, MH algorithms outperform random search because each iteration yields more than one solution.

7.1.3 META-HEURISTIC ALGORITHMS

The critical feature of MH algorithms is their impressive ability to prevent algorithms from converging prematurely. Since algorithms are stochastic, MH operates as a black box, avoiding local optima, and rapidly and effortlessly exploring the search space. The balancing factor between exploration and exploitation must be satisfied to achieve the optimal solution in MH algorithms. Population-based MH algorithms are classified into four types: evolutionary-based (EA), swarm-based (SA), physics-based (PA), and human-based (HA) algorithms (Balakrishnan, Dhanalakshmi, and Khaire 2021). Population-based MH launches their optimization process by generating initial random solutions. Figure 7.2 shows the cataloging of MH algorithms.

- **Evolutionary algorithm**: EA focuses on genetic variation, mutation, and natural selection in evolutionary processes. GA and differential evolution (DE) (Hancer 2018) are some prevalent algorithms in EA.
- **Physics-based algorithms**: PA imitates the characteristics of physical forces such as gravity, friction, and electromagnetic energy. Harmony Search (HS) (Diao and Shen 2012) and SA (Stochino and Gayarre 2019) are the most prominent algorithm in PA.
- **Swarm-based algorithms**: The social behaviors of animals influence SA. PSO, ant colony optimization (ACO), grey wolf optimization (GWO), and WOA are notable examples of SA.
- **Human-based algorithms**: Human psychological behaviors motivate HA. Firework algorithm (Zheng et al. 2015) and mine blast algorithm (Sadollah et al. 2012) are standard algorithms of this category.

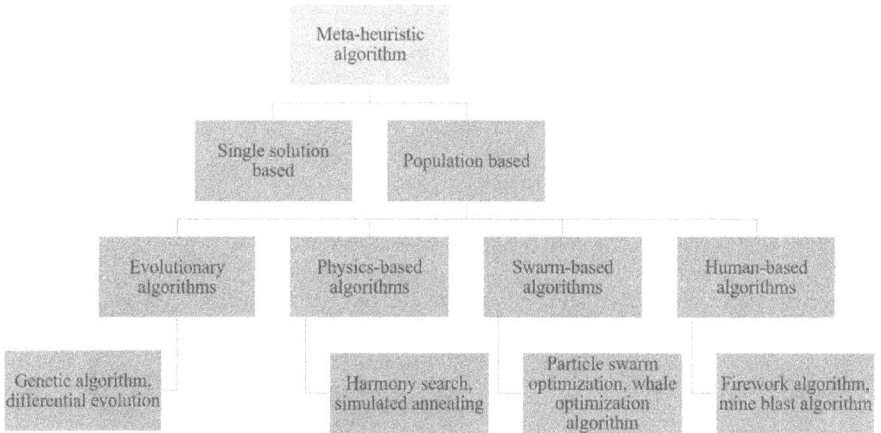

FIGURE 7.2 Classification of MH algorithms.

7.1.4 MOTIVATION

Over the years, MH algorithms have earned an unrivaled reputation in the fields of rigorous problem solving and optimization. However, MH algorithms have their own set of benefits and drawbacks when it comes to solving different problems. Balancing the nature between exploration and exploitation evaluates the performance of the MH algorithm. The researchers favor the hybridization of one or more MH algorithms to improve exploration and extraction capabilities. The No Free Lunch (NFL) rule suggests that when all solutions in a class are added together, the contribution of each solution method is the same. No matter how much the outcomes of various algorithms differ from one another, they're all similar. MPA is a nature-inspired, swarm-based MH algorithm proposed Faramarzi et al. (2020) based on the survival of the fittest theory. The standard MPA outperforms other MH techniques in many engineering applications but fails to satisfy the local optima. In the paper, a hybrid approach of the MPA and SA is proposed to improve the intensification and diversification of conventional MPA. The iMPA effectively improves the predictive model's search capability and avoids the local minima stagnation. The SA technique is used to speed up the search space exploration. The foraging technique, also known as Levy and Brownian movements, deals with predator–prey biological interactions.

7.1.5 CONTRIBUTIONS

The following are the critical contributions made in this work:

- Devised a hybrid approach by combining MPA and SA to augment the exploration, exploitation, and prevent local optima stagnation.
- The predictive ability is evaluated in terms of converging power, selected features, and accuracy.
- The proposed model is validated using three well-known, high-dimensional datasets.

- The proposed model evaluates the selection subset using a k-nearest neighbors (KNN) classifier based on various performance measures such as precision, recall, and F1-score.

7.1.6 ORGANIZATION OF PAPER

The following is a summary of this chapter: Section 7.2 presents a comprehensive overview of related work. Sections 7.3 and 7.4 present preliminaries of standard MPA and SA. Section 7.5 deals with the detailed description of the datasets used in this chapter and the implementation of the proposed iMPA. Simulation outcomes are discussed in Section 7.6, and the conclusion and the future direction of the research work are provided in Section 7.7.

7.2 RELATED WORK

Latest studies show that hybrid algorithms provide superior performance to different problems such as healthcare (Sharma et al. 2020; Pattnayak 2021), medical applications (Thaiyalnayaki 2021), Internet of Things (Jindal, Gupta, and Bhushan 2019), Internet of Health Things (Khamparia et al. 2020), biomedical text processing and food industry (Paramesha, Gururaj, and Jena 2021), feature selection, and other engineering applications. For FS problems, Oh et al. (2004) suggested the first hybrid optimization, a combination of local search and GA. In this method, local search operations with ripple variables are created and incorporated into the hybrid-GAs. The proposed model also shows superior performance in time complexity than the conventional GA. Vasant et al. (2010) offered a hybrid version for global optimization that combines the SA and GA approaches to solve industrial production management problems. The SA is used to enhance the exploitation behavior in the global search space. In terms of computing time and convergence ability, the proposed methods demonstrate significant enhancements. Wu and Lu (2012) suggested a hybrid version of GA and SA, including kernel optimization. They have used Linear, Poly, and Radial Basis Function (RBF), three related kernel functions. The methodology is used to improve GA's local search capability and premature convergence. Abdel-Basset et al. (2021) proposed a hybrid variant of Harris hawks optimization (HHO) based on bitwise and SA to solve the FS problem. Two bitwise operators are used to migrate the best solution to the update stage. The prosed model is evaluated using the KNN with Euclidean distance metric with 24 benchmark datasets and 19 artificial datasets.

In another work, Elgamal et al. (2020) proposed an improved version of HHO that employs SA to solve FS problems, particularly in the medical field. The algorithm offers two enhancements; first, using chaotic maps to enhance the population diversity. Second, solving the problem of local optima issue using SA. Mafarja and Mirjalili (2017) proposed a hybrid version of WOA using SA for FS problems. SA aims to improve exploitation by searching for the most promising regions identified by the WOA algorithm. In other research, Gao et al. (2020) suggested binary equilibrium optimization combined with SA for feature selection problems. Continuous values generated in EO are transformed into a binary using a v-shaped transfer function. The

well-known local search technique (SA) is used to boost the exploitation of the proposed model. The suggested FS system is validated using 18 well-known UCI datasets.

Cui et al. (2020) proposed a hybrid variant of the improved dragonfly algorithm
combined with Maximum Relevance-Minimum Redundancy (mRMR). First, the
model has three enhancement features with a low weight having a slight chance of
being picked into a candidate subset with a small probability of mRMR generating a
promising subset. Second, to balance global and local capacity, dynamic swarming
variables are suggested. Finally, the position updating function incorporates quan-
tum local optimum and global optimum. Abdollahzadeh and Gharehchopogh (2021)
proposed a novel hybridized version of HHO and fruit fly optimization algorithms
for FS problems. The author has presented three different multi-objective feature
selection framework algorithms based on evolutionary algorithms. Al-Tashi et al.
(2019) suggested a modern hybrid optimization algorithm that takes advantage of
GWO and PSO's capabilities. The KNN classifier with Euclidean separation matrices is used as a wrapper-based approach to finding the best solutions.

To address the shortcomings of FS, Faris et al. (2018) suggested an improved
version of SSA. They have created a wrapper FS using SSA as a search technique
in the proposed approach. In addition to the transformation features, the crossover
operator replaces the average operator and boosts the system's exploration behavior.
Zhang et al. (2018) suggested a combination of biogeography-based optimization
(BBO) and GWO to balance the learning model's exploration and exploitation. The
differential mutation and multi-migration operators, and the opposition-based learning approach in BBO and GWO, respectively, are used to increase performance. The
suggested model effectively outperforms all single-objective and clustering optimization benchmark functions. Zheng et al. (2019) proposed a hybrid model named
maximum Pearson maximum distance improved WOA for FS problems.

7.3 MARINE PREDATORS ALGORITHM

The MPA is a population-based MH optimization strategy made up of three distinct
optimization situations:

- **Case 1:** $V \geq 10$ implies that the predators are not in a position to move.
- **Case 2:** When $V \approx 1$, predator and prey move according to Brownian and
  Lévy movements, respectively.
- **Case 3:** $V = 0.1$ implies the movement of the predators based on the Lévy
  flight.

Environmental factors such as eddy formation or fish aggregating devices (FADs)
alter predators' behavior to locate potential prey areas. Marine memory is used to
recognize where they previously found food, which helps update the design space.

7.3.1 MPA FORMULATION

The MH algorithms distribute the initial population uniformly across the search
space. In the first iteration, the top predator searches for the prey and restructures the

Elite matrix when the top predator replaces a better predator. Predators reorganized their positions based on the **Prey matrix**. This optimization method focuses on the entire process of locating the best predators using these two matrix values.

$$Y_o = Y_{min} + rand\left(Y_{max} - Y_{min}\right) \tag{7.1}$$

Constructing an Elite matrix determines the top predators' fitness that contains information about the position of the prey. Equation 7.2 depicts the formation of the Elite matrix.

$$Elite = \begin{bmatrix} Y_{1,1} & \cdots & Y_{1,d} \\ \vdots & \ddots & \vdots \\ Y_{n,1} & \cdots & Y_{n,d} \end{bmatrix}_{n*d} \tag{7.2}$$

Where Y_1 indicates the top predator. Equation 7.3 represents the Prey matrix.

$$Prey = \begin{bmatrix} Y_{1,1} & \cdots & Y_{1,d} \\ \vdots & \ddots & \vdots \\ Y_{n,1} & \cdots & Y_{n,d} \end{bmatrix}_{n \times d} \tag{7.3}$$

7.3.2   MPA Optimization Scenarios

This section contains an in-depth discussion of the three phases of MPA.

7.3.2.1   High-velocity Ratio or Prey Is Moving Faster than Predators

No activities can be seen in the predator when velocity V is greater than 10. Equation 7.4 depicts the mathematical model for high velocity.

While $iter < \dfrac{1}{3} Max\_iter$

$$\overrightarrow{Stepsize_i} = \overrightarrow{R_B} \otimes \left(\overrightarrow{Elite_i} - \overrightarrow{R_B} \otimes \overrightarrow{Prey_i}\right) \quad i = 1,\dots n$$
$$\overrightarrow{Prey_i} = \overrightarrow{Prey_i} + P.\,\overrightarrow{R} \otimes \overrightarrow{Stepsize_i} \tag{7.4}$$

Where R_B is the Brownian movement. $\otimes$ Represents the element-wise multiplication of two vectors. The element-wise multiplication of R_B with prey calculates the next position of the target.

7.3.2.2   Unit Velocity Ratio or Prey and Predators Moving at the Same Speed

Exploration and exploitation are essential when prey and predator are looking for the target simultaneously because, sometimes, the target can also act as potential predators. According to this scenario, half of the population is dedicated to exploitation (prey), while the other half is dedicated to exploration (predators). When the unit velocity V equals one, the target moves according to Lévy, whereas the predator moves according to Brownian motion.

While $\frac{1}{3} Max\_iter < iter < \frac{2}{3} Max\_iter$

Lévy/Exploitation

$$\overrightarrow{Stepsize_i} = \overrightarrow{R_L} \otimes \left(\overrightarrow{Elite_i} - \overrightarrow{R_L} \otimes \overrightarrow{Prey_i} \right) \quad i = 1, \ldots n/2$$
$$\overrightarrow{Prey_i} = \overrightarrow{Prey_i} + P. \overrightarrow{R} \otimes \overrightarrow{Stepsize_i} \tag{7.5}$$

Where R_L is Lévy's movements. The element-wise multiplication of $\vec{R}_L$ and prey mimics the prey movements based on the Lévy movement strategy.

Brownian/Exploration

$$\overrightarrow{Stepsize_i} = \overrightarrow{R_B} \otimes \left(\overrightarrow{R_B} \otimes \overrightarrow{Elite_i} - \overrightarrow{Prey_i} \right) \quad i = n/2, \ldots n$$
$$\overrightarrow{Prey_i} = \overrightarrow{Elite_i} + P.CF \otimes \overrightarrow{Stepsize_i}$$
$$CF = \left(1 - \frac{t}{Max\_iter} \right)^{\left(\frac{2*t}{Max\_iter} \right)} \tag{7.6}$$

7.3.2.3 Low-velocity Ratio or Predators Moving Faster than Prey

The final stage addresses the high exploitation potential.

While $iter < \frac{2}{3} Max\_iter$

$$\overrightarrow{Stepsize_i} = \overrightarrow{R_L} \otimes \left(\overrightarrow{R_L} \otimes \overrightarrow{Elite_i} - \overrightarrow{Prey_i} \right) \quad i = 1, \ldots n$$
$$\overrightarrow{Prey_i} = \overrightarrow{Elite_i} + P. CF \otimes \overrightarrow{Stepsize_i} \tag{7.7}$$

According to the study, predators do not move in the first phase when the velocity is more significant than ten. In the second phase, predators update their position using Brownian motion when the speed equals one. The third phase is where predators move using the Lévy motion.

7.3.3 Eddy Formation or FAD's Effect

As a result of behavioral changes in the MPA, significant problems such as eddy formation or FAD effect can observe. The FAD's products are used to determine the impact of search space falling to local optima. This effect is mathematically derived as follows:

$$\overrightarrow{Prey_i} = \begin{cases} \overrightarrow{Prey_i} + CF \left[\overrightarrow{Y_{min}} + \vec{R} \otimes \left(\overrightarrow{Y_{max}} - \overrightarrow{Y_{min}} \right) \right] \otimes \vec{U} & r \leq FADs \\ \\ \overrightarrow{Prey_i} + \left[FADs\,(1-r)+r \right] * \left(\overrightarrow{Prey_{r1}} - \overrightarrow{Prey_{r2}} \right) & r > FADs \end{cases} \tag{7.8}$$

Where initially, the 0.2 value of FADs represents the effects of FADs on the optimization process. *r1* and *r2* subscript of the prey indicates the random index of the Prey matrix.

7.3.4 MARINE MEMORY

The MPA foraging process is handled by recalling where the predators previously found food using their memories. The elite matrix is revised after the fitness of the matrix is determined, taking into account the impact of prey updates and the use of FADs. The fitness evaluation is completed by comparing the current iteration to the previous iteration; the updated one is replaced when it is better than the previous one.

7.4 SIMULATED ANNEALING

SA is a well-known single-solution MH algorithm based on Kirkpatrick's hill-climbing method proposed in 1983. SA employs a certain probability of accepting a wrong "move" at each iteration to avoid local stagnation of the optimal solutions. This algorithm, like other MH algorithms, generates the initial key at random during each iteration. Based on the fitness function, the current solution is compared to the neighbor solution. If the adjacent solution is better, the present solution is replaced. The Boltzmann probability function $P = e^{-\theta T}$ determines the probability of selecting a worse solution.

7.5 IMPROVED MARINE PREDATORS ALGORITHM

This section includes a brief overview of the datasets used in the study and the model's implementation. Python is used to implement the proposed algorithm.

7.5.1 DATASET

The proposed model's effectiveness is evaluated using three publicly available high-dimensional microarray datasets. The data for this study is obtained from http://csse. szu.edu.cn/staff/zhuzx/Datasets.html (Khaire and Dhanalakshmi 2020). All three datasets used in this study have two classes in the target variables. Table 7.1 provides a detailed overview of the dataset used in the study.

TABLE 7.1
Overview of the Dataset

Dataset	Number of Features	Number of Samples
Central Nervous System (CNS)	7129	60
Colon Cancer	2000	60
Leukemia	7129	72

7.5.2 IMPLEMENTATION

This section goes over the steps involved in the proposed method. The SMOTE-Tomek algorithm has been used to balance the input data. The Gaussian distribution is used to generate the initial population of random search agents during initialization. Equation 7.3 shows the random population matrix. Figure 7.3 depicts a flowchart of the proposed iMPA.

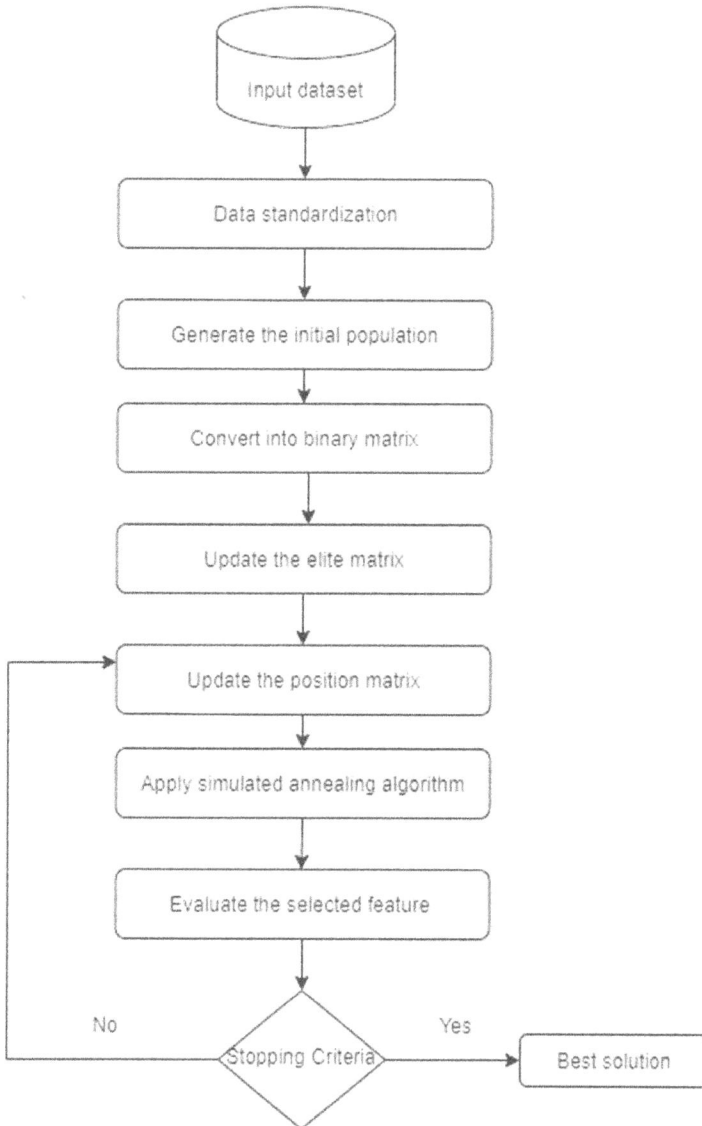

FIGURE 7.3   Flowchart of the proposed iMPA.

For classification, the proposed model employs the sigmoid function. The following equation is used to convert the continuous values of the random search agents to binary values [1 – selected, 0 – not selected].

$$Y_{i,j} = \begin{cases} 1 \text{ if } \dfrac{1}{1+e^{-y_{i,j}}} \geq 0.95 \\ 0 \text{ otherwise} \end{cases} \tag{7.9}$$

Each random search agent's fitness is determined using a standard ML classifier. Equation 7.10 is used to assess the fitness of each predator in the position matrix.

$$fitness(Y_i) = \beta * Err_{x_i} + (1-\beta) * \left(\dfrac{|Y_i|}{n} \right) \tag{7.10}$$

Where β is an arbitrary number in the range of [0, 1]. Then, on each iteration, run the SA algorithm. The proposed model employs a KNN classifier to evaluate the selected subset.

7.6   RESULTS AND DISCUSSION

Equation 7.10 is used to calculate the fitness value of the proposed function in the convergence curve. The algorithm efficiently converges to global minima with larger step sizes during iterations. Figure 7.4 depicts the converging ability of the three microarray cancer datasets. The convergence curve of the proposed approach has been recorded for 20 epochs. The proposed iMPA effectively converges the predictive model to the global minima with significant improvement. Compared to CNS and colon cancer, the proposed iMPA shows better converging outcomes in leukemia. While converging, the model does not show the traces of stagnation in the local minima.

As the model progresses, the proposed model's training and testing accuracy improves to the maximum. For anonymous data, the proposed model yields promising accuracy values. At the end of the 20th epoch, the proposed algorithm had a negligible variance between training and testing accuracy, as shown in Figure 7.5. In CNS, we can observe the more significant difference between train and test accuracy till the 15th epoch. However, in the further iteration proposed approach successfully reduce the gap. For Colon Cancer and Leukemia, the proposed iMPA effectively yields accuracy in the range of [0.82, 1.0], indicating that the proposed model can address the overfitting-underfitting problem in traditional machine learning strategies by effortlessly addressing the bias-variance trade-off.

Figure 7.6 depicts the proposed model's ROC curve. The higher AUC value for datasets indicates that the proposed method can assign a higher probability to a randomly selected real positive sample than a negative sample on average. We iterate the proposed model for 20 epochs and select the top ten features from the initial input dataset based on feature weights and frequency. The KNN classifier is used to validate the selection of parts. The characteristics chosen are

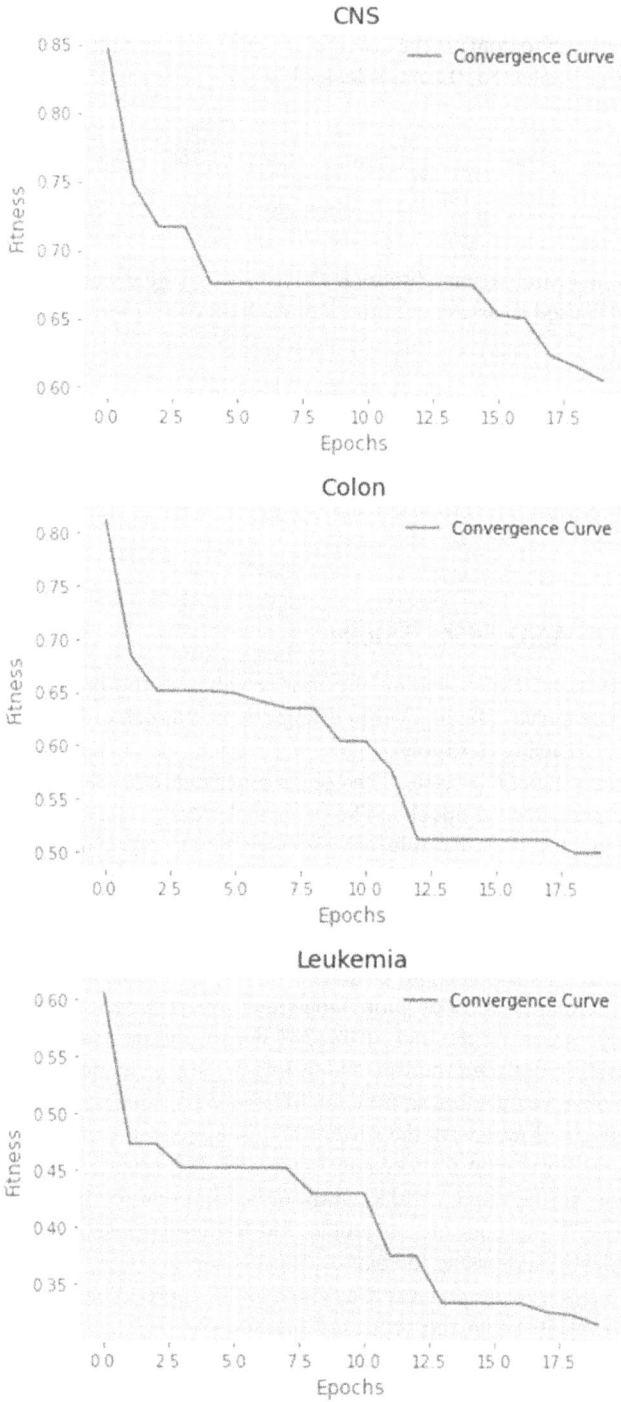

FIGURE 7.4 Convergence curves.

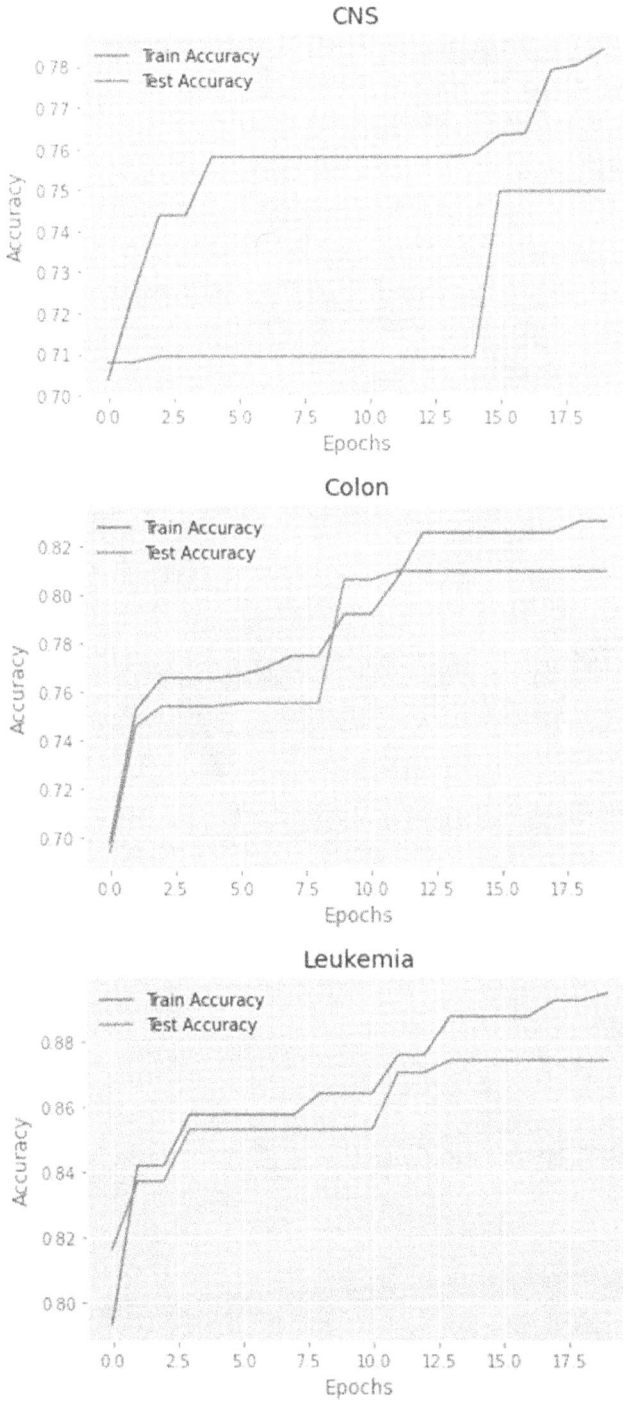

FIGURE 7.5 Training and test accuracy.

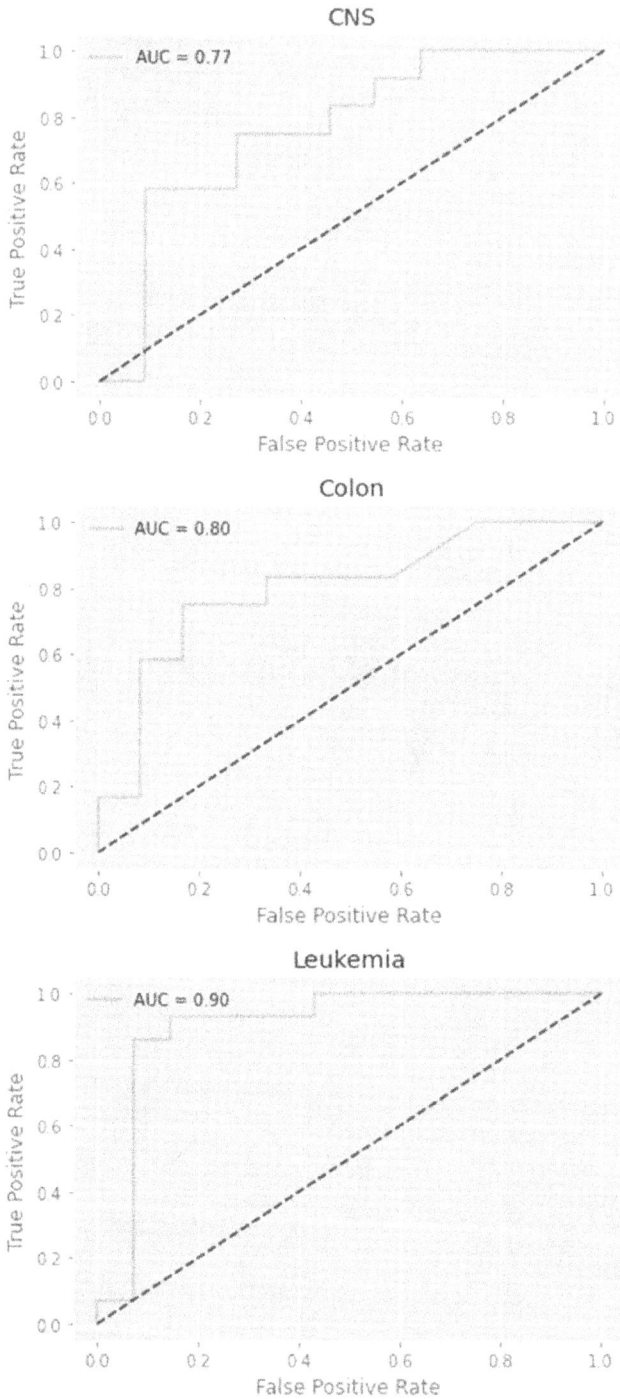

FIGURE 7.6   ROC-AUC curves.

TABLE 7.2

Validation of Features Selected by iMPA

Dataset	Class	Precision	Recall	F1-score	Accuracy
CNS	0	0.55	0.90	0.69	0.61
	1	0.80	0.33	0.47	
Colon	0	0.80	0.67	0.73	0.75
	1	0.71	0.83	0.77	
Leukemia	0	0.81	0.93	0.87	0.86
	1	0.92	0.78	0.85	

the most important predictors of lethal cancer. The higher ROC-AUC curve of the proposed model shows that the features selected by it can provide significant confidence in knowledge discovery and decision making. Moreover, a reduced set of selected features can yield more accurate results than overall features present in the input data.

Tables 7.2 and 7.3 summarize and compare the performance analysis of the predictive models for the selected feature subsets to validate the feature subsets. The predictive model's accuracy, precision, recall, and F1-score measures are used to validate essential features. The comparative analysis of the selected features indicates that the features carefully chosen by the proposed iMPA provide higher confidence and classify the unseen test sample with higher precision. The proposed iMPA outperforms conventional MPA in terms of selecting features and their accuracy.

Tables 7.4 and 7.5 contain a detailed description of the selected features. Both tables include the count of features selected throughout 20 epochs. Comparative analysis of both tables indicates that the proposed iMPA select important features with higher stability, whereas conventional MPA appoints elements with higher deviation. Except for the first features for all datasets, features selected by MPA have a count of less than five. On the other hand, the proposed iMPA picks standard features in every iteration; therefore, it has more stability in selecting the elements.

TABLE 7.3

Validation of Features Selected by Conventional MPA

Dataset	Class	Precision	Recall	F1-score	Accuracy
CNS	0	0.47	0.68	0.55583	0.58
	1	0.75	0.51	0.60714	
Colon	0	0.65	0.54	0.58992	0.68
	1	0.68	0.71	0.69468	
Leukemia	0	0.72	0.78	0.7488	0.75
	1	0.83	0.69	0.75355	

TABLE 7.4

Selected Features by Conventional MPA

CNS		Colon		Leukemia	
Genes	Count	Genes	Count	Genes	Count
z26317_at	13	t51539	17	u29175_at	18
u46746_s_at	5	y00345	13	d42040_s_at	7
k03189_f_at	4	r96070	4	u26173_s_at	4
ab000905_at	3	x67699	4	x16699_at	3
u36621_cds2_at	3	h79136	4	m71243_f_at	3
m23575_f_at	3	control.11	3	j00148_cds2_f_at	3
j04988_at	3	m26383	3	z50853_at	3
x54667_s_at	2	h16991	3	hg1877-ht1917_s_at	2
x79200_s_at	2	d16431	3	m37457_s_at	2
d87002_cds2_at	2	v00520	3	u18550_at	2

TABLE 7.5

Selected Features by Proposed iMPA

CNS		Colon		Leukemia	
Genes	Count	Genes	Count	Genes	Count
hg2714-ht2810_at	17	m86934	20	x02530_at	19
ab000905_at	14	h72965	20	z19002_at	19
u31449_at	14	x82166	19	hg511-ht511_at	19
u31799_at	14	t55117	19	hg4310-ht4580_at	18
u03187_at	13	m55268	19	hg4263-ht4533_at	16
x52003_at	13	r53455	18	d13666_s_at	16
y10141_s_at	13	t72403	18	u90546_r_at	14
u33054_at	13	u12134	17	x02419_rna1_s_at	14
d87002_cds2_at	13	l26405.1	15	j03060_at	14
m68907_s_at	12	t64941	13	l41390_at	11

7.7 CONCLUSION AND FUTURE SCOPE

This chapter proposed an improved version of MPA (iMPA) using hybridization of SA and MPA for feature selection problems in biotechnology. The proposed iMPA searches the global search space efficiently and converges to global optima within specified epochs. iMPA optimizes the parameters of the sigmoid function for the collection of specific cancer-causing features. The proposed model avoids local minima stagnation. The computational complexity of the KNN classifier is reduced by employing the top ten features selected based on their frequency of occurrence in the input data. This chapter has used various performance measures such as precision, recall, F1-score, and ROC-AUC curve to validate the set of significant features. The proposed iMPA outperforms conventional MPA in terms of all performance metrics. Thus, it is understood that the proposed method is better than the existing FS techniques. The proposed algorithm can be implemented for multi-objective optimization using machine learning, and a deep learning environment will be a part of future work. In addition to that, it could be interesting to see how well the suggested iMPA algorithm performs on more complicated scientific and engineering issues, and to increase its complexity without impacting its existing performance.

ACKNOWLEDGMENT

This research is funded by the Department of Science and Technology, Government of India, under the Interdisciplinary Cyber-Physical Systems (ICPS) scheme (Grant no. T-54).

REFERENCES

Abdel-Basset, Mohamed, Weiping Ding, and Doaa El-Shahat. 2021. "A Hybrid Harris Hawks Optimization Algorithm with Simulated Annealing for Feature Selection." *Artificial Intelligence Review* 54 (1): 593–637. https://doi.org/10.1007/s10462-020-09860-3

Abdollahzadeh, Benyamin, and Farhad Soleimanian Gharehchopogh. 2021. "A Multi-Objective Optimization Algorithm for Feature Selection Problems." *Engineering with Computers*. https://doi.org/10.1007/s00366-021-01369-9

Al-Tashi, Qasem, Said Jadid Abdul Kadir, Helmi Md Rais, Seyedali Mirjalili, and Hitham Alhussian. 2019. "Binary Optimization Using Hybrid Grey Wolf Optimization for Feature Selection." *IEEE Access* 7: 39496–508. https://doi.org/10.1109/ACCESS.2019.2906757

Balakrishnan, K., R. Dhanalakshmi, and Utkarsh Mahadeo Khaire. 2021. "Improved Salp Swarm Algorithm Based on the Levy Flight for Feature Selection." *Journal of Supercomputing*. https://doi.org/10.1007/s11227-021-03773-w

Cui, Xueting, Ying Li, Jiahao Fan, Tan Wang, and Yuefeng Zheng. 2020. "A Hybrid Improved Dragonfly Algorithm for Feature Selection." *IEEE Access* 8: 155619–29. https://doi.org/10.1109/ACCESS.2020.3012838

Diao, Ren, and Qiang Shen. 2012. "Feature Selection with Harmony Search." *IEEE Transactions on Systems, Man, and Cybernetics, Part B: Cybernetics* 42 (6): 1509–23. https://doi.org/10.1109/TSMCB.2012.2193613

Eberhart, Russell, and James Kennedy. 1995. "New Optimizer Using Particle Swarm Theory." In *Proceedings of the International Symposium on Micro Machine and Human Science*, 39–43. https://doi.org/10.1109/mhs.1995.494215

Elgamal, Zenab Mohamed, Norizan Binti Mohd Yasin, Mohammad Tubishat, Mohammed Alswaitti, and Seyedali Mirjalili. 2020. "An Improved Harris Hawks Optimization Algorithm with Simulated Annealing for Feature Selection in the Medical Field." *IEEE Access* 8: 186638–52. https://doi.org/10.1109/ACCESS.2020.3029728

Faramarzi, Afshin, Mohammad Heidarinejad, Seyedali Mirjalili, and Amir H. Gandomi. 2020. "Marine Predators Algorithm: A Nature-Inspired Metaheuristic." *Expert Systems with Applications* 152 (August): 113377. https://doi.org/10.1016/j.eswa.2020.113377

Faris, Hossam, Majdi M. Mafarja, Ali Asghar Heidari, Ibrahim Aljarah, Ala' M. Al-Zoubi, Seyedali Mirjalili, and Hamido Fujita. 2018. "An Efficient Binary Salp Swarm Algorithm with Crossover Scheme for Feature Selection Problems." *Knowledge-Based Systems* 154: 43–67. https://doi.org/10.1016/j.knosys.2018.05.009

Gao, Yuanyuan, Yongquan Zhou, and Qifang Luo. 2020. "An Efficient Binary Equilibrium Optimizer Algorithm for Feature Selection." *IEEE Access* 8: 140936–63. https://doi.org/10.1109/ACCESS.2020.3013617

Hancer, Emrah. 2018. "Differential Evolution for Feature Selection : A Fuzzy Wrapper – Filter Approach." *Soft Computing* 23 (13): 5233–48. https://doi.org/10.1007/s00500-018-3545-7

Jindal, Mansi, Jatin Gupta, and Bharat Bhushan. 2019. "Machine Learning Methods for IoT and Their Future Applications." In *Proceedings - 2019 International Conference on Computing, Communication, and Intelligent Systems, ICCCIS 2019*, 430–34. https://doi.org/10.1109/ICCCIS48478.2019.8974551

Paramesha, K., H.L. Gururaj, and Om Prakash Jena. 2021. "Applications of Machine Learning in Biomedical Text Processing and Food Industry." In *Machine Learning for Healthcare Applications*, edited by Sachi Nandan Mohanty, G. Nalinipriya, Om Prakash Jena, and Achyuth Sarkar. Hoboken: Scrivener Publisher-Wiley. https://doi.org/10.1002/9781119792611.ch10

Khaire, Utkarsh Mahadeo, and R. Dhanalakshmi. 2020. "High-Dimensional Microarray Dataset Classification Using an Improved Adam Optimizer (IAdam)." *Journal of Ambient Intelligence and Humanized Computing* 11: 5187–5204. https://doi.org/10.1007/s12652-020-01832-3

Khamparia, Aditya, Prakash Kumar Singh, Poonam Rani, Debabrata Samanta, Ashish Khanna, and Bharat Bhushan. 2020. "An Internet of Health Things-Driven Deep Learning Framework for Detection and Classification of Skin Cancer Using Transfer Learning." *Transactions on Emerging Telecommunications Technologies* 32(7): e3963. https://doi.org/10.1002/ett.3963

Lei, Shang. 2012. "A Feature Selection Method Based on Information Gain and Genetic Algorithm." In *Proceedings - 2012 International Conference on Computer Science and Electronics Engineering, ICCSEE 2012*, 355–58. https://doi.org/10.1109/ICCSEE.2012.97

Mafarja, Majdi M, and Seyedali Mirjalili. 2017. "Hybrid Whale Optimization Algorithm with Simulated Annealing for Feature Selection." *Neurocomputing* 260: 302–12. https://doi.org/10.1016/j.neucom.2017.04.053

Mirjalili, Seyedali, and Andrew Lewis. 2016. "The Whale Optimization Algorithm." *Advances in Engineering Software* 95 (May): 51–67. https://doi.org/10.1016/j.advengsoft.2016.01.008

Muthukrishnan, R., and R. Rohini. 2017. "LASSO: A Feature Selection Technique in Predictive Modeling for Machine Learning." In *2016 IEEE International Conference on Advances in Computer Applications, ICACA 2016*, 18–20. https://doi.org/10.1109/ICACA.2016.7887916

Nag, Kaustuv, and Nikhil R. Pal. 2016. "A Multiobjective Genetic Programming-Based Ensemble for Simultaneous Feature Selection and Classification." *IEEE Transactions on Cybernetics* 46 (2): 499–510. https://doi.org/10.1109/TCYB.2015.2404806

Niranjan Panigrahi, Ishan Ayus, and Om Prakash Jena. 2021. "An Expert System-Based Clinical Decision Support System for Hepatitis-B Prediction & Diagnosis." In *Machine Learning for Healthcare Applications*, edited by Sachi Nandan Mohanty, G. Nalinipriya, Om Prakash Jena, and Achyuth Sarkar. Hoboken: Scrivener Publisher-Wiley. https://doi.org/10.1002/9781119792611.ch4

Oh, Il Seok, Jin Seon Lee, and Byung Ro Moon. 2004. "Hybrid Genetic Algorithms for Feature Selection." *IEEE Transactions on Pattern Analysis and Machine Intelligence* 26 (11): 1424–37. https://doi.org/10.1109/TPAMI.2004.105

Pattnayak, Parthasarathi, and Om Prakash Jena. 2021. "Innovation on Machine Learning in Healthcare Services–An Introduction." In *Machine Learning for Healthcare Applications*, edited by Sachi Nandan Mohanty, G. Nalinipriya, Om Prakash Jena, and Achyuth Sarkar. USA: Scrivener Publisher-Wiley. https://doi.org/10.1002/9781119792611.ch1

Paul, Saurabh, and Petros Drineas. 2016. "Feature Selection for Ridge Regression with Provable Guarantees." *Neural Computation* 28(4): 716–42. https://doi.org/10.1162/NECO_a_00816

Sadollah, Ali, Ardeshir Bahreininejad, Hadi Eskandar, and Mohd Hamdi. 2012. "Mine Blast Algorithm for Optimization of Truss Structures with Discrete Variables." *Computers and Structures* 102: 49–63. https://doi.org/10.1016/j.compstruc.2012.03.013

Sharma, Nikhil, Ila Kaushik, Bharat Bhushan, Siddharth Gautam, and Aditya Khamparia. 2020. "Applicability of WSN and Biometric Models in the Field of Healthcare." *Deep Learning Strategies for Security Enhancement in Wireless Sensor Networks*, 304–29. https://doi.org/10.4018/978-1-7998-5068-7.ch016

Stochino, Flavio, and Fernando Lopez Gayarre. 2019. "Reinforced Concrete Slab Optimization with Simulated Annealing." *Applied Sciences (Switzerland)* 9 (15). https://doi.org/10.3390/app9153161

Patra, Sudhansu Shekhar, Om Praksah Jena, Gaurav Kumar, Sreyashi Pramanik, Chinmaya Misra, and Kamakhya Narain Singh. 2021. "Random Forest Algorithm in Imbalance Genomics Classification." In *Data Analytics in Bioinformatics: A Machine Learning Perspective*, edited by Xiaobo Zhang, Rabinarayan Satpathy, Tanupriya Choudhury, Suneeta Satpathy, and Sachi Nandan Mohanty. River Street, Hoboken: Wiley. https://doi.org/10.1002/9781119785620.ch7

Sundarrajan, Sudharsana, and Mohanapriya Arumugam. 2016. "Weighted Gene Co-Expression Based Biomarker Discovery for Psoriasis Detection List of Abbreviations." *Gene* 593 (1): 225–34. https://doi.org/10.1016/j.gene.2016.08.021

Thaiyalnayaki, K. 2021. "Classification of Diabetes Using Deep Learning and Svm Techniques." *International Journal of Current Research and Review* 13 (1): 146–49. https://doi.org/10.31782/IJCRR.2021.13127

Urbanowicz, Ryan J., Melissa Meeker, William La Cava, Randal S. Olson, and Jason H. Moore. 2018. "Relief-Based Feature Selection: Introduction and Review." *Journal of Biomedical Informatics* 85: 189–203. https://doi.org/10.1016/j.jbi.2018.07.014

Vasant, Pandian. 2010. "Hybrid Simulated Annealing and Genetic Algorithms for Industrial Production Management Problems." *International Journal of Computational Methods* 7 (2): 279–97. https://doi.org/10.1142/S0219876210002209

Wu, Jiansheng, and Zusong Lu. 2012. "A Novel Hybrid Genetic Algorithm and Simulated Annealing for Feature Selection and Kernel Optimization in Support Vector Regression." In *2012 IEEE 5th International Conference on Advanced Computational Intelligence, ICACI 2012*, 999–1003. https://doi.org/10.1109/ICACI.2012.6463321

Zhang, Xinming, Qiang Kang, Jinfeng Cheng, and Xia Wang. 2018. "A Novel Hybrid Algorithm Based on Biogeography-Based Optimization and Grey Wolf Optimizer." *Applied Soft Computing Journal* 67: 197–214. https://doi.org/10.1016/j.asoc.2018.02.049

Zheng, Yu Jun, Xin Li Xu, Hai Feng Ling, and Sheng Yong Chen. 2015. "A Hybrid Fireworks Optimization Method with Differential Evolution Operators." *Neurocomputing* 148: 75–82. https://doi.org/10.1016/j.neucom.2012.08.075

Zheng, Yuefeng, Ying Li, Gang Wang, Yupeng Chen, Qian Xu, Jiahao Fan, and Xueting Cui. 2019. "A Novel Hybrid Algorithm for Feature Selection Based on Whale Optimization Algorithm." *IEEE Access* 7: 14908–23. https://doi.org/10.1109/ACCESS.2018.2879848

8 Survey of Deep Learning Methods in Image Recognition and Analysis of Intrauterine Residues

Bhawna Swarnkar, Nilay Khare,
and Manasi Gyanchandani

CONTENTS

DOI: 10.1201/9781003226147-8

8.1 INTRODUCTION

In childbirth, after the delivery of a fetus from the birth canal of a woman, the placenta is expelled within 3–20 minutes. Placenta is the temporary organ which forms during pregnancy in women's uterus. Basically the functionality of placenta is to supply sufficient oxygen and provide nutrients to fetus as it grows in the womb. It also removes the waste products from the body of the fetus.

Now when it comes to the health of placenta it depends upon various factors, with some of them are under mother's control while others are not. These are as follows: maternal age, water breaking before labor, high blood pressure, twin pregnancy, disorder of blood clotting, any previous uterine surgery, any problem with the placenta in a previous pregnancy, and abdominal trauma.

Placental problems that are more common during pregnancy involve abruption of placenta and low-lying placenta, which causes premature birth of fetus. It is a medical emergency when placenta detaches itself totally or partially from the uterus inner wall, causing insufficient supply of oxygen and nutrients, which results in excessive bleeding from the woman's vagina. Another problem is placenta previa in which the cervix gets covered completely or partially by placenta and is common in the early stages of pregnancy; however, it may get resolved as the uterus grows, but if it does not, then C-section is the only solution. In all these situations the patient suffers vaginal bleeding which is potentially excessive.

Now these come under the conditions which cause complications during pregnancy, but after the delivery of the fetus, residual placenta can create a concern regarding the health of the mother. Retained placenta is the term used for placenta which remains inside the mother's uterus and this postpartum retained placenta has some tissues which are still remaining [1]. Another outlook on remnant placenta is that it is the phenomenon in which placenta's part remains inside the mother's uterus more than half an hour after the child is delivered and it is known as the third stage of labor [2]. Retained placenta is a common complication. In most cases, tiny fragments are the tissues of placenta retained in womb are not easily detected. Postpartum hemorrhage, abdominal infection of uterine cavity, and endometriosis are the main causes of remnant placental tissues. On-time clinical intervention is required which can efficiently and thoroughly administered so as to prevent adherence (state of adhering) which is responsible for painful sensations in the uterus [3]. Reproductive health can be adversely affected because of the risk of intrauterine adhesions, which is also termed secondary amenorrhea and is responsible for risking the quality of a woman's life who is of child-bearing age [4]. Intrauterine adhesions also affect the recovery process of postpartum and medicinal overload. Although, it is not a tough task to detect the postpartum remnant placenta; it is easily diagnosed at the time of child delivery as to whether the placenta is undamaged or not [5]. On time diagnosis plays a significant role in the history of medical science.

There are different perspectives of retained placenta in scientific demonstration. If it is diagnosed as a mild case of postpartum residual placenta, it is demonstrated as secondary anemia, infrequency in vaginal bleeding after childbirth, or it happens in a sudden, occasional way in smaller amounts [6]. It is found in medical check-ups that excessive bleeding can be life-threatening in women with severe complications like poor restoration of the uterus, when the cervix gets remodeled in a loose and soft structure, the softening of a swollen/widened uterus, and patients who have infections in the inner part of the uterine cavity have recognizable delicacy in the lower portion of abdomen. Sometimes proper examination is needed to perform a diagnosis of residual placenta if no such typical symptoms like those mentioned by clinical experts are present, otherwise it can easily be left unnoticed which is likely to harm the reproductive health of the woman. So in order to get rid of such problems, doctors (gynecologists) make use of B-scan ultra-sonography or B-scan.

8.1.1 Medical Imaging Modalities in Gynecology and Obstetrics

Extraction of meaningful information from medical images in order to comprehend the state of an investigated system is the main purpose of clinical experts. On the basis of the pharmaceutical condition and configuration, structure, functioning of various organs, the following imaging modalities are used for diagnostic and treatment purposes in gynecology and obstetrics:

- **Medical thermography:** Also called digital infrared thermal imaging, it is the research technique used for primitive examination and control at the time of treatment of homeostatic imbalance. Its use is experience based, such as in certain tumor types, where they are expected to be vascularized highly, so it could be at a higher temperature as compare with neighboring tissues. In the last stage of brain tumor or breast cancer, where thermal sensors are used in measuring temperature difference is an area where thermography has achieved a great success.
- **Light microscopy:** It is of key importance in the study of anatomical landmarks in various conditions and provides meaningful magnification. This resolution is influenced by diffraction, astigmatism, chromatic aberration, and geometric distortion spherical aberration.
- **Electron microscopy:** It gives a resolving power of and is helpful in exposing the ultra-structures of cells and tissues of the body. Electron microscopy has two types: transmission electron microscope and scanning electron microscope.
- **X-ray imaging:** X-ray comes under the domain of radiography. It is used to study the bone structure of the human body. They are a type of electromagnetic radiation. Tissues ingurgitate radiation in different amounts, which is why our body parts appear in shades of light and dark when under an X-ray machine. It works on frequency and wavelength which is not seen by the naked eye but can penetrate skin to create a picture beneath.
- **Computed tomography (CT):** CT scans are a form of X-rays which produce a three-dimensional (3D) picture of a diagnostic image. After capturing image data, conversion of data into digital form is done by employing the image so that it can get fully scanned. CT scans are considered to be the primary image modality when it comes to identification of problems like postpartum and postoperative complications because of anatomic view of localization. They offer clear visibility of bowel, bladder, and uterus. CT

scans are commonly used in diagnosis of ovarian tumors and sometimes in uterus examinations. Visualization and localization of endometriosis, intra-abdominal, retroperitoneal, hematomas are done by CT scans. CT scans are capable of differentiating types of fluid in comparison with ultrasound. Large pelvic masses, tubo-ovarian abscesses, post-operative complications are also examined by CT scan.

- **Magnetic resonance imaging (MRI):** This method of diagnosis in radiography uses large magnets and radio waves to represent the internal body organ. It gives near-perfect 3D visualization of internal organs and soft tissues in real time with good contrast; hence making the representation of anatomical structures like muscles, joints, brain, spinal cord in much better way. Thus compiled sequences contain uniform combinations of radio frequency and pulsed field gradient, forming the infrastructure of MRI representations. Because of its better contrasting in individual tissues in classification of ovarian tumor detection, MRIs are preferred over CT scans. MRI scans are used in the detection of endometriosis. MRIs can delineate tiny soft tissues, so it is one of the most powerful tools for locating and detecting uterine fibroids. With high contrast resolution there is no risk of being exposed to radiation. Uterine anomalies are well examined with the help of MRI. It has been proven to be the best imaging tool when it comes to reliability in visualizing the complex anatomy of utero vagina.
- **Ultrasound:** It is considered the safest form of image analysis which uses high frequency sound waves to predict the internal body organs. Ultrasound appliances have three main constituents which are monitor, processor, and transducer. Ultrasound is the most used imaging technique for diagnosis of reproductive complications; it is able to produce a cross-section view of the orbit and eyes. B-scan ultrasound enables clinical experts to conveniently, quickly identify images with higher accuracy rate and it is simple to handle.

With the help of B-scan, even the tiny tissues present in the uterus can be scanned clearly, so it is the most preferred imaging tool to scrutinize remnant placental tissues [8]. Ultrasound also provides a clear scan of placental lobules, which are circular-or ring-shaped and have a strong echo [9]. There is a presence of light mass in uterine cavity which does not breach the outer muscular layer of the uterus which can be seen by B-scan and is known as myometrium, unless there is implantation of placental part. Medium and low echoes (irregular ones) are common in women with short-term disease. Necrosis, organization, enhancement of echoes, degeneration of tissues, and rough spots of light are common in women with long-term disease [10]. Accumulation of blood, endometriosis, and inner uterine cavity involution of uterine are also scanned by ultrasound [11].

In this chapter, we mainly discuss deep learning architectures and how these architectures are helping in the diagnosis of disease without much human intervention. This chapter mainly focuses on these deep learning algorithms which are very efficient and accurate in analyzing medical images for classification, segmentation, and detection, which are discussed in this chapter. Also, how features of images get extracted by wavelet transform, gray-level co-occurrence matrix (GLCM), and space pyramid recurrent module, which is rarely used, is also discussed.

These are the major contributions of this chapter, which are arranged as follows. First we discuss the history and show the related work, then deep learning algorithms, which can contribute to the analysis of intrauterine residue, are discussed. This is followed by a review of how these algorithms are being used in different applications and technologies. Then feature extraction methods are discussed, followed by the conclusion.

8.2 RELATED WORK IN MEDICAL IMAGE ANALYSIS AND ITS HISTORY

There was one implementation (i.e. implementation of ML models) in medicine, discussing various antibiotic therapies, which was the MYCIN system produced by Shortliffe [12]. Researchers worked on unsupervised machine learning algorithms but eventually the majority of them conducted their work using supervised machine learning algorithms, especially from 2014 to 2019, mainly convolutional neural network (CNN) [13]. CNN performance has improved with the advancements in hardware like graphics processing units (GPUs), and has been widely used in analyzing medical images.

Artificial neural neuron was first described in 1943 by McCulloch and Pitts [14] and later shown by Rosenblatt [15] in 1958, when it has developed into perception. Basically, layers of connected perceptrons where inputs and outputs are linked together to form a network known as artificial neural network (ANN). And when this ANN has multiple layers, it forms a deep neural network (DNN). DNN is capable of learning features of significantly low level (e.g. outlines and edges) automatically and combines them to make higher level features (e.g. fully formed shapes) in the succeeding layers.

CNNs have their origin in 1982, one of them is proposed by Fukushima, the concept of neocognitron (self organizing neural network for pattern recognition) [16]. But formalization of CNN was done by Lecun et al. [17]. CNNs were used in error back propagation which was described by Rumelhart et al. [18].

Krizhevshy et al. [19] proposed his work using CNNs which won 2012 ImageNet large Scale Visual recognition Challenge (IVSVRC) in which the error rate was 15% in CNN, in which Rectified Linear Unit (RELU) functions in CNN, data augmentation [20]. Since then, widespread use of CNN in image recognition has become a trend.

Venkatesh et al. [35] used predictive models of machine learning and statistical methods for predicting the risk of postpartum hemorrhage. In this chapter, data of 55 candidates was taken for which they used random forest, extreme gradient boosting, and logistic regression techniques. And the performance of the model was measured in terms of C statistics (0.93; 95%), (0.92; 95%), (0.87; 95%), calibration (0.92–0.93, 0.91–0.92, 0.86–0.87), and decision curves, respectively.

Klumpner et al. [36] evaluated the ability of an automated surveillance system and maternal early warning criteria (MEWC) for detection of severely morbid postpartum hemorrhage (sPPH). They took data of 7853 deliveries out of which 120 (1.5%) suffered sPPH. Results were obtained in terms of sensitivity: 60.8% (95% CI, 52.1–69.6); specificity: 82.5% (95%, CI, 81.7–83.4); positive predictive value

(PPV): 5.1% (95%, Cl, 4.0–6.3); and negative predictive value (NPV): 99.3% (95% Cl, 99.1–99.5). And for MEWC characteristics for sPPH the results were sensitivity: 75.0% (95% Cl, 67.3–82.7); specificity: 66.3% (95% Cl, 65.2–67.3); PPV: 3.3% (95% Cl, 2.7–4.0); and NPV 99.4% (95% Cl, 99.2–99.6). So the combined sensitivity of two systems was 83.3% (95% Cl, 75.4–89.5). By this automated system they try to improve the detection of severely morbid postpartum hemorrhage.

Man [37] used trending classification algorithms of machine learning for better the prediction risk of PPH. Dataset was extracted from the electronic health record system with 12 variables which are of high relevance in risk of occurrence of PPH. Comparative analysis is done using logistic regression, decision trees, random forest, k-nearest neighbouring algorithm (KNN), support vector machines (SVMs), ANN results were obtained in terms of precision, recall, and accuracy. Out of all the algorithms, random forest predictions were the most accurate result at 89%.

8.3   MACHINE LEARNING (DEEP LEARNING) ARCHITECTURES

There has been a dramatically increasing number of papers using deep learning architectures, the most dominant of which is CNN. which is discussed in this section along with other architectures.

8.3.1   CONVOLUTIONAL NEURAL NETWORK

One of the most researched algorithms in deep learning is CNN for medical image analysis [13]. The reason behind this is that the spatial relationship is preserved by CNN when input images are filtered. In the context of radiology, spatial relationship between input images has a significant role. It helps to better identify two different things in the smallest tissues, for example, we can determine where normal placental tissues interfaces with cancerous tissues. Basic functionality of CNN is to take input images of raw pixels and transform them into layers: convolutional layer, RELU layer, and pooling layer. CNN makes a fully connected layer that assigns probabilities or class scores, which makes better classification of input into highest probability class.

1. **Convolution layer:** Operation of two functions can be termed as convolution. Whenever any image is analyzed by it, there are two functions, one of them consist of pixel values (e.g. input values) at some position in any image and the other is a kernel (or filter). Each of them can be shown as an array of numbers. Now, computation between these two functions can be done by the dot product, resulting in an output. Then the filter will be shifted towards the position which comes next in that image, which is known as stride length.

   Feature Map (or activation map) is produced by repeating the same computation until the entire image is covered. In this feature map, filter is tightly activated and it "sees" features like a dot, a curved-edge, or a straight line. In image recognition when any picture of a face/brain/uterus is fed into CNN, lines and edges which are low level features are discovered by filters, initially. Then these features in subsequent layers progressively build up to high-level features which are nose, eyes, and ears, they act as feature maps and become input for the next layer in CNN. Convolution makes use of three innate principles to execute computationally effective machine learning algorithm: parameter sharing (weight sharing), sparse connections, and equivalent (or invariant) representation [21].

Neurons in CNN have sparse connections, which means not all inputs are connected to the next layer, whereas in other neural networks every input neuron is connected to its preceding neuron in succeeding layer which is not similar to some other neural networks. CNN algorithm efficiency is increasing because it has small receptive fields, meaningful features can be learnt moderately, and the number of weights to be calculated can be reduced radically. Memory storage requirements for CNNs are reduced by using fixed weights for each filter across various locations in the whole image, known as parameter sharing. This quality makes it different from other fully connected neural networks where weights between layers are numerous, as it is only used once and then discarded. The quality of equivariant representation arises by parameter sharing. This implies that feature map translations are the results of corresponding input translations.

The * symbol is convolution operation, when input I(t) is convolved with kernel K(t) then feature map is defined by O(t) as shown in equation 8.1:

$$O(t) = (I * K)(t) \tag{8.1}$$

The discretized convolution, when t can only take integer values, is shown by equation 8.2.

$$O(t) = \sum I(x).K(t-x) \tag{8.2}$$

Above equation shows one-dimensional convolution operation, now for two-dimensional (2D) operation with input I (x, y) and kernel (m, n) is given by equation 8.3.

$$O(t) = \sum\sum I(m, n).K(x-m, y-n). \tag{8.3}$$

Now when the kernel is flipped by commutative law, above equation is written as:

$$O(t) = \sum\sum I(x-m, y-n).K(m, n). \tag{8.4}$$

When cross-correlation function is implemented which is same as of convolution but without flipping the kernel, equation becomes:

$$O(t) = \sum\sum I(x+m, y+n).K(m, n). \tag{8.5}$$

2. **RELU layer:** An activation function which sets all negative input values to zero is known as RELU layer. Training and calculation become accelerated and simplified. It is helpful in avoiding the vanishing gradient problem. Its equation can be written as:

$$\mathbf{f}(\mathbf{a}) = \mathbf{max}(\mathbf{0}, \mathbf{a}).\qquad(8.6)$$

Here a is input to the neuron. Some other activation functions are sigmoid, tanh, leaky RELUs, randomized RELUs, and parametric RELUs.

3. **Pooling layer:** This is placed between the convolution and RELU layers. Pooling layer's functionality is to cut the data's dimensionality and thus reduce the number of parameters. It can help reduce the problem of overfitting. Pooling layers include max pooling, average pooling, and L2 normalization pooling layers, spatial pyramid pooling, and spectral pooling. Max pooling usually takes the largest value of input by discarding other values within the filter. It produces a strongest activation function over a neighborhood. The logic behind this is that the relative location of one feature to another is more important than that of exact location.

4. **Fully connected layer:** This is the last layer in CNN. In this layer, each and every neuron in preceding layers is connected to every other neuron. Depending on what level of feature extraction is needed, there can be one or more connected layer just like convolution, RELU, pooling layers. Fully connected layer computes the probability score for the classification task into the different classes which are available as its input and takes the output from the preceding layers (convolution, RELU, or pooling layers).

RELU layer works on the features that are most strongly activated so that its class can be easily determined. For instance, on histological glass slide, cancerous cells have a higher DNA-to-cytoplasm ratio when compared with non-cancerous cells. CNN would be more likely to predict the presence of cancerous cells if features of DNA were strongly detected from the previous layer. CNN has the ability to learn significant associations from the training data, by using training methods of standard neural network which uses back propagation [10] and stochastic gradient descent.

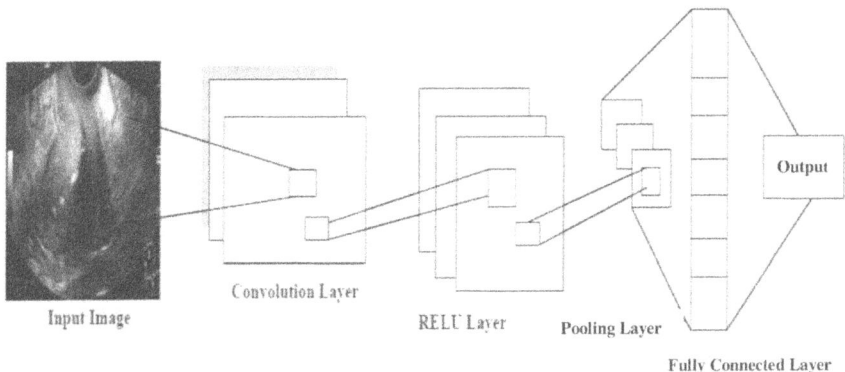

FIGURE 8.1   Feature extraction of intrauterine residue through CNN.

8.3.2 TRANSFER LEARNING (WITH CNN)

In transfer learning, the building and training of CNN from scratch is not required, in fact it uses a pre-trained and pre-built model. The basic concept of transfer learning is simple: First a model gets trained on a large dataset which is smaller. For example, in image recognition with a CNN, if transfer learning is used, the first few convolution layers of network are frozen and training of the last few layers will be done to make a prediction. The idea behind using only the last few layers is the ability of these layers to predict specific features within an image, like lips and forehead, with great accuracy whereas the first few layers are convolution layers and are capable of extracting general low-level features like edges, patterns, and gradients. Transfer learning includes training the machine learning algorithm on unrelated or partly related datasets in addition to the labeled training dataset to remove the barrier of insufficient training. Except the last fully connected layer, weights can be applied to all layers of CNN. Although transfer learning with CNN is applied in making various predictions, it is mainly used in medical image analysis. CNN

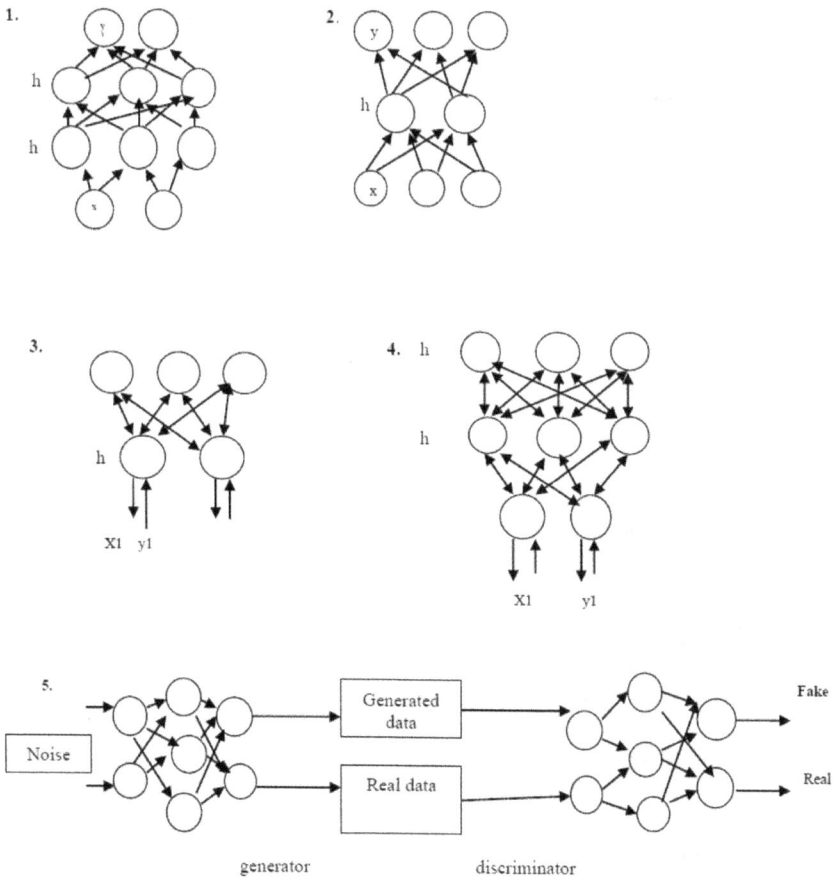

FIGURE 8.2 Deep learning architectures: 1. RNN, 2. Auto-encoder, 3.RBM, 4. DBNs, 5. GANs.

architectures in conjunction with transfer learning is explored by Shin et al. [23] for detection of enlarged thoraco-abdominal lymph node presence. It also makes use of other classifications of post-delivery intrauterine remnants.

8.3.3 RECURRENT NEURAL NETWORK

Another ANN is recurrent neural networks (RNNs)in which output from the preceding layer is treated as an input for the next layer. It is mostly used in analysis of sequential data and natural language processing. RNN has evolved into gated recurrent units and long short-term memory. Most important feature of RNN is hidden state, it remembers information of sequence being followed. RNN has a memory for remembering all the calculations which have been performed. The same parameters for each input are used to produce the output. Mainly RNN has been used in the segmentation of images. RNN has great predictive power, so many researchers have making use of it for prediction of the likelihood of successful IVF. RNNs are also being used to detect endometriosis. In medical image analysis RNN is mainly used in segmentation tasks.

8.3.4 DEEP BELIEF NETWORKS AND RESTRICTED BOLTZMANN MACHINE

A restricted Boltzmann machine is a shallow feed forward network, like other neural networks. In the restricted Boltzmann machine, forward and backward connection have restrictions in that they all share the same weights. The restricted Boltzmann machine has a fully connected node with two layers, with both types of connection, forward and backward (cycle). Whenever computation is done in a network, a gradient update is performed, affecting the connections both forward and backward.

Deep belief networks (DBNs) are made up of restricted Boltzmann machines which are connected sequentially. It is a graphical representation which is generative in nature. Generative means it can produce all possible values, generated for the case at that time.

8.3.5 AUTO-ENCODERS

Auto-encoders are neural networks which learn data in unsupervised manner. Auto-encoders aim to reduce dimensionality by training the network. In medical image analysis these features are of great significance where the data to be trained is limited. Long-Yi-Guo et al. [24] proposed the composite features of multi-omics data, which is produced by de-noising auto-encoder being used for generation of low-dimensional features which were fed as an input into k-means for clustering to classify ovarian cancer.

An auto-encoder consists of two parts: encoder (ϕ) and decoder (f) which maps input (X) to code space (F), which are mathematically expressed as, $\phi{:}X{\rightarrow}F$, $f{:}F{\rightarrow}X$ and we aim to achieve encoder and decoder parameter such that ϕ, $f = \arg \max_{\phi, f}\|X = (\phi \circ f)X\|$. Code-space, which is also named latent space, can be defined as basic neural network as, $z = \sigma(Wx + b)$ and x can be generated from z as $x = \sigma'(W'z + b')$ where, σ', W', b' differs from σ, W, b depending upon the design of the network.

8.3.6 GENERATIVE ADVERSARIAL NETWORKS

When a generative modeling is used with deep learning methods it is referred to as generative adversarial network (GNN). It works on automatic discovering and learning the patterns in input data in a way that model can be used to generate new examples from the original dataset. Although GNNs are unsupervised in approach, they can train a generative model by framing the problem as a supervised learning problem with two sub-models: generator model and discriminator model. They provide a path to sophisticated domain-specific data augmentation.

8.4 MEDICAL IMAGE ANALYSIS (TECHNOLOGIES AND APPLICATIONS)

8.4.1 IMAGE FEATURE DESCRIPTION BASED ON DEEP LEARNING

In image recognition, features play a crucial role. When we use methods to change the value of the pattern we recognize in any image, this step is referred to as feature extraction. Features are of many types: color, texture, different shape, and spatial relation. In deep learning, multiple linear functions are used to be complex nonlinear function, which shows a strong learning capability of essential features of any given dataset, by training deep learning network structure.

A deep learning algorithm is constructed with n number of layers, where input to each layer is a result obtained from preceding layers and all these layers are interconnected by weight matrix. By this input data, a sequence of hierarchical features can be obtained.

8.4.2 ANALYSIS OF GENERATIVE MODEL

A self-learning model is simple and applies in clustering algorithms, but these models do not perform well with generalization in the initial training phase when they have to deal with a small amount of data. In most deep learning algorithms, discriminative models have been used. Models which induce the conditional probability in accordance with Bayes formula is the generative model. It has high optimization and models complex relations between observed and hidden variables.

8.4.3 LOW-DENSITY SEPARATION METHOD IN SEMI-SUPERVISED

An extension to SVM is the direct push SVM which works on the principle of direct push learning. Classifiers can be used out of training samples. It has labeled as well as unlabeled data. Its aim is to find a separating hyper-plane to maintain maximum gap between labeled and unlabeled data. SVM, direct push SVM, and Gaussian process are low-density methods with separation.

8.5 APPLICATIONS

The area of computer vision has the conclusive aim of using systems to mutate learning and human vision. Analysis of any image lies between processing and computer vision.

8.5.1 CLASSIFICATION

Classification is one of the first contributions of deep learning to the analysis of medical images. Classification requires a huge dataset with known ground truth to train on different cases. Optimum classification involves the accuracy in classification, performance, and computational resources. Some classification techniques are ANN, SVM, KNN, and Fuzzy C-means (FCM).

8.5.2 SEGMENTATION

It is a great challenge to differentiate the organs of interest and extract them from the background in algorithm development. The segmented region is of great importance because steps to be taken are guided by segmentation in the whole analysis. It can be done in three ways: manual segmentation, semi-automatic segmentation, and fully automatic segmentation.

8.5.3 DETECTION

Detection, also known as computer aided detection (CAD), refers to software used for pattern recognition which distinguishes suspicious features on the image to reduce false negative readings. The processes of classification and localization come together in order to detect and this is known as detection.

8.5.4 LOCALIZATION

Localization of anatomical structures such as organs or landmarks, has been an essential task. Localization requires parsing of 3D volumes and to solve 3D data parsing several approaches have been processed in deep learning. Localization is most commonly used in fully automatic end-to-end applications using supervised and unsupervised learning models.

8.5.5 REGISTRATION

Registration refers to a spatial alignment of images and is a common function in determining one-to-one correspondence between the coordinates of two or more images. In the process of registration, alignment to second implant placement is made for a reference image. Registration in medical images has potential applications which are reviewed by researchers.

8.6 RECOGNITION OF IMAGE BASED ON FEATURE EXTRACTION IN DEEP LEARNING

Features extraction is important step in medical image analysis. Some of the features of extraction techniques are discussed as follows.

8.6.1 FEATURE EXTRACTION OF IMAGE BY USING WAVELET TRANSFORM

This is one of the transform-based feature extraction methods. Discrete wavelet transform (DWT) is ideal for de-noising and comprising signals images as it helps represent images with fear coefficient. Analyzing image frequencies at various scales is done using wavelet. Wavelet coefficients from the MRI scans of the brain are extracted. Information of frequency of signal function is quite important for the purpose of classification is localized by wavelet transform.

When we apply 2D-DWT, it gets decomposed into two region of interest (ROI) levels, from which we get four sub-bands named as Low-Low, Low-High, High-High, High-Low; represented by LL, LH, HH, and HL, respectively.

As a result of this decomposition of image, we are able to see in detail high- and low-level content of frequency in image. In wavelet approximation, low-frequency position of an image is represented by LL1, LL2 at first and second level, respectively. Similarly, LH1, LH2, HH1, HL2 are representations of high-frequency levels of image. In these frequency levels, representation of horizontal, vertical, and diagonal is given in detail. Here we have used image of low frequency. So LL1 shows the original image approximation, it further undergoes decomposition of second level approximation and image details. This process will be repeated until the desired level of resolution is obtained.

Now from sub-band, components of spatial frequency were extracted in the process of decomposition. For better analysis of images, we have used both LL and HH, because HH has higher performance in comparison to LL, to obtain text features of brain tumor images. The components of different frequency and each component studied with resolution matched to its scale and expressed is as:

$$\textbf{DWT } d(s) = \begin{cases} P_{ij} = \sum d(s) h \times i(s - 2\,ij) \\ P_{ij} = \sum d(s) l \times i(s - 2ij) \end{cases} \tag{8.7}$$

Here signal d(s) has component attribute corresponding to which is represented by Pi, j coefficients correspond to the wavelet function, and d i, and j represent the approximated signal components. The h(s) and l(s) are functions referring to high-pass and low-pass filters coefficient in the equation, respectively, while wavelet scale and translation factor are represented by parameters i and j.

8.6.1.1 Cyclic Network Design

8.6.2 FEATURE EXTRACTION OF IMAGE BY USING GRAY-LEVEL CO-OCCURRENCE MATRIX

Human eyes are unable to see variation between normal and malignant tissues, so it is done by texture analysis. It chooses the effective quantitative features for improving accuracy which helps in early diagnosis. Texture analysis has two steps: first order and second order analysis. First order statistical textural analysis gray level frequencies are measured at random positions of the image and information of features are extracted from image intensity histogram. Correlation between image pixels is also considered. In second order analysis, the information of features is obtained by calculating the gray levels probability at any distance chosen randomly and over entire image orientations.

Extraction of statistical features is done by using gray-level co-occurrence matrix (GLCM), also known as gray-level spatial dependence matrix (GLSDM). Gray-level pixel values have spatial relation between them which is defined by the approach known as GLSDM. GLCM is a 2D histogram where frequency of event p occurs

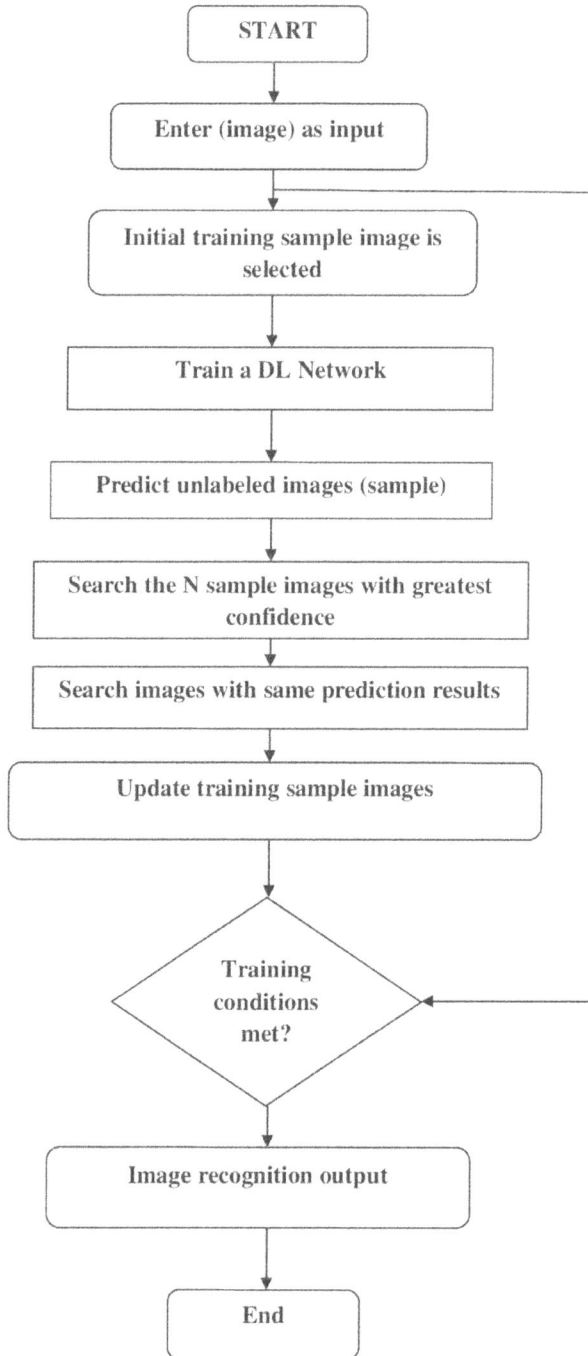

FIGURE 8.3   Flowchart of image recognition.

with event q represented by (p, q)th elements, and is used to calculate how often a pixel with intensity p occurs in relation with another pixel q at a certain distance S and orientation. By this method, GLCM helps in finding the textural features such as homogeneity, entropy, correlation, energy, and contrast from low- and high-level sub-bands of the first four levels of wavelet decomposition.

8.6.3 SPACE PYRAMID RECURRENT MODULE

Space pyramid recurrent module acquires the structure of spatial pyramid. In spatial pyramid structures, convolution operation is performed and the image is converted into features of various sizes. In the convolution layer when the size of features is smaller, extraction of categorical information becomes easy. And, contrastingly, when the feature size is large, the location is easily extracted by convolution layer. Dimensional features are easily differentiated by adding circular convolution network into spatial pyramid loop module.

Spatial pyramid recurrent module works as follows: It is connected to base network, where resultant features become input for its first layer, with both category and location information. This approach helps in improving image recognition.

8.7 CONCLUSION

In this survey chapter, we discussed common placental problems and intrauterine residues, and how they can affect the health of patients. We also discussed how deep learning algorithms are helpful in on-time, efficient, accurate diagnosis. We discussed various image modalities that are being used in the treatment of intrauterine residues and how they play a significant role in diagnosis. Then this chapter briefly presented various deep learning architectures which are capable of medical image recognition, classification, and segmentation tasks. It showed how deep learning method of generative modeling and low density-based methods are capable of describing features in medical image analysis and their applications in various steps of image analysis, such as in segmentation, classification, localization, and detection. Lastly we discussed feature extraction in deep learning which are based on GLCM, Wavelet transform, and space pyramid recurrent module, which provide solutions for extracting semantic and categorical information.

8.8 FUTURE SCOPE AND CHALLENGES

Forming algorithms that are accessible as software in the public domain and integrating them into larger libraries are essential steps in medical image analysis. These analyzing technologies are capable of figuring out three pillars, which would be even better, as follows:

- An algorithm which is adaptable to numerous tasks in analyzing images;
- An unambiguous process which is supported by proper appliances in order to improve the configuration of a particular function;
- A valid setup with numerous measures that permit algorithms to be tested on an image database.

For resulting algorithms, it is important to satisfy the important conditions which are required for the subsequently developing process in terms of better accuracy, memory consumption, and computation time. Another challenge is demand of using more heterogenous image data.

REFERENCES

[1] Q. Zhu, B. Du, and P. Yan, "Boundary-weighted domain adaptive neural network for prostate MR image segmentation," IEEE Trans. Med. Imag., vol. 39, no. 3, pp. 753–63, Mar. 2020.

[2] M. Mehdipour Ghazi, B. Yanikoglu, and E. Aptoula, "Plant identification using deep neural networks via optimization of transfer learning parameters," Neurocomputing, vol. 235, pp. 228–35, Apr. 2017.

[3] J. Bi, H. Yuan, and M. Zhou, "Temporal prediction of multiapplication consolidated workloads in distributed clouds," IEEE Trans. Autom. Sci. Eng., vol. 16, no. 4, pp. 1763–73, Oct. 2019.

[4] M. Gao, U. Bagci, L. Lu, A. Wu, M. Buty, H.-C. Shin, H. Roth, G. Z. Papadakis, A. Depeursinge, R. M. Summers, Z. Xu, and D. J. Mollura, "Holistic classification of CT attenuation patterns for interstitial lung diseases via deep convolutional neural networks," Comput. Methods Biomech. Biomed. Eng., Imag. Vis., vol. 6, no. 1, pp. 1–6, Jan. 2018.

[5] A. Karargyris, J. Siegelman, D. Tzortzis, S. Jaeger, S. Candemir, Z. Xue, K. C. Santosh, S. Vajda, S. Antani, L. Folio, and G. R. Thoma, "Combination of texture and shape features to detect pulmonary abnormalities in digital chest X-rays," Int. J. Comput. Assist. Radiol. Surg., vol. 11, no. 1, pp. 99–106, Jan. 2016.

[6] A. Nibali, Z. He, and D. Wollersheim, "Pulmonary nodule classification with deep residual networks," Int. J. Comput. Assist. Radiol. Surg., vol. 12, no. 10, pp. 1799–808, Oct. 2017.

[7] C. Qin, D. Yao, Y. Shi, and Z. Song, "Computer-aided detection in chest radiography based on artificial intelligence: A survey," Biomed. Eng. OnLine, vol. 17, no. 1, pp. 1–23, Dec. 2018.

[8] M. Anthimopoulos, S. Christodoulidis, L. Ebner, A. Christe, and S. Mougiakakou, "Lung pattern classification for interstitial lung diseases using a deep convolutional neural network," IEEE Trans. Med. Imag., vol. 35, no. 5, pp. 1207–1216, May 2016.

[9] E. Elyan and M. M. Gaber, "A _ne-grained random forests using class decomposition: An application to medical diagnosis," Neural Comput. Appl., vol. 27, no. 8, pp. 2279–88, Nov. 2016.

[10] S. Shen, S. X. Han, D. R. Aberle, A. A. Bui, and W. Hsu, "An interpretable deep hierarchical semantic convolutional neural network for lung nodule malignancy classification," Expert Syst. Appl., vol. 128, pp. 84–95, Aug. 2019.

[11] Y. Li, C. Huang, L. Ding, Z. Li, Y. Pan, and X. Gao, "Deep learning in bioinformatics: Introduction, application, and perspective in the big data era," Methods, vol. 166, pp. 4–21, Aug. 2019.

[12] E. H. Shortliffe, Computer-Based Medical Consultations: MYCIN, vol. 2. New York, NY: Elsevier, 1976.

[13] G. Litjens et al. (Jun. 2017). "A survey on deep learning in medical image analysis." [Online]. Available at: https://arxiv.org/abs/1702.05747

[14] W. S. McCulloch and W. Pitts, "A logical calculus of the ideas immanent in nervous activity," Bull. Math. Biol., vol. 5, no. 4, pp. 115–33, 1943.

[15] F. Rosenblatt, "The perceptron: A probabilistic model for information storage and organization in the brain,"Psychol. Rev., vol. 65, no. 6, pp. 365–86, 1958.

[16] D. H. Hubel, and T. N. Wiesel, "Receptive fields, binocular interaction and functional architecture in the cat's visual cortex," J. Physiol., vol. 160, no. 1, pp. 106–54, 1962.

[17] K. Fukushima, and S. Miyake, "Neocognitron: A self-organizing neural network model for a mechanism of visual pattern recognition," in Competition and Cooperation in Neural Nets. Berlin, Germany: Springer, pp. 267–85, 1982.

[18] Y. LeCun et al., "Backpropagation applied to handwritten zip code recognition," Neural Comput., vol. 1, no. 4, pp. 541–51, 1989.

[19] D. E. Rumelhart, G. E. Hinton, and R. J. Williams, "Learning representations by back-propagating errors," Nature, vol. 323, pp. 533–56, Oct. 1986.

[20] A. Krizhevshy, I. Sutskever, and G. E. Hinton, "ImageNet classi_cation with deep convolutional neural networks," in Proc. Adv. Neural Inf. Process. Syst., pp. 1097–105, 2012.

[21] I. Goodfellow, Y. Bengio, and A. Courville, *Deep Learning*. Cambridge, MA: MIT Press, 2016.

[22] O. Russakovsky et al., "ImageNet large scale visual recognition challenge," Int. J. Comput. Vis., vol. 115, no. 3, pp. 211–52, Dec. 2015.

[23] H.-C. Shin et al., "Deep convolutional neural networks for computer aided detection: CNN architectures, dataset characteristics and transfer learning," IEEE Trans. Med. Imag., vol. 35, no. 5, pp. 1285–98, May 2016.

[24] Long-Yi Guo, Ai-Hua Wu, Yong-xia Wang, Li-ping Zhang, Hua Chai, Xue-Fang Liang, "Deep learning-based ovarian cancer subtypes identification using multi-omics data," BioData Mining, vol. 12, 2020.

[25] R. Ashraf, M. Ahmed, S. Jabbar, S. Khalid, A. Ahmad, S. Din, and G. Jeon, "Content based image retrieval by using color descriptor and discrete wavelet transform," J. Med. Syst., vol. 42, no. 3, p. 44, Mar. 2018.

[26] H. Xie, D. Yang, N. Sun, Z. Chen, and Y. Zhang, "Automated pulmonary nodule detection in CT images using deep convolutional neural networks," Pattern Recognit., vol. 85, pp. 109–19, Jan. 2019.

[27] Y. Li, S. Wang, R. Umarov, B. Xie, M. Fan, L. Li, and X. Gao, "DEEPre Sequence-based enzyme EC number prediction by deep learning," Bioinformatics, vol. 34, no. 5, pp. 760–69, Mar. 2018.

[28] A. S. Qureshi, A. Khan, A. Zameer, and A. Usman, "Wind power prediction using deep neural network based meta regression and transfer learning," Appl. Soft Comput., vol. 58, pp. 742–55, Sep. 2017.

[29] E. Elyan and M. M. Gaber, "A genetic algorithm approach to optimizing random forests applied to class engineered data," Inf. Sci., vol. 384, pp. 220–34, Apr. 2017.

[30] J. Kawahara, C. J. Brown, S. P. Miller, B. G. Booth, V. Chau, R. E. Grunau, J. G. Zwicker, and G. Hamarneh, "BrainNetCNN: Convolutional neural networks for brain networks; towards predicting neurodevelopment," NeuroImage, vol. 146, pp. 1038–49, Feb. 2017.

[31] G. Litjens, T. Kooi, B. E. Bejnordi, A. A. A. Setio, F. Ciompi, M. Ghafoorian, J. A. W. M. van der Laak, B. van Ginneken, and C. I. Sánchez, "A survey on deep learning in medical image analysis," Med. Image Anal., vol. 42, pp. 60–88, Dec. 2017.

[32] S. Zhou, Q. Chen, and X. Wang, "Active deep learning method for semi-supervised sentiment classification," Neurocomputing, vol. 120, pp. 536–46, Nov. 2013.

[33] Z. Zou, S. Tian, X. Gao, and Y. Li, "MlDEEPre: Multi-functional enzyme function prediction with hierarchical multi-label deep learning," Frontiers Genet., vol. 9, p. 714, Jan. 2019.

[34] K. Kamnitsas, C. Ledig, V. F. J. Newcombe, J. P. Simpson, A. D. Kane, D. K. Menon, D. Rueckert, and B. Glocker, "Efficient multi-scale 3DCNN with fully connected CRF for accurate brain lesion segmentation," Med. Image Anal., vol. 36, pp. 61–78, Feb. 2017.

[35] K. K. Venkatesh, R. A. Strauss, C. A. Grotegut, R. P. Heine, N. C. Chescheir, Jeffrey S. A. Stringer, D. M. Stamilio, K. M. Menard, and J. E. Jelovsek, "Machine learning and statistical models to predict postpartum hemorrhage," Obstetrics Gynecol., vol. 135, pp. 935–43, April. 2020.

[36] T. T. Klumpner, J. A. Kountanis, S. R. Meyer, J. Ortwine, M. E. Bauer, A. Carver, A. M. Piehl, R. Smith, G. Mentz, and K. K Tremper, "Use of a novel electronic maternal surveillance system and the maternal early warning criteria to detect severe postpartum hemorrhage," Obstetric Anesthesia Digest, vol. 131, pp. 857–65(9), Jan 2020.

[37] Zhauhui Man. Comparative study of machine learning models to predict PPH. Nov, 2019. https://doi.org/10.17615/fcpv-1085

9 A Comprehensive Survey on Breast Cancer Thermography Classification Using Deep Neural Network

Amira Hassan Abed, Essam M. Shaaban,
Om Prakash Jena, and Ahmed A. Elngar

CONTENTS

9.1 INTRODUCTION

Worldwide cancer statistics report that breast cancer disease is one of the most deadly types of cancer, after cellular breakdown in the lungs [1]. In 2018, two billion new breast cancer cases were accounted around the world and 627,000 deaths. According to a research [2], breast cancer patient endurance is heavily linked to tumor size during the diagnosis phase, indicating a 98% chance of patient survival if the size is lesser than 10 mm. According to a parallel study, 70% of bosom disease cases are identified when the malignancy is 30 mm in size [3]. When a tumor is larger than 20 mm in diameter, it is usually detectable during screening [4]. As a result, boosting early cancer disease detection is crucial for encouraging early treatment. Early treatment might be useful after detection by screening assessments, for example, clinical breast examination (CBE) and breast

DOI: 10.1201/9781003226147-9

169

self- examination (BSE). CBE is a standard clinical assessment performed by medical services experts to distinguish bosom injuries, while BSE is performed by a person to notice actual changes and presence of bosoms. The act of BSE engages women to assume liability for their wellbeing [5].

Screening strategies generate clinical images of bosoms. The analyses of these images are regularly done by specialists. Several studies mentioned that the low analytic precision of thermograms resulted from specialists' weak capabilities and skills in deciphering such images. The development of different illnesses and restricted human capabilities has propelled analysts and medical experts to utilize computer-aided innovation to encourage breast thermography-based analysis and accordingly limit blunders. Thus, a computer-assisted framework is required to automatically characterize thermograms into typical and abnormal classes. Thinking about this necessity, the number of studies toward proposing a computer-assisted system for examining clinical images has been consistently increasing. Numerous computer-aided strategies for examination have been implemented to help medical teams in deciphering the clinical images. Over the last few years, critical effort has concentrated on the improvement of DL models. Since these are openly accessible, they employed effectively, utilizing networks with pre-training. For breast cancer identification, numerous existing studies depend on DL utilizing mammograms [6–8], histology pictures [9], tomosyntheses [10], and ultrasound pictures [11] have demonstrated acceptable accuracies.

However, hardly any investigations have added to non-obtrusive thermal imaging of bosoms utilizing the deep neural organization (DNN) procedure. Taking existing restricted assets, the research on the issue is still in its early phases. Thus, critical effort is needed to create a dependable computer-aided system to empower the early recognition of breast disease. This requires an investigation of significant past, new and vital future exploration studies on thermal imaging and DL for bosom malignant identification and ought to be considered of foremost significance. Through our work, we survey current advancement in breast disease identification utilizing DL and thermography as a non-obtrusive methodology. Different machine learning techniques in healthcare analysis and solutions related to genomics classification and clinical diagnosis of healthcare issues are reported [12–15].

This work is coordinated as follows. Section 9.2 presents the background of breast cancer. Section 9.3 defines thermography and explains its role in breast cancer. Section 9.4 describe about breast thermograms using deep learning classification. Section 9.5 is a review on breast cancer using thermographs and deep learning, and Section 9.6 concludes the work.

9.2 BACKGROUND OF BREAST CANCER

Breast cancer is one of the most widely publicized cancers worldwide. Breast. This kind of cancer has been found in both males and females; moreover, its recurrence with females is high in comparison to males. This is straightforwardly considered based on the fundamental difference between the breast in the two

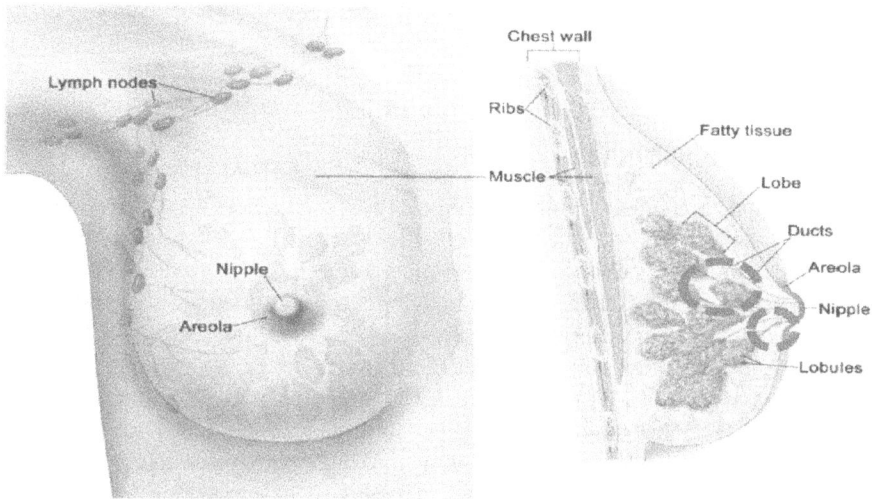

FIGURE 9.1   Common breast cancer locations.

sexes, as hazardous microorganisms are discovered in milk production centers, labia majora, and milk flowing tunnels and canals, as a result of repetitive inspections. Figure 9.1 depicts an anatomical view of the female bosom with a variety of frequently occurring breast cancer sites. Breast cancer might progress for a variety of reasons, some of which are unknown. In any event, the odd enlargement of living cells is among the confirmed bosom malignant behaviors. Though some genes are crucial for cell division and growth, those genetic traits fail to detect anomalies for a myriad of purposes.

This prompts a fast development and propagation of dead cells that cannot be split or increased in size, generating a type of tumor. The generated tumor is classed as harmful in the case of the prevalence over the breast and assaults its encompassing with tissues; when it stays involved in specific tissues, similar to conduits and lobules, it is ordered as non-intrusive tumor. It is critical to recall that cancer cells would spread to any part of the human body; in breast malignancy, they move across the lymph or blood. In the last phase, the bosom disease is assumed in its high-level phase and abscission mediation, known as biopsy, is typically requested.

It is enthusiastically prescribed that patients have to take care of the bosom cancer before it converts to this high-level stage. For this particular explanation, breast cancer screening techniques and devices are developed for detection purpose following the standard methodology. These techniques differ in their procedures, applications, and results, yet there is no preferred technique for physicians.

Frequently, doctors require the screening using various techniques to affirm the acquired outcomes. In any case, a point that can be considered is the concomitant of the shielding technique. New headway in the automated operation has animated scientists to re-investigate screening techniques for upgrade purposes. These days, it is very conceivable to discover a re-examination of previously non-proficient breast shielding strategies and adjusting to the accessible handling and clustering methods to deliver extensive outcomes.

9.3 THERMOGRAPHY

Thermography is a prescient method for observing the state of plant hardware constructions and frameworks not simply electrical gear. It utilizes instrumentation to view infrared energy outflows (surface temperature) to decide working conditions. Infrared thermography (IRT), thermal imaging, and thermal video are instances of infrared imaging areas. Thermographic cameras are a tool for distinguishing radiation in the long-infrared scope of the electromagnetic range (approximately 9,000–14,000 nanometers or 9–14 μm) and create thermograms, which are photographs of the radiation. The dark radiative cooling law states that anything with a temperature above absolute zero emits infrared radiation, making it possible for thermography to see human current circumstances with or without visible illumination.

The consignment of radiation generated by every organism increases with temperature; consequently, thermography allows us to perceive seasonal variation. Thermal entities stand out well against cooler substrates during screening using thermal imaging cameras; people and certain other warm-blooded organisms become easily visible against the climate, day or night. As a result, thermography is particularly beneficial to the military and various users of espionage equipment.

9.3.1 THERMOGRAPHY IN BREAST CANCER DIAGNOSIS

Thermography has a variety of novel uses. Several methods are for early discovery of cancer by recognizing early indications of disease, ten years sooner than different techniques, for example, mammography [16]. Another novel capability of thermography is assessment procedures for malignancy treatment. Anticipating the future state of a patient with the use of thermography [17]. It has been reported that 44% of individuals with abnormal thermograms had been diagnosed with breast cancer five years following thermography [17].

Thermography likewise indicated that there is a 24% chance of survival in three years after determining that a specific patient has a high-level malignancy, where this likelihood for tumors at prior levels was near 80% [17]. The affectability of mammography in more youthful individuals or females with thick bosom tissue will be diminished. Yet, thermography is freedom to the patients' ages and the thickness of bosom cancers. Thermography can detect breast cancer symptoms one year earlier than mammography in 70% of individuals [17]. The size of undetectable tumors in mammography is around 1.66 cm, but the size is limited to 1.28 cm in thermography. In comparison to a regular thermogram, an anomalous thermogram can predict the jeopardize of breast cancer 22 times better. Furthermore, the anomalous thermograms are ten times more meaningful. Thermal picture examination can be gathered by thermobiology in five primary classes: TH1 – "normal uniform non-vascular", TH2 – "vascular ordinary uniform", TH3 – "vague (questionable)", TH4 – "abnormal", and TH5 – "extremely abnormal". Classified pictures are shown in Figure 9.2 [18].

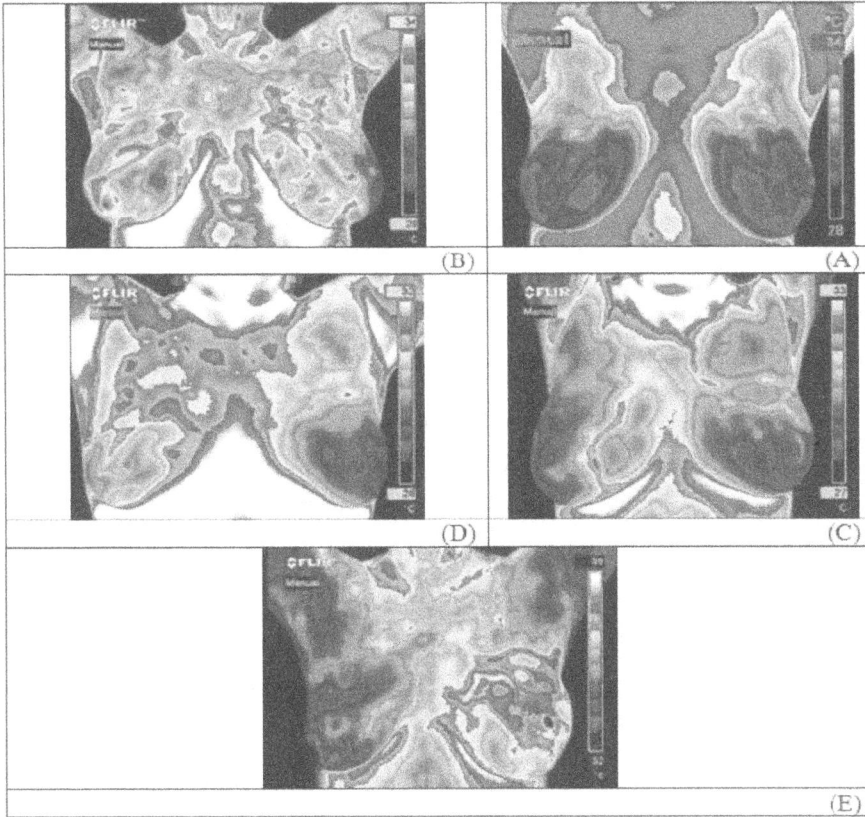

FIGURE 9.2   (a)-(e) Different classes based on thermobiology [see [18]].

9.4   BREAST THERMOGRAMS USING DEEP LEARNING CLASSIFICATION

The neural networks (NNs) are roused by how neurons in the human cerebrum process. Each neuron in the human brain is interconnected and information streams through every one. In NNs, neurons get input and play out many activities with "weights" and "biases." The strength of the connection between two hubs is indicated by the weight. Outside values that increase or decrease the net input of the activation work are known as biases. In each layer, hubs are the individual preparation units. A neuron structure based on mathematical assumption is shown in Figure 9.3.

It can learn from data with two objectives: to comprehend the data streaming process and its explication, and to foresee future impressions. A probabilistic accuracy rate is not required for foreseeing future solutions. Regardless, clinical information interpretations place a premium on accuracy. When it comes to detecting breast cancer, 100% precision is necessary to ensure that the judgement is made on a firm foundation. The NN is a vast concurrent circulatory processor composed of basic processing units that have a particular fondness for reliable data, making it

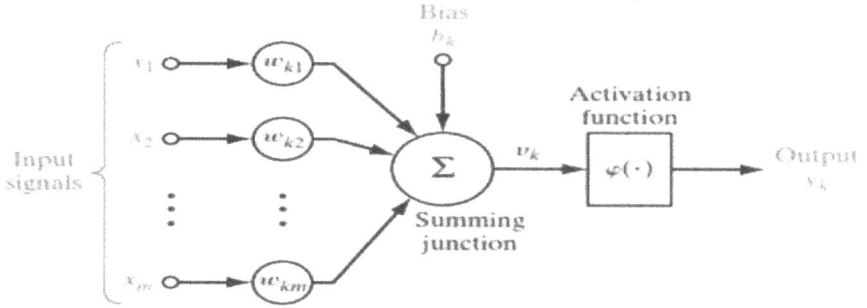

FIGURE 9.3   The neuron structure based on mathematical assumption.

extremely easy to utilize. The NN algorithm allows for the learning of subjective medical image values. Consequently, it is suitable for interpretations of bosom thermograms characterization.

A CNN is a DNN technique in which it processes the input pictures by allotting various accessible weights and biases to locate significant features which separate one picture from another. Thus, the classification output can be seen as the yield. Figure 9.4 supports the overall CNNs building for the classification of the bosom thermograms in two sets, normal and cancer. Three significant contemplations should be focused: "dataset readiness in picture pre-preparing", "feature learning", and "classification". The classification may be double ("normal and cancer"), or many classes, for example, solid, generous, and harmful. In the accompanying part, we survey the ideas and related endeavors in CNN usage for classification breast thermogram.

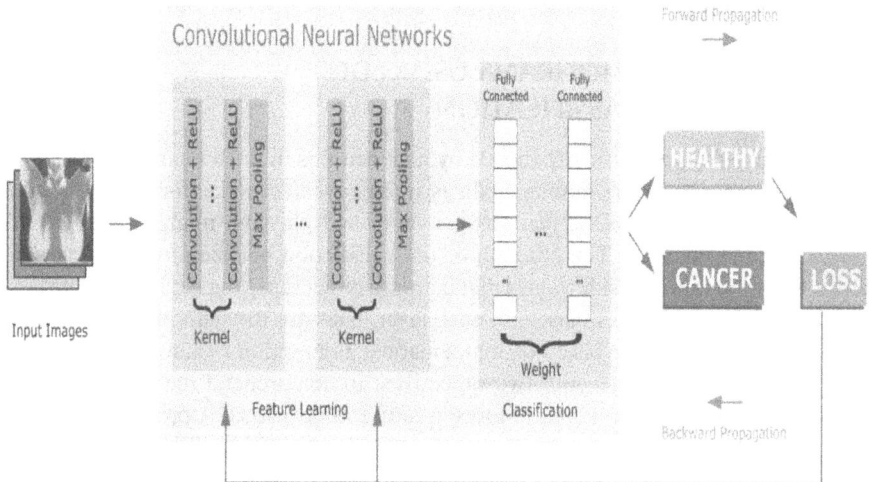

FIGURE 9.4   Proposed CNN method for premature breast thermograms detection.

9.4.1 PREPROCESSING IMAGES PROCESS

Preprocess of Images is a significant process to enhance the features of images, by stifling undesirable information and upgrading significant features of images to improve the NN algorithm performance. Preprocessing Images process is vital for NNs as the accomplishment of the learning interaction relies upon the features gaining from input Images. For the most part, Preprocessing of Images incorporates mean deduction, standardization, PCA brightening, and neighborhood contrast standardization. Furthermore, many algorithms are utilized for bosom thermograms pre-preparing incorporate resizing, segmentation of the region of interest (ROI), and expansion.

9.4.2 CONVOLUTIONAL NEURAL NETWORKS

In most cases, neural networks are used to detect and identify objects in image input data. Overall, CNNs are similar to other NNs in that they have weight, predilection, and beginning work when gathering inputs. Regardless, CNNs enable features extrication to describe patterns from high-dimensional data sources. Convolution is the name given to this interaction, which is implemented in a "convolutional layer" (Feature Extraction Layer). As seen in Figure 9.4, CNN contains two important layers: feature extrication and completely connected networks, which are explained in the subsections below.

9.4.2.1 Feature Extraction Layer

The feature extraction layer is in charge of encoding input data to generate features (images). As a result, one picture is coded as a feature map comprising numbers that define picture characters. Convolution and pooling are the two implementation aspects of this layer. The convolution portion is structured as a filter (kernel) of a certain size. Because there are three shade channels (RGB) in the bosom thermograms, there are three filters for each channel. The convolution layer's output is a feature map, which is then transferred to the pooling layer. One layer of assumed step size is included in the pooling layer. One channel with a defined step size is included in the pooling layer. Inputs are up-tested in the convolutional layer, but feature maps are down-tested in the pooling layer. Max pooling and average pooling are the two most common types of pooling initiation works. In max pooling, the utmost estimation of the feature maps is chosen, whereas in average pooling, the average estimation of the feature maps is chosen.

CNNs repeat the convolution and max pooling procedures until they perceive the image's features in the learning features phase. The convolution cycle in CNN is seen in Figure 9.5 using bosom thermograms as input data. Because the inputs contain three colors (RGB), the kernel volume also has three separate two-dimensional kernels. Each passage is associated with a single kernel. The kernel's size is determined by the number of feature maps available.

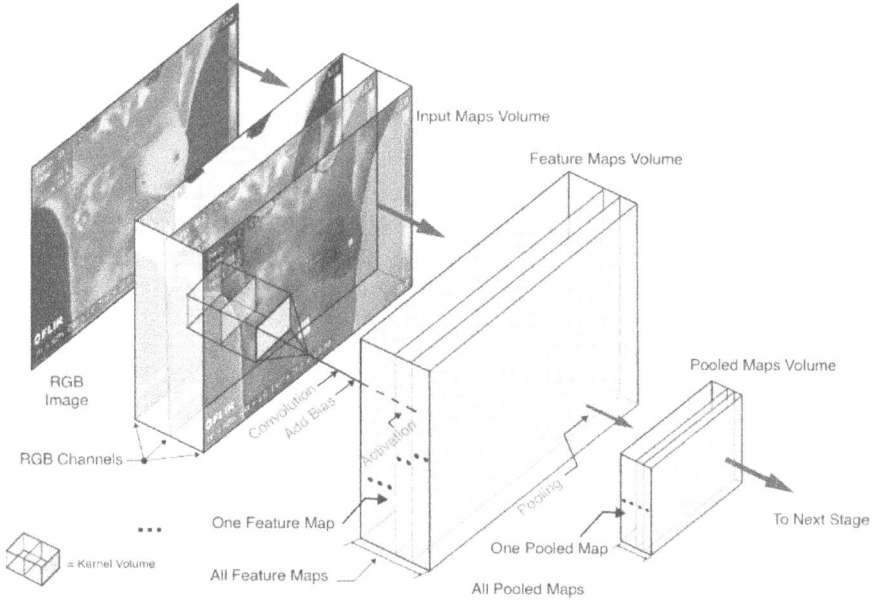

FIGURE 9.5   Conception of convolutional phases of a cancerous breast thermograms [see [19]].

9.4.2.2   Fully Connected Layer

The convolutional layer produces feature maps in the form of a multi-level array. In this vein, it's critical to level or reform a one-dimensional array from feature elements before using it as a contribution for the fully associated layer. As a result, fully associated layers are convolutional layers having a -1 1 filter size. A totally associated layer, also known as a thick layer, is one in which each input is linked to each output using learnable weights. When features are determined by convolutional layers and down-examined by pooling layers, they are planned to the network's final yields, by a subset of entirely associated layers. In most cases, the final entirely associated layer has the same number of resultant hubs as classes [20].

9.4.3   IMAGE CLASSIFICATION

Classifying images is defining the way toward grouping pictures as indicated with visual substance. The training process for NNs includes perceiving thermograms of breasts with identified labels, for example, normal and up-normal. This test is called the supervised learning [21]. During the classification of an item into various classes, CNNs regularly settle on a decision based on probabilistic perspective, which is named inference. This indicates that probabilities are nothing but an array of numbers somewhere in the range of 0 and 1. One type of resulting model with the Softmax function that determines the possibility of an event being appropriated. In CNNs, the Softmax function computes the likelihood of a resultant picture over the conceivable target classes.

9.5   REVIEW ON BREAST CANCER USING THERMOGRAPHS AND DEEP LEARNING

Samir and Shivajirao [22] introduced an impressive proof in which thermography is a significant and underestimate technique. They utilized a novel machine learning approach (CNN) over conventional artificial intelligence methods to characterize bosom disease using warm pictures. They utilized two pre-trained transfer learning models, VGG16 and InceptionV3, to optimize execution of their gauge CNN model and outcome obtained from the InceptionV3 model is better than that of VGG16. In the same year Ekici and Jawzal [23] created programming for early identification of bosom malignancy, which utilizes picture preparing methods and calculations to break down thermal breast images to distinguish the indications of the cell deterioration in these pictures. Utilizing this new technique, the features will be separated from the warm pictures caught using thermal cameras, and could be utilized to group the breast pictures as ordinary or abnormal through utilizing convolutional neural networks (CNNs) streamlined based on Bayes algorithm. In another investigation by Hossein et al. [24] they introduced a new strategy dependent on a computer-supported diagnosis innovation for the early discovery of sickness in patients with asymptomatic breast malignancy. Since in thermography the areas with high temperatures are inclined to physiological issues, the designed method depends on the factual examples of the worm districts of the breast. Along these lines, they attempted to distinguish irregular warmth patterns by introducing fitting features in thermal images depending on a progression of patient pictures and DNN methods for enhancing the precision of finding variations in bosom cancer.

Iqbal et al. [25] introduced a complete report for the early discovery of bosom cancer. They investigated the prescient exactness of various CNN designs: resnet18, resnet34, resnet50, resnet152, VGG16, and VGG19, to group patients with bosom cancer versus normal utilizing thermographies. They have indicated that Resnet lingering models show amazing outcomes in the arrangement of carcinoma from thermographies, particularly Resnet18, Resnet34, and Resnet50. Furthermore, expanding the quantity of layers does not optimize the approval exactness, when contrasted with the outcomes obtained for Resnet152. Resnet structures show a better presentation than VGG models. Oliveira and Grassano [26] introduced a novel procedure relying on an inceptionV3 coupled with k-Nearest Neighbors (InceptionV3-KNN) and a specific segment that they named StageCancer. These methods prevail to order breast cancer into four phases (T1: non-obtrusive bosom disease; T2: the tumor matches 2 cm; T3: when the tumor is larger than 5 cm; and T4: the full bosom is covered by malignant growth). They detailed that it is the first occasion when that such classification is finished utilizing warm pictures of the bosoms. Their outcomes guarantee that infrared imaging combined with a ground-breaking PC Help Gadget (computer-aided design) can prompt an exact tumor finder.

Juan Pablo et al. [27], they propose a computerized examination to survey the abilities of DNNs for bosom thermogram classifications. All pictures were ordered with seven diverse deep learning pre-prepared structures. The DNNs VGG16 demonstrated the best execution, accomplishing an accuracy of 91.18%. The outcomes recommend that bosom disease thermography related to DNN can be utilized as subordinate to mammography for pre-screening, despite the fact that there are still bogus positives. Information growth has appeared to expand exactness of DNN with a restricted dataset, for example, for their situation. Fernández-Ovies et al. [28] introduced a CNN-based technique for bosom disease analysis utilizing warm pictures. They indicated that an all-around delimited dataset split strategy is required to diminish the inclination and over-fitting through the preparation stage; in this manner their exploratory outcomes affirm that. Furthermore, their paper passes on the primary cutting-edge benchmark of CNN models, for example, ResNet, SeResNet, VGG16, Inception, Inception ResNetV2, and Xception for the dataset from Mastology Research with Infrared Image (DMR-IR) dataset. Similarly, this investigation builds up the primary CNN hyper-boundaries streamlining in a thermography dataset for bosom disease, where the top CNN model accomplished 92% exactness. They showed that the compromise between database size and data enlargement procedures is critical in classification assignments lacking adequate information.

Iqbal et al. [25] introduced the framework of thermography-based application-explicit Advanced Back End processor for a shrewd screening tool. Thermal pictures of the chest taken by infrared cameras are pre-prepared to specify the districts of interest. To ensure productive equipment, texture features are deliberately chosen, which are then taken off to a double classifier, dependent on trained linear support vector machine and CNN to choose the decision boundary. The presented framework accomplishes proficient equipment usage by misusing developed classifier. In 2018, Matheus and Lucas [26] built a supervised strategy for dissecting infrared thermography of bosoms for exact classification utilizing CNN that does not depend on selected features. They propose four procedures to decide how the unique convention fits better in a CNN algorithm. The outcomes demonstrated that their DL approach utilizing the shaded picture dataset gave great execution not as grayscale dataset for "static protocol" and those CNNs got outcomes for the two conventions: static and dynamic. They expect that since substantially more data about temperature is put into the shading set and CNN features catch patterns in a more productive way than selected feature selection. Following this investigation, Dalmia et al. [29] indicated that the division of problem areas in a thermal image is an intense issue generally because of the inaccessibility of large thermography datasets on bosoms, the absence of standardized information, and the reliance of caught warm pictures on mood, enthusiasm, and actual condition of the subject. In this study, they investigate different CNN models for semantic segmentation beginning with naive patch-based classifiers to more refined ones including a few varieties of the encoder–decoder network for recognizing the areas of interest in the warm pictures. The author suggested the importance of the utilization of multi-layered CNN for identification of areas of interest in infrared bosom warm pictures. Other works related to breast cancer thermography are reported concisely in Table 9.1.

TABLE 9.1
Review on Breast Cancer Thermography using Deep Learning

References	Task	Technique	Acquisition Protocol	Image Dimensions	Dataset	Accuracy (%)	CNN Models
[7]	Classification	FC-NNs	Dynamic protocol	3D image	2400 images of DDSM	97	FC-NNs
[22]	Classification	CNN	Static & Dynamic	3D image	1140 images of DMR-IR dataset	93.1	VGG16, Baseline, Inception-V3
[23]	Classification	CNN	Dynamic protocol	2D image	3895 images of visual lab dataset	96.7	Bayes optimization
[30]	Classification	CNN	Dynamic protocol	2D image	680 images of visual lab dataset	95.8	ReLU
[31]	Classification	CNN	Static & Dynamic	3D image	1140 images of DMR-IR dataset	91.32	TensorFlow
[24]	Classification	DNN	Dynamic protocol	2D image	1,960 images from Vision Lab	96.77	Sparse
[32]	Classification	DNN	Dynamic protocol	2D image	1062 images from Vision Lab	91.8	InceptionV3-KNN
[28]	Classification	CNN	Dynamic protocol	3D image	2,411 images from Vision Lab	96	ResNet 18, ResNet 34, ResNet 50, ResNet 152, VGG16 & VGG19
[25]	Classification	CNN	Dynamic protocol	3D image	7800 images from Vision Lab	91.8	VGG16 & VGG19
[33]	Classification	CNN	Static protocol	3D image	37 images of DMR-IR dataset	93.42	SMO classifier
[34]	Classification	CNN	Static & Dynamic	3D image	1140 images of DMR-IR dataset	94	ResNet101, DenseNet, MobileNetV2 & ShuffleNetV2
[35]	Classification	CNN	Static protocol	2D image	173 images of DMR-IR dataset	91.18	AlexNet, GoogLeNet, ResNet-50, ResNet-101, InceptionV3, VGG16 & VGG19
[27]	Classification	CNN	Dynamic protocol	2D image	1140 images of DMR-IR dataset	92	ResNet, SeResNet, VGG16, Inception, InceptionResNetV2 and Xception
[26]	Classification	CNN	static & dynamic	2D image	1017 images of DMR-IR dataset	95	ResNet 50, VGG16 & VGG19
[29]	Classification	CNN	Dynamic protocol	2D image	750 images of visual lab dataset	92.1	U-Net, V-Net, VGGNet & InputCascade CNN

9.6 CONCLUSION

Early breast cancer recognition remains fundamental to bosom disease control. Bosom self-assessment is prescribed by the World Health Organization to raise awareness in women about bosom malignancy hazards. Thermography is designed for performing an early localization via screening technique, and we accept that it gives a promising improvement for a self-screening strategy which would identify bosom malignancy at an early stage. An outline of breast thermograms may demonstrate that the early indications of bosom cancer can be seen through distinguishing the lopsided thermal conveyances between the bosoms.

The lopsided thermal distribution on bosom thermograms would be assessed using computer-aided innovation, which can limit mistakes. Our review has demonstrated that the present NN models have prompted an optimization in classification exactness of breast cancer thermograms, especially in distinguishing among normal and harmful cases. Nevertheless, the NNs model performance should be improved. Future research would see more efforts in improving bosom thermogram classification. This will need delegate datasets, preparing enlarged ROIs, allocating kernels, and executing "lightweight" CNN models. Accomplishment of these goals will abbreviate the time relating to convolution calculation and increment precision rates. A free detection technique utilizing thermography can then be built for self-bosom detection tool at a beginning phase without requiring actual inclusion of tissues.

REFERENCES

[1] IAFR Cancer. Global Cancer Observatory [Online]. Available: http://gco.iarc.fr/ Accessed: Feb. 3, 2021.
[2] C. Nickson and A.M. Kavanagh, "Tumour size at detection according to different measures of mammographic breast density," *J. Med. Screening*, vol. 16, no. 3, pp. 140–46, Sep. 2009.
[3] S.A. Narod, "Tumour size predicts long-term survival among women with lymph node-positive breast cancer," *Current Oncol.*, vol. 19, no. 5, pp. 249–53, Sep. 2012.
[4] OncoLink Team, Jan. 2021. All About Breast Cancer. [Online]. Available: https://www.oncolink.org/cancers/breast/all-about-breast-cancer
[5] *Breast Cancer: Prevention and Control.* World Health Organization, Geneva, Switzerland, 2019.
[6] H. Chougrad, H. Zouaki, and O. Alheyane, "Deep convolutional neural networks for breast cancer screening," *Comput. Methods Programs Biomed.*, vol. 157, pp. 19–30, Apr. 2018.
[7] M.A. Al-Masni, M.A. Al-Antari, J.-M. Park, G. Gi, T.-Y. Kim, P. Rivera, E. Valarezo, M.-T. Choi, S.-M. Han, and T.-S. Kim, "Simultaneous detection and classification of breast masses in digital mammograms via a deep learning YOLO-based CAD system," *Comput. Methods Programs Biomed.*, vol. 157, pp. 85–94, Apr. 2018.
[8] J. Arevalo, F.A. González, R. Ramos-Pollán, J. L. Oliveira, and M.A.G. Lopez, "Representation learning for mammography mass lesion classification with convolutional neural networks," *Comput. Methods Programs Biomed.*, vol. 127, pp. 248–57, Apr. 2016
[9] D. Bardou, K. Zhang, and S. M. Ahmad, "Classification of breast cancer based on histology images using convolutional neural networks," *IEEE Access*, vol. 6, pp. 24680–93, 2018.

[10] X. Zhou, T. Kano, H. Koyasu, S. Li, T. Hara, X. Zhou, M. Matsuo, and H. Fujita, "Automated assessment of breast tissue density in non-contrast 3D CT images without image segmentation based on a deep CNN," *Proc. SPIE*, vol. 10134, Mar. 2017, Art. no. 101342Q.

[11] H. Li, J. Weng, Y. Shi, W. Gu, Y. Mao, Y. Wang, W. Liu, and J. Zhang, "An improved deep learning approach for detection of thyroid papillary cancer in ultrasound images," *Sci. Rep.*, vol. 8, no. 1, pp. 1–12, Dec. 2018.

[12] S.S. Patra, O.P. Jena, G. Kumar, S. Pramanik, C. Misra, and K.N. Singh, "Random Forest Algorithm in Imbalance Genomics Classification." In: *Data Analytics in Bioinformatics: A Machine Learning Perspective*, Wiley Scrivener Publication, 2021. https://doi.org/10.1002/9781119785620.ch7.

[13] P. Pattnayak and O.P. Jena, "Innovation on Machine Learning in Healthcare Services-An Introduction." In: *Machine Learning for Healthcare Applications*, pp. 1–14, Wiley Scrivener Publisher, 2021. https://doi.org/10.1002/9781119792611.ch1

[14] N. Panigrahi, I. Ayus and O.P. Jena, "An Expert System-Based Clinical Decision Support System for Hepatitis-B Prediction and Diagnosis." In: O. P. Jena, S.N. Mohanty, G. Nalinipriya and A. Sarkar (Eds.)*Machine Learning for Healthcare Applications*, pp. 57–75, Wiley Scrivener Publisher, 2021. https://doi.org/10.1002/9781119792611.ch4

[15] K. Paramesha, H.L Gururaj, and O.P. Jena, "Applications of Machine Learning in Biomedical Text Processing and Food Industry." In: *Machine Learning for Healthcare Applications*, pp. 151–67, Wiley Scrivener Publisher, 2021. https://doi.org/10.1002/9781119792611.ch10

[16] A. Hassan, M. Nasr, and W. Saber, "The future of Internet of Things for anomalies detection using thermography", *International Journal of Advanced Networking and Applications (IJANA)*, vol. 11, no. 1, pp. 4142–49 (2019).

[17] G. Ahmad, Z. Iman, G. Hossein, and H. Javad, "A review of the dedicated studies to breast cancer diagnosis by thermal imaging in the fields of medical and artificial intelligence sciences," *Biomedical Research*, vol. 27, no. 2, pp. 543–52, 2016.

[18] Thermobiological, 2016. Available at: http://www.breastthermography.com/breast_thermography_ proc.htm

[19] R. C. Gonzalez, "Deep convolutional neural networks [lecture notes]," *IEEE Signal Process. Mag.*, vol. 35, no. 6, pp. 79–87, Nov. 2018.

[20] R. Yamashita, M. Nishio, R. K.G. Do, and K. Togashi, "Convolutional neural networks: An overview and application in radiology," *Insights Image*, vol. 9, no. 4, pp. 611–29, Aug. 2018.

[21] O. Simeone, "A brief introduction to machine learning for engineers," *Found. Trends Signal Process*, vol. 12, nos. 3–4, pp. 200–431, 2018.

[22] Y. Samir and J. Shivajirao, "Thermal infrared imaging based breast cancer diagnosis using machine learning techniques," *Multimedia Tools and Applications*, 2020. https://doi.org/10.1007/s11042-020-09600-3

[23] S. Ekici and H. Jawzal, "Breast cancer diagnosis using thermography and convolutional neural networks," *Medical Hypotheses*, 2020 Apr, 137, pp. 109542. https://doi.org/10.1007/s11042-020-09600-310.1016/j.mehy.2019.109542

[24] H. Zadeh, A. Fayazi, B. Binazir, and M. Yargholi, "Breast cancer diagnosis based on feature extraction using dynamic models of thermal imaging and deep autoencoder neural networks," *Journal of Testing and Evaluation* 49, 2020, https://doi.org/10.1520/JTE20200044

[25] H. Iqbal, B. Majeed, U. Khan and M. A. Bin Altaf, "An Infrared High Classification Accuracy Hand-held Machine Learning based Breast-Cancer Detection System," *2019 IEEE Biomedical Circuits and Systems Conference (BioCAS)*, pp. 1–4, Nara, Japan, 2019. https://doi.org/10.1109/BIOCAS.2019.8918687

[26] M. Oliveira and L. Grassano, "Convolutional Neural Networks for Static and Dynamic Breast Infrared Imaging Classification," *2018 31st SIBGRAPI Conference on Graphics, Patterns and Images (SIBGRAPI)*, pp. 174–81, Parana, Brazil, 2018. https://doi.org/10.1109/SIBGRAPI.2018.00029

[27] Z. Juan Pablo, A. Zein, B. Khaled, M. Safa, and Z. Noureddine, "A CNN-based methodology for breast cancer diagnosis using thermal images." *Computer Methods in Biomechanics and Biomedical Engineering: Imaging & Visualization*, pp. 1–15, 2020. https://doi.org/10.1080/21681163.2020.1824685

[28] F.J. Fernández-Ovies, S. Alférez-Baquero, E.J. de Andrés-Galiana, A. Cernea, Z. Fernández-Muñiz, and J.L. Fernández-Martínez, Detection of Breast Cancer Using Infrared Thermography and Deep Neural Networks. In: Rojas I., Valenzuela O., Rojas F., and Ortuño F. (eds), *Bioinformatics and Biomedical Engineering. IWBBIO 2019. Lecture Notes in Computer Science*, Pp 513-524 vol. 11466, 2019, Springer Publisher, Cham. https://doi.org/10.1007/978-3-030-17935-9_46

[29] A. Dalmia, S.T. Kakileti, and M. Geetha, "Exploring Deep Learning Networks for Tumour Segmentation in Infrared Images." *14th Quantitative InfraRed Thermography Conference*, 25 – 29 June 2018, Berlin, Germany, 2018. https://doi.org/10.21611/qirt.2018.052

[30] S. Mishra, A. Prakash, S. K. Roy, P. Sharan, and N. Mathur, "Breast Cancer Detection using Thermal Images and Deep Learning," *2020 7th International Conference on Computing for Sustainable Global Development (INDIACom)*, pp. 211–216, New Delhi, India, 2020. doi: https://doi.org/10.23919/INDIACom49435.2020.9083722

[31] M. Farooq and P. Corcoran, "Infrared Imaging for Human Thermography and Breast Tumor Classification using Thermal Images," *2020 31st Irish Signals and Systems Conference (ISSC)*, pp. 1–6, Letterkenny, Ireland, 2020. doi: 10.1109/ISSC49989.2020.9180164

[32] M. Sebastien., O. Krejcar, P. Maresova, A. Selamat, and K. Kuca, Novel Four Stages Classification of Breast Cancer Using Infrared Thermal Imaging and a Deep Learning Model. In: Rojas I., Valenzuela O., Rojas F., and Ortuño F. (eds), *Bioinformatics and Biomedical Engineering. IWBBIO 2019. Lecture Notes in Computer Science*, vol. 11466, Springer, Cham, 2019. https://doi.org/10.1007/978-3-030-17935-9_7

[33] S. Tello-Mijares, F. Woo, and F. Flores, "Breast cancer identification via thermography image segmentation with a gradient vector flow and a convolutional neural network." *Journal of Healthcare Engineering*, 2019, Article ID 9807619. https://doi.org/10.1155/2019/9807619

[34] R. Roslidar, K. Saddami, F. Arnia, M. Syukri, and K. Munadi, "A Study of Fine-Tuning CNN Models Based on Thermal Imaging for Breast Cancer Classification," *2019 IEEE International Conference on Cybernetics and Computational Intelligence (CyberneticsCom)*, pp. 77–81, Banda Aceh, Indonesia, 2019. https://doi.org/10.1109/CYBERNETICSCOM.2019.8875661

[35] J. Torres-Galván, E. Guevara and F. J. González, "Comparison of Deep Learning Architectures for Pre-Screening of Breast Cancer Thermograms," *2019 Photonics North (PN)*, pp. 1–2, Quebec City, QC, Canada, 2019. https://doi.org/10.1109/PN.2019.8819587

10 Deep Learning Frameworks for Prediction, Classification and Diagnosis of Alzheimer's Disease

Nitin Singh Rajput, Mithun Singh Rajput, and Purnima Dey Sarkar

CONTENTS

10.1 INTRODUCTION

Alzheimer's disease (AD) is one of the significant and common appearances of progressive dementia. Pathogenesis of AD is represented by two attributes: development of extra-cellular senile plaquette made up of insolvable amyloid beta peptide along with intraneural gathering of neuro-fibrillary entangles of accumulated hyperphosphorylated tau [1]. It also causes gliosis, defined as a widespread modification of glial cells [2]. These hallmarks are significant advents of AD; although, the ultimate situation of this disorder remains imperceptible. It is anticipated that worldwide one out

DOI: 10.1201/9781003226147-10

183

of eighty-five individuals will be touched by this disease by the year 2050 [3]. Thus, in order to have an effective management and to retard or avert the disease progression, excessive efforts are underway to come up with strategies for early detection, classification, and diagnosis of AD. Particularly progressive neuroimaging and other techniques *viz.* magnetic-resonance-imaging (MRI), positron-emission-tomography (PET), computed-tomography (CT), microscopy, X-ray, etc. are commonly used to recognize anatomical as well as molecular biomarkers pertaining to this disease [4]. Speedy advancement in neuroimaging technologies has complicated the process of amalgamating extensive, multi-dimensional multimodal data related to neuroimaging. Consequently, attention has been shooting up rapidly in computer-based ML techniques aiming at integrative investigations for AD.

ML comes under the umbrella of artificial intelligence (AI), which studies multi-faceted associations among variables in data and these algorithms have been categorized as supervised, unsupervised, and reinforcement learning [5]. So as to solicit ML algorithms, pre-processing phases and proper architectural design must be ensured [6]. Sorting studies with the aid of ML usually requires feature mining, feature assortment, reduction in dimensions of data, and choice of classification algorithm based on the features. Such requirements could be fulfilled with focused knowledge and optimization, which may lack in reproduction and may be time-consuming [6]. With purpose of removing these limitations, DL, a special class of ML techniques, has been employed in AD research. DL is a subclass of ML, which acquires features from a hierarchical learning method where depictions are inevitably revealed from raw data [7]. DL algorithms engage numerous, deep layers made up of perceptron algorithm that apprehends both low-level and high-level data depictions, permitting them to acquire more affluent notions of inputs [7]. This precludes the necessity of manually engineered structures and permits DL structures to automatically discover formerly unknown models apart from simplifying various types of data. Modified versions of such algorithms have been effectively used in the area of medicine and other engineering fields [8].

In neurodegenerative disease research, DL uses first-hand data, acquired by neuroimaging, to produce features via on-the-fly learning and it has been gaining valuable consideration in the context of extensive, multidimensional analysis of medical images. For instance, DL methods, like convolutional neural networks (CNN), are used to show faster growth in comparison to prevailing ML approaches [9]. DL techniques are performing a progressive vital part in neurological research, addressing complications in various sub-domains. Initially, sorting the images and partitioning was the focus point of DL advancement. Such functions are exclusively suited to DL due to many neuroimaging data obtained by manual analysis. Gradually, DL techniques are applied to efficient brain mapping along with related areas, with the aid of neuroimaging data for various tasks like early detection and classification. Lately, DL-based diagnostic studies taking select data types, laboratory outcomes, and images into account are used to pinpoint AD risk. Considering these facts, in this chapter, we discuss the various models for scrutiny of neuroimaging data using DL approaches for the early prediction, classification, and diagnosis of AD.

Figure 10.1 illustrates the generalized scheme for early detection, classification, and diagnosis of AD. This scheme is employed for various datasets such as MRI, PET, CT, and cerebro-spinal fluid (CSF) to study the outcomes. In this chapter, select studies, which are following the technique specified in Figure 10.1, have been taken

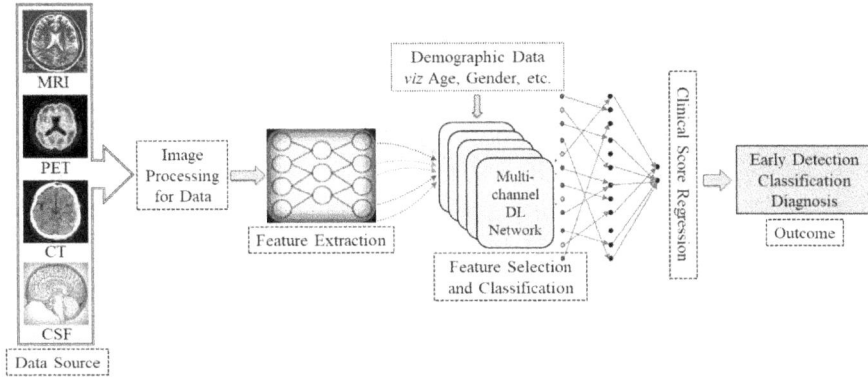

FIGURE 10.1   Illustration of DL framework for detection, classification, and diagnosis of AD.

into account. Here, images from various sources are pre-processed and then feature extraction, selection, and classification are performed using DL methods and, after that, the outcome is considered to detect, classify, and diagnose AD.

10.2   DL-BASED PREDICTION OF AD

It is a multifaceted and challenging job to envisage the early incidence of an ailment, hence to overcome such a challenge, in the previous few decades various investigators of eminent fields provided various applications of ML techniques in healthcare systems for early prediction and classification of numerous diseases [10]. Early detection is crucial for tangible management of AD, and ML has been used in the past for the auxiliary diagnosis of AD. However, most prevailing technologies need manual parameter setting, show only single view data, and emphasize only two-class (i.e. dementia or not) classification complications [11]. Therefore, it is conceivable to develop more efficacious and precise automatic prediction and diagnosis methods for AD and mild cognitive impairment by integrating complementary information of different modalities.

A multi-view clustering model has been proposed by Zhang et al. [11] that improves the AD prediction as well as screening and classifying various AD stages based upon symptoms. The consensus multi-view clustering (CMC) constructed on non-negative matrix factorization and has the capacity to fully extract data structures with limited medical images. This framework does not require manual setting of parameters and do not require approaches that indicate relations among various entities. This model also attains a representation comprising common features, and corresponding information of multi-view data [11].

Kim et al. [12] combined in silico and DL-based investigations and proposed a potential tactic for recognizing the clinical usefulness of critical AD-specific single-nucleotide variants (SNVs) in prediction of AD. The researchers used a DL-based exon splicing prediction tool, proficient with human genome arrangements and projected 14 splicing sites in human phospholipase c gamma-1 (PLCγ1) gene. It was found that one of these entirely harmonized with an SNV in exon 27 of PLCγ1 gene in an AD mouse model, thus exon splicing utilized DL in AD prediction [12].

An integrated framework comprising DL, feature assortment, unpremeditated interpretation, and analysis of genetic-imaging data has been developed by Liu et al. [13] in order to predict and further study AD. This resulted in enhanced precision in prediction, identification of brain loci impairment due to disease, and knowledge of pathways from genetic variations to AD with the aid of image intervention [13]. In order to predict the subset of patients with mild cognitive decline who would head toward development of AD, an innovative multimodal data combination framework containing DL of characteristics of sMRI and dynamic functional connectivity (dFC) based mining of fMRI features have been fabricated. The multimodal (sMRI-fMRI) blending of data confirmed a significant enhancement in performance in comparison with the unimodal investigations with the fMRI and sMRI modalities. As such, the discoveries highlight the advantages of merging multiple neuroimaging data modes via data fusion, validate the projecting value of the tested DL and dFC features and contend in favor of exploration of similar approaches to learn neuroanatomical and functional alterations in the neuroimaging data [14]. Prediction and early diagnosis of AD based on electroencephalogram (EEG) signal-based investigations has gained valuable attention in the diagnostic field. Kim and Kim [15] proposed a classifier based on DNN using the relative power to fully achieve and reunite the features via its own learning structure. In comparison to shallow neural networks, the DNN improved AD early prediction and diagnosis, and also empowered result interpretation, as the relative power attributes have been used as the domain knowledge [15]. Clinical scores have been obtained from MRI data for early prediction of AD based on a DL model that combines a joint learning-based feature selection built upon standardization of correntropy – feature encoding based on deep polynomial network and support vector regression [16].

Table 10.1 summarizes various DL frameworks for the early prediction of AD using multiple datasets. It shows the outcome for early prediction of AD considering various schemes and select datasets.

10.2.1 Prediction of Amyloidogenicity

Brain amyloids are a specific kind of protein mass that are typical features of AD and exhibit a specific diffraction-like pattern during X-ray. Some experimental procedures allow identifying these peptides; however, they are expensive and tedious and hence unsuitable for genome-wide investigations and need alternative prediction models [2].

Wojciechowski and Kotulska [17] proposed a new structure-based technique combined with ML tactics for predicting amyloidogenicity, termed PATH (Prediction of Amyloidogenicity by THreading). It has been demonstrated that relating existing structures of amyloidogenic fragments improves prediction performance of AD [17]. Several ML techniques are employed on various steady classes of query peptide, using their energy terms. Also, these methods give insights into possibly the most steady structural group of peptides when kept open in a crystallizing environment [17].

Scoring schemes that are semi-quantitative in nature, like the Consortium to Establish a Registry for Alzheimer's Disease (CERAD) created on ML tactics, have produced numerical results for whole slide images, which were linked with semi-quantified results derived by people for AD pathology [27]. Vizcarra et al. [18]

TABLE 10.1

Deep Learning Models in Early Prediction of Dementia of the Alzheimer Type

Method	Dataset	Imaging/ Technique	Number of Subjects (n)	Outcome	Reference
NMF-based CMC	ADNI	MRI	1870	Accuracy 5% higher than existing method (WRMK)	[11]
PATH	Protein Data Bank	Modeller 9.21	1080 hexapeptides	AUC of 0.87	[17]
CNN	Data from individuals	CERAD	40	Measurable differentiation among groups (p < 0.05)	[18]
CNN	ADNI	MRI	509	Accuracy rate 0.84	[19]
SlideNet	Data from individuals	PET	2	AUC greater than 0.85 for all cases	[20]
CNN	ADNI	MRI	785	AUC of 0.92	[21]
DBN	ADNI	FDG-PET	109	Accuracy of 83.9%	[22]
DCNN	ADNI	DTI	151	Prediction accuracy 0.7463 at 24 m	[13]
SNN	ADNI and BIOCARD	MRI	3566	Sensitivity 0.82 and specificity 0.97	[23]
MRNN	ADNI	MRI, PET and other biological markers	1618	Accuracy 81%	[24]
ResNet	ADNI	sMRI-fMRI data fusion framework	134	Significant outperform (p < 0.001)	[14]
CNN	ADNI and AIBL	MRI	2146	Concordance index greater than 0.70	[25]
CTDE	ADNI	MRI	805	R value for MMSE at 36 m is 0.85	[16]
DNN	Data from individuals	EEG	20	Correct classification rate (CCR) more than 50%	[15]
MSH-ELM	ADNI	MRI, FDG-PET, and CSF biomarkers	202	Accuracy of 96.10%	[26]

confirmed these ML algorithms by means of CNNs and showed that the pathological heterogeneity might modify the outcome parameters of the algorithm. Their findings authenticate CNN models as reliable and robust in scenarios like cohort disparities and deliver additional concept proving for futuristic investigations to include ML techniques into neuro-pathological applications [18].

10.2.2 PREDICTION OF TAU PROTEIN ABNORMALITY

Accumulation of anomalous tau type protein entities in brain regions is a compulsive attribute of AD and is the finest predictor of neural damage and clinical deterioration [28]. Ample PET data tracers aimed at tau protein are available for research purposes. However, authentication of these data tracers in contradiction to direct recognition of tau protein accumulation in brain tissue leftovers is inadequate due to methodological limitations. In order to decrypt the existence and positioning of tau abnormalities and validate PET tau tracers, a convolutional neuronal network SlideNet has been designed to process large datasets. This computational method aims at creating a quantitative, three-dimensional (3D) tau density map and exhibits an outcome of great efficacy with an AUC of 0.89 [20]. A multimodal sparse hierarchical extreme learning machine (MSH-ELM) system was implicated on volume and mean intensity obtained from Fluoro-Deoxy-Glucose-PET (FDG-PET), MRI, and CSF features (viz. tau and amyloid beta) by means of a sparse Extreme Learning Machine Auto Encoder (sELM-AE). The MSH-ELM method exhibited an accuracy of 96.10% in distinguishing healthy individual to that of AD patient [26].

10.2.3 PREDICTION OF TRANSITION FROM MILD COGNITIVE IMPAIRMENT TO AD

Some mild cognitive impairment clinically progresses to AD, while others have a tendency to remain steady and do not develop to AD. Hence, to discriminate a patient with light cognitive impairments that holds a chance of growing AD, personalized and effective strategies are required. Among numerous DL schemes which are functional in evaluating variations in the brain that emerge at structural levels during MRI, CNN has added acceptance because of its excellent competence in automatic process of feature learning by employing diversified multi-layer perceptron.

In order to detect early changes or ascertaining the possibility of converting light cognitive decline in AD, Pan et al. [19] developed a classifier unit by integrating CNN with EL, which could be implied on MRI data. A variety of CNN-based schemes are developed by using a bunch of MRI scan datasets which are unified into a single ensemble and the performance is assessed using stratified fivefold cross validation scheme. CNN-EL technique is capable of detecting the most distinguishable brain locus having generalization capacity of the ensemble technique for effective early capturing of neural disparities for AD development [19]. Spasov et al. [21] investigated a new DL framework, formed on dual-learning and an ad-hoc layer to distinguish 3D densities, which aims at categorizing patients with mild cognitive impairment who might be at high risk of developing AD in the next three years. This DL technique combines demographic, structural MRI, neuropsychological, and APOe4 genetic data to form the input and provides an outcome with 86.00% accuracy [21]. Similarly, with the aid of FDG-PET scans, Shen et al. [22] developed a deep belief network (DBN) based method to recognize persons with mild cognitive impairment phase and pre-indicative AD. It also identifies and segregates them from other persons who only have mild cognitive impairment. The classification accuracy was found to be more than 80% [22].

Recently, asymmetries in anatomical shape and volume of brain were realized in the course of AD, which could possibly be utilized as pre-clinical imaging bio-markers to predict and discriminate AD with light cognitive impairment. In order to utilize the discrimination influence of whole brain volume asymmetry, MRICloud pipeline – a DL model using Siamese neural networks (SNN) – has been used by Liu et al. [23]. SNN found to be effectively functional to the discrimination of normal people, patients with mild cognitive decline, and symptomatic cases of AD with the help of the kernel normalized whole brain anatomical volumetric asymmetry encoding features [23]. Lee et al. [24] showed the applicability of multimodal recurrent neural network (MRNN) while predicting conversion of mild cognitive impairment to AD. The developed scheme integrates longitudinal multi-domain data which combines longitudinal CSF and cognitive performance biomarkers with cross-section of neuro-imaging biomarkers gained from AD neuro-imaging initiative (ADNI). This model yielded an accuracy of up to 75% [24].

10.3   DL-BASED CLASSIFICATION OF AD

Sensing a medical anomaly is typically measured to be a composite task performed by domain specialists and physicians. DL is a time-saving technique exhibiting stable, precise, and reproducible outcomes by automating labor-intensive procedures. Moreover, there is a substantial quantity of data in medicine, the blending of which with a trivial sample size of pathological cases makes vital practice of DL tactics for classifying the ailment [29]. Dementia is generally classified based on the global deterioration scale (GDS) which is subjected to the worth of cognitive decline and divides AD into seven stages. In GDS, early dementia is represented by the fourth stage and middle dementia comes under the fifth and sixth stages [30]. In order to facilitate the communication among medical professionals and the families in dementia research, another scale termed the clinical dementia rating (CDR) is used. Various parameters like memory, problem solving, judgment, orientation, and hobbies have been assessed and CDR scores are assigned [31]. Ambiguity among neurons and shortcomings in communication gives rise to detect planning and judgment [32]. This process requires time, ample efforts and domain experts to extract features. Hence, for classification and precise diagnosis of AD, many computer-aided diagnosis systems (CADS) have been set up [33] (Table 10.2).

Today, efforts are being made to extract the features from medical images (X-ray, microscopy, MRI, PET, CT etc.) by establishing DL techniques and models to classify dementia [34]. The basis of these DL techniques is binary classification, which clearly distinguishes whether the person is bearing AD or not [35]. Object detection and image classification have gained ample progress by a huge number of labeled datasets. For instance, implication of CNNs in automatic feature extraction of medical images has been used by many models for AD classification [36].

10.3.1   CLASSIFICATION USING MRI DATA

Lately, a lot of ML techniques have been modified and used to deem fit and classify the dementia of the Alzheimer type. Hu et al. [37] collected a big unit of 3D T1-weighted structural MRI data from neuroimaging in frontotemporal dementia (NIFD) and ADNI, the two openly accessible databases. Researchers gave training to a DL-founded network, which is directly created using first-hand T1 images to categorize Alzheimer's disease and frontotemporal dementia. In this process an outcome of 91.83% accuracy has been received [37]. Suh et al. [38] used a dataset of T1-weighted MRI to develop a two-step algorithm using CNN and differentiated AD from light cognitive impairment having sensitivity as high as 68% and having

TABLE 10.2

Deep Learning Models in Classification of Dementia of the Alzheimer Type

Method	Dataset	Imaging/ Technique	Number of Subjects (n)	Outcome	Reference
DL (Backpropagation algorithm)	ADNI and NIFD	MRI	4099	Accuracy of 91.83%	[37]
XGBoost	ADNI and OASIS	MRI	2727	Sensitivity of 68.00% and specificity of 70.00%	[38]
FCN	ADNI, AIBL, FHS, NACC	MRI	1483	Accuracy of 75.00% to 95.00% for various dataset	[39]
SCNN inspired by OxfordNet architecture	OASIS	MRI	382	Accuracy of 99.05%	[40]
CNN and 3D DenseNet	ADNI	MRI	449	Accuracy of 88.90%	[41]
CNN	Data from individuals	MRI	48	Accuracy of 73.00%	[42]
VCNN	ADNI	MRI	695	Accuracy of 86.60%	[36]
DM2L	ADNI MIRIAD, AIBL	MRI	1984	AUC of 0.986	[43]
ResNet-50	OASIS	MRI	4139	Accuracy of 99.34%	[44]
CNN	Data from individuals	MRI	196	Accuracy of 97.65%	[45]
3LHPM-ICA	Data from individuals	rs-fMRI	34	Accuracy of 95.59%	[46]
3D CNN	ADNI	PET	300	Accuracy of 90.80%	[47]
2D deep CNN	Data from individuals	PET (18F-florbetaben scans)	430	Accuracy of 97.90%	[48]
CNN	Data from individuals	PET	160	Accuracy of 89.32%	[50]
CNN	ADNI	MRI and FDG-PET	1884	Accuracy of 85.00% to 95.00% for both dataset	[49]
CNN and RNN	ADNI	FDG-PET	339	Accuracy of 91.20%	[51]
DL algorithm	ADNI	MRI and PET	202	Accuracy of 91.40%	[52]

specificity around 70%. Moreover, Oh et al. [36] distinguished AD with light cognitive impairment with the aid of volumetric CNN and transfer learning in ADNI dataset using MRI with an accuracy of 86.60%.

A new DL-based framework has been developed by integrating a fully convolutional network (FCN) and a conventional multi-layer perceptron. It produces visualizations of AD risk, with higher resolutions. It could now be utilized to estimate the AD grade [39]. Moreover, aiming at reducing the dependencies on big scale datasets, Mehmood et al. [40] developed a Siamese Convolutional Neural Network (SCNN) which is based on VGG16 architecture to classify various stages of AD in better manner, that is, between no dementia and AD. In another study, attributes of the multi-task CNN and DenseNet have been utilized to automate hippocampal segmentation and classify the AD using structured MRI data [41]. A six-layer CNN model has been utilized by Wada et al. [42] based on MRI feature analysis to classify AD and distinguish it from dementia with Lewy body with an accuracy of 73.00%. Using a deep multi-task multi-channel learning (DM2L) scheme, Liu et al. [43] identified anatomical landmarks from MRI scans with the aid of data-driven algorithm and established a combined classification and regression framework for diagnosis of AD. Similar studies have been conducted by Fulton et al. [44], Wang et al. [45], and Qiao et al. [46] that extract data from MRI scans and utilize DL architecture for classification of AD.

10.3.2 Classification Using PET Data

Jo et al. [47] analyzed PET images using a DL framework, which integrates 3D CNN with layer-wise relevance propagation (LRP) algorithms to classify and detect AD with an accuracy of 90.80%. 18F-florbetaben scans were evaluated through DL-based models, which were trained by means of 2D PET images. It was found that DL was advantageous with high accuracy for clinical diagnosis and differentiation of AD with normal ones and in subjects who necessitate vigorous surveillance among equivocal cases [48]. In view of correctly identifying the virtual strength of MRI and FDG-PET, a research was taken up. It also classifies the dementia of the Alzheimer type in the ADNI dataset. The study was found to be beneficial with great accuracy. It also deliberates how the select data types might be influenced in imminent AD study using DL [49]. Iizuka et al. [50] differentiated among dementia of Lewy body to that of the Alzheimer type using DL-based PET analysis. Similar studies conducted by Liu et al. [51] and Li et al. [52] extract data from PET scans and classify AD using DL techniques.

Table 10.2 discuss various DL frameworks for classification of AD using multiple datasets. It contains the outcomes of select methods applied on different datasets to classify dementia of the Alzheimer's type.

10.4 DL-BASED DIAGNOSIS OF AD

Proper and early diagnosis of neurodegenerative progressions in the human brain is thought vital for initiating treatment and appropriate care. This may comprise sensing anatomical and functional cerebral alterations, for instance variations in the level of asymmetricity between the right and left hemispheres, and fluctuation in metabolites. With the speedy expansion of expertise in neuroimaging, it has become the utmost spontaneous and unfailing technique for the supplementary diagnosis of AD. Deviations in imaging data can be noticed by using a computing algorithm to diagnose dementia in the early stage and its various phases. It could help to screen the advancement of the disease [53] (Table 10.3).

TABLE 10.3

DL Models in Diagnosis of Dementia of the Alzheimer Type

Method	Dataset	Imaging/ Technique	Number of Subjects (n)	Outcome	Reference
CNN	ADNI	MRI	750	Accuracy of 90.50%	[54]
WSL-based DL (ADGNET)	KACD and ROAD	MRI	12800	Sensitivity of 99.69%	[55]
FCN	ADNI	fMRI	170	Accuracy of 85.20%	[56]
ANN and SVM-DA	Data from individuals (CSF)	Raman Spectroscopy	38	Sensitivity and specificity more than 80%	[83]
DMFNet	ADNI	MRI and PET	500	Accuracy of 95.21%	[72]
CNN	ADNI	MRI and DTI	406	Accuracy of 93.50%	[57]
TL (ResNet)	ADNI and OASIS	MRI	2179	Accuracy of 86.05%	[63]
3DAN	ADNI	MRI	1832	Accuracy of 72.00%	[60]
CNN	ADNI	MRI	1075	Accuracy of 97.01%	[61]
DNN	ADNI	MRI	801	Accuracy of 71.18%	[58]
RSBN	ADNI	fMRI	170	Accuracy more than 55% for various methods	[66]
3D CNN	ADNI	MRI	315	Accuracy of 98.06%	[59]
DL (multimodal fusion)	ADNI	MRI	72	Accuracy of 83.30%	[60]
SVM	ADNI	FDG-PET	466	Accuracy of 91.50%	[70]
CNN architecture Inception V3	ADNI	18F-FDG PET	1002	specificity of 82% and sensitivity of 100%	[71]
DL, RF, XGBoost	EMIF-AD	CSF metabolites	883	AUC greater than 0.85 for all	[84]
DNN	ADNI	MRI, PET and SNP	805	Accuracy of 90.00%	[74]
LUPI	ADNI	MRI and PET	103	Accuracy more than 85% for various algorithm	[75]
3D CNN	ADNI	MRI and FDG-PET	731	Accuracy of 87.46%	[78]
DNN	ADNI	MRI and FDG-PET	1242	Accuracy of 86.40%	[79]
MM-SDPN	ADNI	MRI and PET	202	Accuracy more than 95.00% for various classifiers	[76]
DNN	ADNI	MRI, PET and SNP	805	Accuracy of 65.00%	[74]
AAL (DL)	ADNI	MRI, PET and CSF and blood markers	818	Accuracy of 90.00%	[77]
SVMs, MLPs, RBNs, and DBNs	Data from individuals	Kinematic acquisition and assessment	108	Accuracy more than 70.00%	[85]

10.4.1 Diagnosis Using MRI Data

Herzog and Magoulas [54] proposed a low-cost method comprising a data dispensation pipeline that utilizes features of brain asymmetries, mined from the MRI dataset, to investigate organizational variations and to classify the pathology by make use of ML. This data-processing framework provides an outcome with great efficacy [54]. Weakly supervised learning (WSL) is a sub-class of supervised ML methods which utilizes actual feature illustration from inadequate or lower quality observations. Liang and Gu [55] proposed a WSL-based computer-aided AD diagnostic technique using ADGNET framework, which comprises a support network and a task network to sort and reform concurrent images for identifying and categorizing AD with the help of bounded annotations [55]. Functional connectivity networks oversee inter-region connections that restrict a service to diagnose brain diseases. In order to overcome from the disadvantage, a sliding window is utilized to produce R-fMRI subseries. Connections between such subseries are now employed to form a sequence of dynamic FCN, aiding AD diagnosis [56].

A study evaluating the influence of having multiple scans for each subject has been carried out by Marzban et al. [57] and suggests the proper drive to ascertain the robustness of the scheme. In this, MRI and diffusion tensor imaging (DTI) techniques indicating diffusion maps and volumes of grey matter have been used to obtain datasets and DL was employed for the objective of classification of AD [57]. Moreover, Lee et al. [58] proposed a novel model for MRI-based diagnosis of AD that scientifically blends region-, voxel- and patch-based techniques into a combined scheme [58]. Also, a novel and robust technique has been developed using 3D CNN topology to diagnose AD with the help of MRI data. This method utilizes Sobolev gradient-based optimization for every parameter of choice and provides an outcome of 98.06% accuracy [59]. Bi et al. [60] developed a novel multimodal data fusion technique for AD diagnosis, and additionally presents an innovative ML pipeline of data union, feature selection, sorting, and disease-producing feature extraction [60]. Similarly, many other researchers utilized DL and ML frameworks to analyze MRI data for the diagnosis of AD using various models (Bi et al. [61]; Jin et al. [62]; Puente-Castro et al. [63]; Basheera and Ram [64]; Cui et al. [65]; Ju et al. [66]; Esmaeilzadeh et al. [67]; Kam et al. [68]; and Li and Liu [69]).

10.4.2 Diagnosis Using PET Data

FDG-PET apprehends the metabolic movement of the brain. It is testified to recognize variations associated with AD before beginning of alterations in the structure. The low-level imaging features are the drawback of computer-aided AD diagnosis with the help of 18F-FDG PET imaging. This causes hurdles in attaining adequate classification accuracy or lack clinical implication. Hence, Li et al. [70] discovered a novel framework grounded on high-order features of radiomics mined from 18F-FDG PET brain images, which could be utilized for AD diagnosis. Similarly, CNN of InceptionV3 architecture was trained on 18F-FDG PET by Ding et al. [71] and obtained a high accuracy in diagnosis of AD.

10.4.3 Multimodal Diagnosis Using MRI and PET Data

An improved performance can be achieved by multimodal image classification if compared with single-modal image classification of AD. With the aid of select information, multimodal neuroimage classification of AD exhibits better performance compared to the single-modal classification. Based on attention mechanism, Zhang and Shi [72] developed a hierarchical multimodal fusion framework which can restrictively cite features from MRI data and PET data and subdue irrelevant information. Multimodality neuroimaging data like MRI and PET deliver valued information regarding brain anomalies while genetic data (single nucleotide polymorphism (SNP)) provide evidence of AD risk factors for patients. Used altogether, these data improve the efficacy in AD diagnosis, hence a three-stage DL and fusion model (combining MRI, genetic, and PET data) has been proposed comprising extraction of higher level features considering every modality solely, combining data and learning approaches [73]. Moreover, another three-stage DL model and a fusion model have been proposed by Zhou et al. [74] comprising MRI, PET, and SNP data.

Li et al. [75] proposed a learning using privileged information (LUPI) based computer-aided diagnosis framework for AD, in which data were moved from the supplementary PI to a diagnosis modality. In another study, multimodal stacked deep polynomial networks (MM-SDPNs) were used for AD diagnosis that consists of two-stage SDPNs. The first one is used for feature representation after which the data will be provided to the next SDPN for fusing multimodal neuroimaging data [76]. Another AD diagnostic method has been developed based on DL architectures practiced on brain areas mentioned by the automated anatomical labeling (AAL). Gray scale images from each area of brain are divided into 3D sub-images conferring to the sections defined by the AAL complete map. These sub-images are utilized for training of various DBN. Then, a group of DBN is constituted in which the end estimate is made by a voting mechanism that provides a potentially strong classification framework in which discriminatory structures are figured in an unsupervised manner [77]. Similarly, many other researchers utilized DL and ML framework for analyzing multimodal data for the diagnosis of AD using various models (Huang et al. [78]; Lu et al. [79]; Thung et al. [80]; Suk et al. [81]; and Suk et al. [82]).

10.4.4 Diagnosis Using Other Datasets

A novel, accurate, fast, and inexpensive method using Raman spectroscopy blended with ML tactics has been invented by Ryzhikova et al. [83] for AD diagnosis. For differentiation purposes, two methods viz. support vector machine discriminant analysis (SVM-DA) along with ANN are used. The method was found to be advantageous in detecting very small but specific disparities for AD, in the early phases of the disease [83]. Some studies have been proposed for testing metabolites action in blood to diagnose and classify AD in comparison with CSF biomarkers. DL along with Random Forest (RF) is utilized by Satmate et al. [84] to diagnose AD with the help of plasma metabolites. These modalities were internally authenticated with the aid of nested cross validation (NCV). Costa et al. [85] made comparisons between MLPs, SVMs, DBNs, and RBNs based on diseased of AD, who is exposed to select progressively difficult postural tasks (total seven) composed of 18 kinematic variables. Considering decision-making space which completely depends on postural kinematics, accuracy of AD diagnosis was found vary between 71.7% and 86.1% [85].

Table 10.3 represents various DL frameworks to diagnose dementia of the Alzheimer type. It shows the size of the datasets and the results for select frameworks that are considered for diagnosis of AD.

10.5 LIMITATIONS AND CHALLENGES IN DL-BASED DETECTION, CLASSIFICATION, AND DIAGNOSIS OF AD

Advances in technology will improve the healthcare services [86] through inferences of biomedical test processing with superior analytics [87, 88] and other domains like genomics classification [89] and food industry [90]. Prevailing ML and DL models are proficient in scoring AD classification, prediction, and diagnosis, but exhibit some limitations, such as:

1. immense computational resources are needed in order to train DL architecture on large numbers of medical images;
2. as the standard data can be costly and bounded with privacy ethics matters, it is burdensome to obtain standard training datasets and ample amount of such datasets is required in order to train model appropriately; and
3. a more precise, focused and monotonous regulation of various parameters is required throughout training the model on medical imaging as any error may result in overfitting complications and disturb the overall execution of the model [40].

Focusing on DL-based diagnosis of AD, in addition to aforementioned limitations, current techniques may have two shortcomings. Primarily, they mostly concentrate on the prediction or classification of AD using controlled learning schemes. They also require categorized information to instruct the frameworks. However, such frameworks are expensive and prove cumbersome in collecting sufficient AD data in actual executions. Subsequently, multi-view learning (learning with multiple views) is rarely considered for MRI data. While learning with multiple views could completely study the operative features and advance the accuracy in calculating data. Also, inspiration for multi-view data grouping comes from the fact that various views have diverse significance together with their own early comprehension. Thus, it becomes essential to produce multi-view MRI data and to evolve unsupervised learning schemes in view of self-regulating diagnose of AD [11].

Considering ample developments, significant challenges still persist as a barrier to the incorporation of DL techniques in the clinical scenery. Though technical issues close to the interpretability and generalizability of frameworks are potential domains for researchers, further problems like data privacy, approachability, and possession rights shall necessitate discussions in the healthcare system and society to conclude that they will be advantageous to all concerned collaborators. The improvement of data quality, precisely, might prove to be distinctively appropriate aim, address by means of DL techniques which had already confirmed efficiency in image processing and analysis [90]. Incapacitating these shortcomings will necessitate the hard work of interdisciplinary squads of physicians, engineers, computer scientists, ethicists, and legal experts. It is one of the ways by which humans could actually understand the prospective uses of DL in medicine to improve the proficiency of frontline workers and improve the degree of care to patients.

10.6 CONCLUSION

AD is a growing neurodegenerative ailment manifested by decay in brain functions with no proper management. Since it is crucial to avert the progression of disease, efficient, self-learning techniques are required to predict and diagnose it. The nature of ample dimensions of neural data, extracted mainly from neuroimaging with computer-aided algorithms, brings out the conception of accurate computer-aided diagnostic systems. DL, a high-tech ML tactic, has outperformed contemporary ML techniques in recognizing entangled structures in multi-dimensional data which is complex in nature. Structural alterations in the brain could be detected by DL techniques which could be utilized to detect features with information related to AD. Automated classification could also be applied for early detection during prodromic stages of the disease.

In this chapter, based on close scrutiny of the existing literature, a wide-ranging investigation of recent automated approaches to classify AD, algorithm-based neuroimaging procedures for dementia diagnosis, and systematic explanation of the most recent DL schemes for early prediction of AD have been presented. Also, progression monitoring of dementia of the Alzheimer type using medical image analysis and DL algorithms have been discussed. The focus was mainly on DL techniques and collective methods, along with some other ML techniques. The research inference, hurdles, and the future instructions pertaining to the study have also been emphasized. Significant research issues in the integration of DL tools in the clinical scenery and the problems for embarking on overcoming current challenges are also noted.

DL holds the capability to deeply modify the practice of medicine. Researchers have gathered data from different sources like hospitals, research laboratories and online repositories (AIBL, BIOCARD, EMIF-AD, FHS, KACD, NACC, NIFD, MIRIAD and ROAD). It is perceived that MRI and PET information and CNN could be effectively employed in order to predict and diagnose AD. In a partial accessible neuroimaging data set, fusion methods have exhibited accuracies of up to 96%, 99% and 99.5% for AD prediction, classification and diagnosis respectively.

DL approaches, which are the deeper version of neural networks, continue to advance in performance and seem to hold promise for diagnostic classification of AD using multimodal neuroimaging data. This is true because DL aims to understand the data representations in better ways, which can be built into any type of ML techniques. Research on AD that uses DL is still budding, refining performance by fusing additional data, increasing transparency that increases understanding of specific disease-associated attributes. In the future, DL methods in the hybridizing of nature-inspired systems should be considered for research in view of more efficacious presentation in the prediction, classification, and diagnosis of neurological disorders.

REFERENCES

[1] Pascoal, Tharick A, Sulantha Mathotaarachchi, Monica Shin, et al. "Synergistic inter-action between amyloid and tau predicts the progression to dementia." *Alzheimer's Dementia* 13 (2017): 644–53.

[2] Rajput, Mithun Singh, Nilesh Prakash Nirmal, Devashish Rathore, and Rashmi Dahima. "Dimethyl fumarate exerts neuroprotection by modulating calcineurin/NFAT1 and NFκB dependent BACE1 activity in Aβ1-42 treated neuroblastoma SH-SY5Y cells." *Brain Research Bulletin* 165 (2020): 97–107.

[3] Salehi, Ahmad Waleed, Preety Baglat, and Gaurav Gupta. "Alzheimer's disease diag-nosis using deep learning techniques." *Int. J. Eng. Adv. Technol* 9, no. 3 (2020): 874–80.

[4] Veitch, Dallas P., Michael W. Weiner, Paul S. Aisen, Laurel A. Beckett, Nigel J. Cairns, Robert C. Green, and Danielle Harvey et al. "Understanding disease progression and improving Alzheimer's disease clinical trials: Recent highlights from the Alzheimer's Disease Neuroimaging Initiative." *Alzheimer's & Dementia* 15, no. 1 (2019): 106–52.

[5] Jindal, Mansi, Gupta Jatin, and Bhushan Bharat. "Machine learning methods for IoT and their future applications". In *2019 International Conference on Computing, Communication and Intelligent Systems (ICCCIS)*, pp. 430–34. IEEE, 2019.

[6] Samper-González, Jorge, Ninon Burgos, Simona Bottani, Sabrina Fontanella, Pascal Lu, Arnaud Marcoux, Alexandre Routier et al. "Reproducible evaluation of classifi-cation methods in Alzheimer's disease: Framework and application to MRI and PET data." *NeuroImage* 183 (2018): 504–21.

[7] LeCun, Yann, Yoshua Bengio, and Geoffrey Hinton. "Deep learning." *Nature* 521, no. 7553 (2015): 436–44.

[8] Sharma, Nikhil, Ila Kaushik, Bharat Bhushan, and Siddharth Gautam. "Applicability of WSN and biometric models in the field of healthcare". In *2020 Deep Learning Strategies for Security Enhancement in Wireless Sensor Networks*, pp. 304–29, IGI Global, India, 2020.

[9] Jo, Taeho, Kwangsik Nho, and Andrew J. Saykin. "Deep learning in Alzheimer's dis-ease: diagnostic classification and prognostic prediction using neuroimaging data." *Frontiers in Aging Neuroscience* 11 (2019): 220.

[10] Khamparia, Aditya, Prakash Kumar Singh, Poonam Rani, Debabrata Samanta, Ashish Khanna, and Bharat Bhushan. "An internet of health things-driven deep learning framework for detection and classification of skin cancer using transfer learning." *Transactions on Emerging Telecommunication Technologies* Sp. Issue (2020): e3963.

[11] Zhang, Xiaobo, Yan Yang, Tianrui Li, Yiling Zhang, Hao Wang, and Hamido Fujita. "CMC: A consensus multi-view clustering model for predicting Alzheimer's disease progression." *Computer Methods and Programs in Biomedicine* 199 (2021): 105895.

[12] Kim, Sung-Hyun, Sumin Yang, Key-Hwan Lim, Euiseng Ko, Hyun-Jun Jang, Mingon Kang, Pann-Ghill Suh, and Jae-Yeol Joo. "Prediction of Alzheimer's disease-specific phospholipase c gamma-1 SNV by deep learning-based approach for high-throughput screening." *Proceedings of the National Academy of Sciences* 118, no. 3 (2021).

[13] Liu, Yuanyuan, Zhouxuan Li, Qiyang Ge, Nan Lin, and Momiao Xiong. "Deep Feature Selection and Causal Analysis of Alzheimer's Disease." *Frontiers in Neuroscience* 13 (2019): 1198.

[14] Abrol, Anees, Zening Fu, Yuhui Du, and Vince D. Calhoun. "Multimodal data fusion of deep learning and dynamic functional connectivity features to predict Alzheimer's disease progression." In *2019 41st Annual International Conference of the IEEE Engineering in Medicine and Biology Society (EMBC)*, pp. 4409–13. IEEE, 2019.

[15] Kim, Donghyeon, and Kiseon Kim. "Detection of early stage Alzheimer's disease using EEG relative power with deep neural network." In *2018 40th Annual International Conference of the IEEE Engineering in Medicine and Biology Society (EMBC)*, pp. 352–55. IEEE, 2018.

[16] Yang, Mengya, Peng Yang, Ahmed Elazab, Wen Hou, Xia Li, Tianfu Wang, Wenbin Zou, and Baiying Lei. "Join and Deep Ensemble Regression of Clinical Scores for Alzheimer's Disease Using Longitudinal and Incomplete Data." In *2018 40th Annual International Conference of the IEEE Engineering in Medicine and Biology Society (EMBC)*, pp. 1254–57. IEEE, 2018.

[17] Wojciechowski, Jakub W., and Małgorzata Kotulska. "pAtH-prediction of Amyloidogenicity by threading and Machine Learning." *Scientific Reports* 10, no. 1 (2020): 1–9.

[18] Vizcarra, Juan C, Marla Gearing, Michael J Keiser, et al. "Validation of machine learning models to detect amyloid pathologies across institutions." *Acta Neuropathology Communications* 8, (2020): 59.

[19] Pan, Dan, An Zeng, Longfei Jia, Yin Huang, Tory Frizzell, and Xiaowei Song. "Early detection of Alzheimer's disease using magnetic resonance imaging: A novel approach combining convolutional neural networks and ensemble learning." *Frontiers in Neuroscience* 14 (2020): 259.

[20] Alegro, Maryana, Yuheng Chen, Dulce Ovando, Helmut Heinser, Rana Eser, Daniela Ushizima, Duygu Tosun, and Lea T. Grinberg. "Deep learning for Alzheimer's disease: Mapping large-scale histological tau protein for neuroimaging biomarker validation." *BioRxiv* (2020): 698902.

[21] Spasov, Simeon, Luca Passamonti, Andrea Duggento, Pietro Liò, Nicola Toschi, and Alzheimer's Disease Neuroimaging Initiative. "A parameter-efficient deep learning approach to predict conversion from mild cognitive impairment to Alzheimer's disease." *Neuroimage* 189 (2019): 276–87.

[22] Shen, Ting, Jiehui Jiang, Jiaying Lu, Min Wang, Chuantao Zuo, Zhihua Yu, and Zhuangzhi Yan. "Predicting Alzheimer Disease from mild cognitive impairment with a deep belief network based on 18F-FDG-PET Images." *Molecular Imaging* 18 (2019): 15–36.

[23] Liu, Chin-Fu, Shreyas Padhy, Sandhya Ramachandran, Victor X. Wang, Andrew Efimov, Alonso Bernal, Linyuan Shi et al. "Using deep Siamese neural networks for detection of brain asymmetries associated with Alzheimer's disease and mild cognitive impairment." *Magnetic Resonance Imaging* 64 (2019): 190–99.

[24] Lee, Garam, Kwangsik Nho, Byungkon Kang, Kyung-Ah Sohn, and Dokyoon Kim. "Predicting Alzheimer's disease progression using multi-modal deep learning approach." *Scientific Reports* 9, no. 1 (2019): 1–12.

[25] Li, Hongming, Mohamad Habes, David A. Wolk, Yong Fan, and Alzheimer's Disease Neuroimaging Initiative. "A deep learning model for early prediction of Alzheimer's disease dementia based on hippocampal magnetic resonance imaging data." *Alzheimer's & Dementia* 15, no. 8 (2019): 1059–70.

[26] Kim, Jongin, Boreom Lee. "Identification of Alzheimer's disease and mild cognitive impairment using multimodal sparse hierarchical extreme learning machine." *Human Brain Mapping* 39, no. 9 (2018): 3728–41.

[27] Al-Janabi, Shaimaa, André Huisman, Paul J. Van Diest. "Digital pathology: current status and future perspectives." *Histopathology* 61, no. 1 (2012): 1–9.

[28] Rajput, Mithun Singh, Nilesh Prakash Nirmal, Devashish Rathore, and Rashmi Dahima. "Dimethyl Fumarate Mitigates Tauopathy in Aβ-Induced Neuroblastoma SH-SY5Y Cells." *Neurochemical Research* 45, no. 11 (2020): 2641–52.

[29] Kumar, Santosh, Bharat Bhusan, Debabrata Singh, Dilip kumar Choubey. "Classification of Diabetes using Deep Learning." In *2020 International Conference on Communication and Signal Processing*, pp. 651–55. IEEE, 2020.

[30] Maqsood, Muazzam, Faria Nazir, Umair Khan, Farhan Aadil, Habibullah Jamal, Irfan Mehmood, and Oh-young Song. "Transfer learning assisted classification and detection of Alzheimer's disease stages using 3D MRI scans." *Sensors* 19, no. 11 (2019): 2645.

[31] O'Bryant, Sid E., Stephen C. Waring, C. Munro Cullum, James Hall, Laura Lacritz, Paul J. Massman, Philip J. Lupo, Joan S. Reisch, and Rachelle Doody. "Staging dementia using Clinical Dementia Rating Scale Sum of Boxes scores: a Texas Alzheimer's research consortium study." *Archives of Neurology* 65, no. 8 (2008): 1091–95.

[32] Sarraf, Saman, Ghassem Tofighi, and Alzheimer's Disease Neuroimaging Initiative. "DeepAD: Alzheimer's disease classification via deep convolutional neural networks using MRI and fMRI." *BioRxiv* (2016): 070441.

[33] Hosseini-Asl, Ehsan, Robert Keynton, and Ayman El-Baz. "Alzheimer's disease diagnostics by adaptation of 3D convolutional network." In *2016 IEEE International Conference on Image Processing (ICIP)*, pp. 126–30. IEEE, 2016.

[34] Hosny, Ahmed, Chintan Parmar, John Quackenbush, Lawrence H. Schwartz, and Hugo J.W.L. Aerts. "Artificial intelligence in radiology." *Nature Reviews Cancer* 18, no. 8 (2018): 500–10.

[35] Khagi, Bijen, Goo-Rak Kwon, and Ramesh Lama. "Comparative analysis of Alzheimer's disease classification by CDR level using CNN, feature selection, and machine-learning techniques." *International Journal of Imaging Systems and Technology* 29, no. 3 (2019): 297–310.

[36] Oh, Kanghan, Young-Chul Chung, Ko Woon Kim, Woo-Sung Kim, and Il-Seok Oh. "Classification and visualization of Alzheimer's disease using volumetric convolutional neural network and transfer learning." *Scientific Reports* 9, no. 1 (2019): 1–16.

[37] Hu, Jingjing, Zhao Qing, Renyuan Liu, Xin Zhang, Pin Lv, Maoxue Wang, Yang Wang, Kelei He, Yang Gao, and Bing Zhang. "Deep learning-based classification and voxel-based visualization of frontotemporal dementia and Alzheimer's disease." *Frontiers in Neuroscience* 14 (2020): 1468.

[38] Suh, C.H., W.H. Shim, S.J. Kim, J.H. Roh, J-H. Lee, M-J. Kim, S. Park et al. "Development and validation of a deep learning–based automatic brain segmentation and classification algorithm for Alzheimer disease using 3D T1-weighted volumetric images." *American Journal of Neuroradiology* 41, no. 12 (2020): 2227–34.

[39] Qiu, Shangran, Prajakta S. Joshi, Matthew I. Miller, Chonghua Xue, Xiao Zhou, Cody Karjadi, Gary H. Chang et al. "Development and validation of an interpretable deep learning framework for Alzheimer's disease classification." *Brain* 143, no. 6 (2020): 1920–33.

[40] Mehmood, Atif, Muazzam Maqsood, Muzaffar Bashir, and Yang Shuyuan. "A deep Siamese convolution neural network for multi-class classification of Alzheimer disease." *Brain Sciences* 10, no. 2 (2020): 84.

[41] Liu, Manhua, Fan Li, Hao Yan, Kundong Wang, Yixin Ma, Li Shen, Mingqing Xu, and Alzheimer's Disease Neuroimaging Initiative. "A multi-model deep convolutional neural network for automatic hippocampus segmentation and classification in Alzheimer's disease." *NeuroImage* 208 (2020): 116459.

[42] Wada, Akihiko, Kohei Tsuruta, Ryusuke Irie, Koji Kamagata, Tomoko Maekawa, Shohei Fujita, Saori Koshino et al. "Differentiating Alzheimer's disease from dementia with Lewy bodies using a deep learning technique based on structural brain connectivity." *Magnetic Resonance in Medical Sciences* 18, no. 3 (2019): 219.

[43] Liu, Mingxia, Jun Zhang, Ehsan Adeli, and Dinggang Shen. "Joint classification and regression via deep multi-task multi-channel learning for Alzheimer's disease diagnosis." *IEEE Transactions on Biomedical Engineering* 66, no. 5 (2019): 1195–206.

[44] Fulton, Lawrence V., Diane Dolezel, Jordan Harrop, Yan Yan, and Christopher P. Fulton. "Classification of Alzheimer's disease with and without imagery using gradient boosted machines and ResNet-50." *Brain Sciences* 9, no. 9 (2019): 212.

[45] Wang, Shui-Hua, Preetha Phillips, Yuxiu Sui, Bin Liu, Ming Yang, and Hong Cheng. "Classification of Alzheimer's disease based on eight-layer convolutional neural network with leaky rectified linear unit and max pooling." *Journal of MedicalSsystems* 42, no. 5 (2018): 1–11.

[46] Qiao, Jianping, Yingru Lv, Chongfeng Cao, Zhishun Wang, and Anning Li. "Multivariate deep learning classification of Alzheimer's disease based on hierarchical partner matching independent component analysis." *Frontiers in Aging Neuroscience* 10 (2018): 417.

[47] Jo, Taeho, Kwangsik Nho, Shannon L. Risacher, and Andrew J. Saykin. "Deep learning detection of informative features in tau PET for Alzheimer's disease classification." *BMC Bioinformatics* 21, no. 21 (2020): 1–13.

[48] Son, Hye Joo, Jungsu S. Oh, Minyoung Oh, Soo Jong Kim, Jae-Hong Lee, Jee Hoon Roh, and Jae Seung Kim. "The clinical feasibility of deep learning-based classification of amyloid PET images in visually equivocal cases." *European Journal of Nuclear Medicine and Molecular Imaging* 47, no. 2 (2020): 332–41.

[49] Punjabi, Arjun, Adam Martersteck, Yanran Wang, Todd B. Parrish, Aggelos K. Katsaggelos, and Alzheimer's Disease Neuroimaging Initiative. "Neuroimaging modality fusion in Alzheimer's classification using convolutional neural networks." *PloS one* 14, no. 12 (2019): e0225759.

[50] Iizuka, Tomomichi, Makoto Fukasawa, and Masashi Kameyama. "Deep-learning-based imaging-classification identified cingulate island sign in dementia with Lewy bodies." *Scientific Reports* 9 (2019): 8944.

[51] Liu, Manhua, Danni Cheng, Weiwu Yan, and Alzheimer's Disease Neuroimaging Initiative. "Classification of Alzheimer's disease by combination of convolutional and recurrent neural networks using FDG-PET images." *Frontiers in Neuroinformatics* 12 (2018): 35.

[52] Li, Feng, Loc Tran, Kim-Han Thung, Shuiwang Ji, Dinggang Shen, and Jiang Li. "A robust deep model for improved classification of AD/MCI patients." *IEEE Journal of Biomedical and Health Informatics* 19, no. 5 (2015): 1610–16.

[53] Lazli, Lilia, Mounir Boukadoum, and Otmane Ait Mohamed. "A survey on computer-aided diagnosis of brain disorders through MRI based on machine learning and data mining methodologies with an emphasis on Alzheimer disease diagnosis and the contribution of the multimodal fusion." *Applied Sciences* 10, no. 5 (2020): 1894.

[54] Herzog, Nitsa J., and George D. Magoulas. "Brain asymmetry detection and machine learning classification for diagnosis of early Dementia." *Sensors* 21, no. 3 (2021): 778.

[55] Liang, Shuang, and Gu Yu. "Computer-aided diagnosis of Alzheimer's disease through weak supervision deep learning framework with attention mechanism." *Sensors* 21, no. 1 (2021): 220.

[56] Lei, Baiying, Shuangzhi Yu, Xin Zhao, Alejandro F. Frangi, Ee-Leng Tan, Ahmed Elazab, Tianfu Wang, and Shuqiang Wang. "Diagnosis of early Alzheimer's disease based on dynamic high order networks." *Brain Imaging and Behavior* 15, no. 1 (2021): 276–87.

[57] Marzban, Eman N., Ayman M. Eldeib, Inas A. Yassine, Yasser M. Kadah, and Alzheimer's Disease Neurodegenerative Initiative. "Alzheimer's disease diagnosis from diffusion tensor images using convolutional neural networks." *PloS One* 15, no. 3 (2020): e0230409.

[58] Lee, Eunho, Jun-Sik Choi, Minjeong Kim, Heung-Il Suk, and Alzheimer's Disease Neuroimaging Initiative. "Toward an interpretable Alzheimer's disease diagnostic model with regional abnormality representation via deep learning." *NeuroImage* 202 (2019): 116113.

[59] Goceri, Evgin. "Diagnosis of Alzheimer's disease with Sobolev gradient-based optimization and 3D convolutional neural network." *International Journal for Numerical Methods in Biomedical Engineering* 35, no. 7 (2019): e3225.

[60] Bi, Xia-an, Ruipeng Cai, Yang Wang, and Yingchao Liu. "Effective diagnosis of Alzheimer's disease via multimodal fusion analysis framework." *Frontiers in Genetics* 10 (2019): 976.

[61] Bi, Xiuli, Shutong Li, Bin Xiao, Yu Li, Guoyin Wang, and Xu Ma. "Computer aided Alzheimer's disease diagnosis by an unsupervised deep learning technology." *Neurocomputing* 392 (2020): 296–304.

[62] Jin, Dan, Bo Zhou, Ying Han, Jiaji Ren, Tong Han, Bing Liu, Jie Lu et al. "Generalizable, reproducible, and neuroscientifically interpretable imaging biomarkers for Alzheimer's disease." *Advanced Science* 7, no. 14 (2020): 2000675.

[63] Puente-Castro, Alejandro, Enrique Fernandez-Blanco, Alejandro Pazos, and Cristian R. Munteanu. "Automatic assessment of Alzheimer's disease diagnosis based on deep learning techniques." *Computers in Biology and Medicine* 120 (2020): 103764.

[64] Basheera, Shaik, and M. Satya Sai Ram. "Convolution neural network–based Alzheimer's disease classification using hybrid enhanced independent component analysis based segmented gray matter of T2 weighted magnetic resonance imaging with clinical valuation." *Alzheimer's & Dementia: Translational Research & Clinical Interventions* 5 (2019): 974–86.

[65] Cui, Ruoxuan, and Manhua Liu. "Hippocampus Analysis by Combination of 3-D DenseNet and Shapes for Alzheimer's Disease Diagnosis." *IEEE Journal of Biomedical and Health Informatics* 23, no. 5 (2018): 2099–107.

[66] Ju, Ronghui, Chenhui Hu, and Quanzheng Li. "Early diagnosis of Alzheimer's disease based on resting-state brain networks and deep learning." *IEEE/ACM Transactions on Computational Biology and Bioinformatics* 16, no. 1 (2017): 244–57.

[67] Esmaeilzadeh, Soheil, Dimitrios Ioannis Belivanis, Kilian M. Pohl, and Ehsan Adeli. "End-to-end Alzheimer's disease diagnosis and biomarker identification." In *International Workshop on ML in Medical Imaging*, pp. 337–345. Springer, Cham, 2018.

[68] Kam, Tae-Eui, Han Zhang, and Dinggang Shen. "A novel deep learning framework on brain functional networks for early MCI diagnosis." In *International Conference on Medical Image Computing and Computer-Assisted Intervention*, pp. 293–301. Springer, Cham, 2018.

[69] Li, Fan, Manhua Liu, and Alzheimer's Disease Neuroimaging Initiative. "Alzheimer's disease diagnosis based on multiple cluster dense convolutional networks." *Computerized Medical Imaging and Graphics* 70 (2018): 101–110.

[70] Li, Yupeng, Jiehui Jiang, Jiaying Lu, Juanjuan Jiang, Huiwei Zhang, and Chuantao Zuo. "Radiomics: a novel feature extraction method for brain neuron degeneration disease using 18F-FDG PET imaging and its implementation for Alzheimer's disease and mild cognitive impairment." *Therapeutic Advances in Neurological Disorders* 12 (2019): 1756286419838682.

[71] Ding, Yiming, Jae Ho Sohn, Michael G. Kawczynski, Hari Trivedi, Roy Harnish, Nathaniel W. Jenkins, Dmytro Lituiev et al. "A deep learning model to predict a diagnosis of Alzheimer disease by using 18F-FDG PET of the brain." *Radiology* 290, no. 2 (2019): 456–64.

[72] Zhang, Tao, and Mingyang Shi. "Multi-modal neuroimaging feature fusion for diagnosis of Alzheimer's disease." *Journal of Neuroscience Methods* 341 (2020): 108795.

[73] Zhou, Tao, Kim-Han Thung, Xiaofeng Zhu, and Dinggang Shen. "Effective feature learning and fusion of multimodality data using stage wise deep neural network for dementia diagnosis." *Human Brain Mapping* 40, no. 3 (2019): 1001–16.

[74] Zhou, Tao, Kim-Han Thung, Xiaofeng Zhu, and Dinggang Shen. "Feature learning and fusion of multimodality neuroimaging and genetic data for multi-status dementia diagnosis." In *International Workshop on Machine Learning in Medical Imaging*, pp. 132–40. Springer, Cham, 2017.

[75] Li, Yan, Fanqing Meng, and Jun Shi. "Learning using privileged information improves neuroimaging-based CAD of Alzheimer's disease: a comparative study." *Medical & Biological Engineering & Computing* 57, no. 7 (2019): 1605–16.

[76] Shi, Jun, Xiao Zheng, Yan Li, Qi Zhang, and Shihui Ying. "Multimodal neuroimaging feature learning with multimodal stacked deep polynomial networks for diagnosis of Alzheimer's disease." *IEEE Journal of Biomedical and Health Informatics* 22, no. 1 (2018): 173–83.

[77] Ortiz, Andres, Jorge Munilla, Juan M. Gorriz, and Javier Ramirez. "Ensembles of deep learning architectures for the early diagnosis of the Alzheimer's disease." *International Journal of Neural Systems* 26, no. 07 (2016): 1650025.

[78] Huang, Yechong, Jiahang Xu, Yuncheng Zhou, Tong Tong, Xiahai Zhuang, and Alzheimer's Disease Neuroimaging Initiative. "Diagnosis of Alzheimer's disease via multi-modality 3D convolutional neural network." *Frontiers in Neuroscience* 13 (2019): 509.

[79] Lu, Donghuan, Karteek Popuri, Gavin Weiguang Ding, Rakesh Balachandar, and Mirza Faisal Beg. "Multimodal and multiscale deep neural networks for the early diagnosis of Alzheimer's disease using structural MR and FDG-PET images." *Scientific Reports* 8, no. 1 (2018): 1–13.

[80] Thung, Kim-Han, Pew-Thian Yap, and Dinggang Shen. "Multi-stage diagnosis of Alzheimer's disease with incomplete multimodal data via multi-task deep learning." In *Deep Learning in Medical Image Analysis and Multimodal Learning for Clinical Decision Support*, pp. 160–68. Springer, Cham, 2017.

[81] Suk, Heung-Il, Seong-Whan Lee, and Dinggang Shen. "Deep sparse multi-task learning for feature selection in Alzheimer's disease diagnosis." *Brain Structure and Function* 221, no. 5 (2016): 2569–87.

[82] Suk, Heung-Il, Seong-Whan Lee, Dinggang Shen, and Alzheimer's Disease Neuroimaging Initiative. "Hierarchical feature representation and multimodal fusion with deep learning for AD/MCI diagnosis." *NeuroImage* 101 (2014): 569–82.

[83] Ryzhikova, Elena, Nicole M. Ralbovsky, Vitali Sikirzhytski, Oleksandr Kazakov, Lenka Halamkova, Joseph Quinn, Earl A. Zimmerman, and Igor K. Lednev. "Raman spectroscopy and machine learning for biomedical applications: Alzheimer's disease diagnosis based on the analysis of cerebrospinal fluid." *Spectrochimica Acta Part A: Molecular and Biomolecular Spectroscopy* 248 (2021): 119188.

[84] Stamate, Daniel, Min Kim, Petroula Proitsi, Sarah Westwood, Alison Baird, Alejo Nevado Holgado, Abdul Hye et al. "A metabolite-based machine learning approach to diagnose Alzheimer-type dementia in blood: Results from the European Medical Information Framework for Alzheimer disease biomarker discovery cohort." *Alzheimer's & Dementia: Translational Research & Clinical Interventions* 5, no. 1 (2019): 933–38.

[85] Costa, Luís, Miguel F. Gago, Darya Yelshyna, Jaime Ferreira, Hélder David Silva, Luís Rocha, Nuno Sousa, and Estela Bicho. "Application of machine learning in postural control kinematics for the diagnosis of Alzheimer's disease." *Computational Intelligence and Neuroscience* 2016 (2016), 1186–200.

[86] Pattnayak, Parthasarathi, and Om Prakash Jena. "Innovation on machine learning in healthcare services–an introduction." *2021 Machine Learning for Healthcare Applications* 1 (2021): 1–15.

[87] Goyal, Sukriti, Nikhil Sharma, Bharat Bhushan, Achyut Shankar, and Martin Sagayam. "IoT enabled technology in secured healthcare: applications, challenges and future directions." *2021 Cognitive Internet of Medical Things for Smart Healthcare. Studies in Systems, Decision and Control* 311 (2021): 25–48.

[88] Panigrahi, Niranjan, Ishan Ayus, and Om Prakash Jena. "An expert system-based clinical decision support system for hepatitis-B prediction & diagnosis." *2021 Machine Learning for Healthcare Applications* 4 (2021): 57–75.

[89] Patra, Sudhanshu Shekhar, Om Prakash Jena, Gaurav Kumar, Sreyashi Pramanik, Chinmaya Misra, and Kamakhya Narain Singh. "Random forest algorithm in imbalance genomics classification." *2021 Data Analytics in Bioinformatics* 7 (2021): 173–90.

[90] Paramesha, K., H.L. Gururaj, and Om Prakash Jena. "Applications of machine learning in biomedical text processing and food industry." *2021 Machine Learning for Healthcare Applications* 10 (2021): 151–67.

11 Machine Learning Algorithms and COVID-19
A Step for Predicting Future Pandemics with a Systematic Overview

Madhumita Pal, Ruchi Tiwari, Kuldeep Dhama, Smita Parija, Om Prakash Jena, and Ranjan K. Mohapatra

CONTENTS

DOI: 10.1201/9781003226147-11

11.1 INTRODUCTION

After the birth of SARS-CoV-2 from the Huanan Seafood wholesale market of Wuhan in China in December 2019, the deadly virus has spread very quickly around the whole world and become the major cause of serious health concern worldwide (Mohapatra et al. 2020a, 2020b; Mohapatra and Rahman 2021). This deadly pathogen is responsible for the ongoing and never-ending COVID-19 pandemic and on March 11, 2020, the World Health Organization (WHO) has declared a global pandemic due to this (Dhama et al. 2020a). This pathogenic viral infection is believed to have originated from animals such as pangolins and bats, however, bats are suspected to be the major source (Mohapatra et al. 2021b). The widespread propagation of this disease has caused nearly three million deaths worldwide to date due to rapid human-to-human transmission. It is also responsible for more than 20.5 million years of life loss globally and has radically changed the common practice of our normal life (Arolas et al. 2021).

SARS-CoV-2 is mainly transmitted through the respiratory aerosols/droplets and fecal-oral route (Chan et al. 2020). Although several other means of transmission have been identified, human-to-human transmission mainly occurs by direct and indirect contacts (i.e. contaminated objects/surfaces/fomite) (Mohapatra et al. 2021a). Moreover, the airborne transmission and hospital-associated transmissions were also reported as a predominant mode of virus spread (Morawska and Cao 2020; Wang et al. 2020a; Zhang et al. 2020a). The most common COVID-19 symptoms are respiratory infections such as cough, shortness of breath, fever, followed by pneumonia. Apart from this, SARS-CoV-2 also affects kidneys, heart, nervous system, and finally progresses to multiple organ damage (Dhama et al. 2020b). It may cause severe complications among immunocompromised persons having diabetes and cardiovascular disorders (Arumugam et al. 2020).

Moreover, this pandemic has devastated the stock and financial markets, and the global economy dramatically (Lenzen et al. 2020; Nicola et al. 2020). The efficient rate of human-to-human transmission makes it challenging to prevent community transmission and to formulate the evidence-based proper infection control strategies to save health workers, children, and old-aged individuals (Kucharski et al. 2020). Moreover, no approved drugs are available to combat SARS-CoV-2 and hence, scientists, doctors, and researchers are trying days and nights to find a solution to combat SARS-CoV-2 and its emerging variants (Mohapatra et al. 2020c, 2021c; Sah et al. 2021). Hence, the accurate prediction of the disease will help in providing high-quality healthcare services and may reduce the disease severity and mortality. Timely actions are needed for the accurate prediction of the disease to provide high-quality healthcare service management.

Artificial neural networks (ANNs), Internet of Things (IoT), and ML techniques may provide valuable suggestions in numerous fields, such as agriculture, environmental science, food industry (Paramesha et al. 2021), and classification of diabetes (Kumar et al. 2020), chronic diseases (Reddy and Imler 2017), skin cancer (Khamparia et al. 2020), epidemiology, public health, and smart healthcare systems (Uddin et al. 2019; Hassanien et al. 2021; Panigrahi et al. 2021; Patra et al. 2021; Pattnayak and Jena 2021). Furthermore, some researchers have explained the challenges related to the use of various ML techniques in order to extract the results with good efficiency (Jindal et al. 2019; Rana et al. 2019). Kumar et al. (2020) have investigated deep learning (DL) models for the classification of diabetes and the results were compared with Naïve Bayes (NB) and Random Forest (RF) algorithms. In this overview, we have discussed different ML techniques for the automotive detection, prediction, and diagnosis of COVID-19 outbreak which may help to increase the survival rate of patients.

This chapter is organized into five sections as follows: The introductory section describes the current understanding of the disease and outlines how ANN, IoT, and different ML techniques are helpful to provide valuable suggestions in numerous fields. Section 11.2 explains the theoretical concept of several ML techniques with the performance measurement parameters. The detailed methodology of the study is illustrated in Section 11.3. Further, Section 11.4 discusses how ML techniques are currently used for the prediction and accurate diagnosis of COVID-19 for the better healthcare services. Finally, Section 11.5 summarizes and offers a conclusion with suggestions for further improvements in this direction.

11.2 DIFFERENT ML TECHNIQUES

ML is the part of AI and is an automated learning process which learns from its past experience. ML models extract features from large databases, then preprocess and classify them. ML models analyze a large number of datasets and make decisions based on past data (Fatima et al. 2020). ML techniques are grouped into four categories (Figure 11.1):

- Supervised learning
- Unsupervised learning
- Semi supervised learning
- DL

11.2.1 SUPERVISED LEARNING

Machine requires labeled data for future prediction in supervised learning. It is mainly used for solving classification and regression problems. ANN, logistic regression (LR), RF, support vector machine (SVM), k-nearest neighbor (K-NN), and NB come under supervised learning algorithms.

11.2.1.1 Artificial Neural Networks

ANN is the most powerful supervised ML algorithm commonly used for feature extraction in data mining. It contains three layers namely input layer, hidden

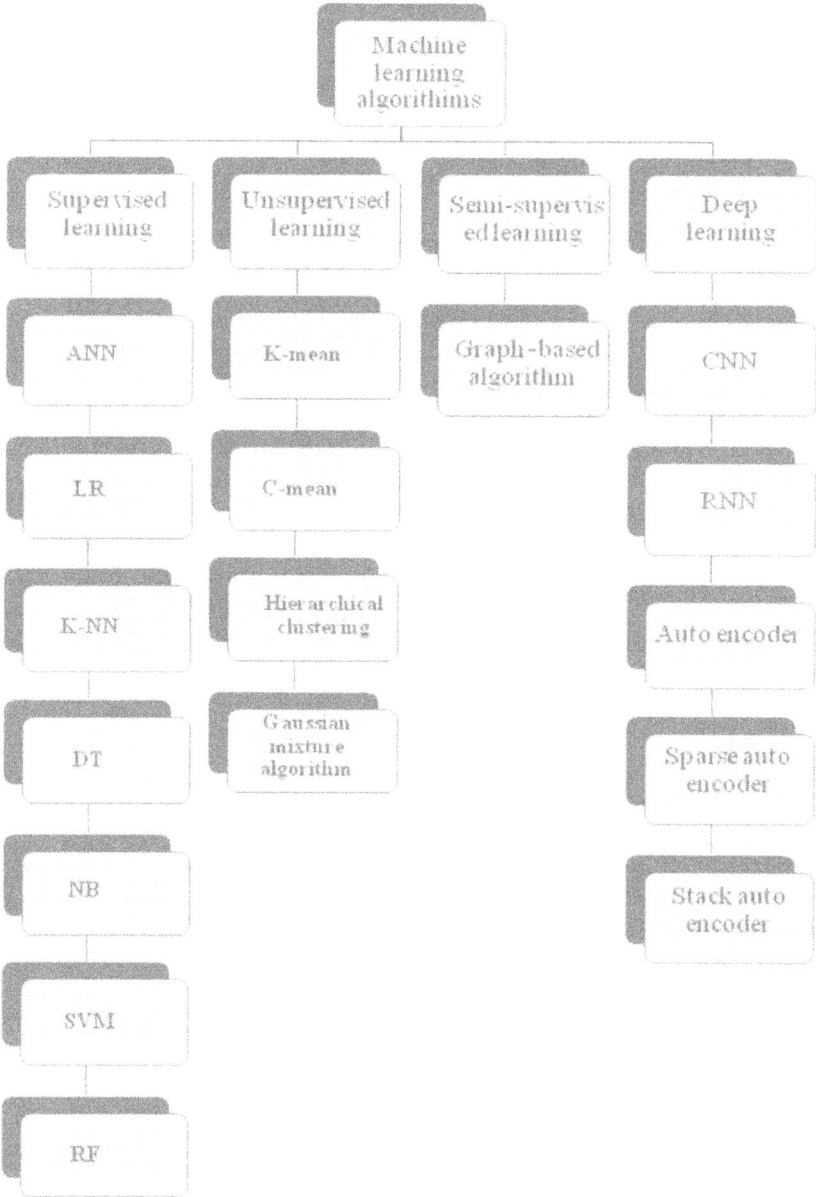

FIGURE 11.1   Several used ML techniques.

layer, and output layer (Uzun and Tezel 2012; Singhal and Pareek 2018). Several types of activation functions are employed in hidden layer for nonlinear mapping. There are two perceptron types of ANNs. One is simple ANN used for binary classification; another one is multilayer perceptron used for complex regression and classification problems. The equation for prediction of a single neuron in forward propagation path is:

$$\text{Output} = a_{i+} \sum_{k=1}^{m_y} w_{ik} y_i \qquad (11.1)$$

W_{ij} = weight propagated from i/p to o/p. a_j bias value, b_i input value.
   The activation function which are commonly used in the ANN are:

$$\text{sigmoid} = \frac{1}{1+e^{-x}} \qquad (11.2)$$

$$\text{Tanh} = \frac{e^{x}-e^{-x}}{e^{x}+e^{-x}} \qquad (11.3)$$

$$\text{RELU} = \{0, \text{for } y \leq 0 \text{ y, for } y > 0 \qquad (11.4)$$

11.2.1.2   Logistic Regression

LR is a supervised algorithm is mainly used for binary classification problems. It gives discrete outcome (Ahmad and Yusoff 2013). The equation that represents Logistics regression model is:

$$Y(x) = \frac{e^{x}}{1+e^{x}} \qquad (11.5)$$

X is the input variable.

11.2.1.3   K-Nearest Neighbor

K-NN is a supervised learning algorithm used for solving classification as well as regression problems, but is mainly used for feature classification of similar featured data (Imandoust and Bolandraftar 2013). Different distant metrics are used for finding the neighbor for classification such as Euclidean distance and Manhattan distance.

$$\text{Euclidean distance } \text{dist}(a, b) = \sqrt{\sum_{1=1}^{m} (a_i - b_i)^2} \qquad (11.6)$$

11.2.1.4   Decision Tree

This algorithm is based on a classification and regression tree. It contains smaller data samples of larger datasets (Sharma and Kumar 2016).

11.2.1.5   Naïve Bayes

NB is a supervised ML algorithm used for solving classification problem. It is based upon Naïve Bayes probability theorem (Wu et al. 2015; Ibrahim et al. 2017). Consider M is the set of training samples and y is the tuple with z features that are expressed as y= {C$_1$, C$_2$, C$_3$, ... C$_z$}. Suppose there are k classes represented as D$_1$, D$_2$, D$_3$. For the tuple y, the classifier forecast class belongingness of y with highest posterior probability conditioned on y. This classifier predicts that y belongs to Dj class if,

$$p\left(D_j|y\right) > p\left(D_k|y\right) \text{ for } 1 \le k \le n, j \ne k. \tag{11.7}$$

p(D$_i$|X) is called maximum posteriori hypothesis.

As per Bayes theorem,

$$p\left(D_j|y\right) = p\left(y|D_j\right)p\left(D_j\right)/p\left(y\right) \tag{11.8}$$

If all the feature values are independent of each other then,

$$P\left(y|D_i\right) = \Pi p\left(y|D_j\right) \tag{11.9}$$

where y is the tuple with feature z.

11.2.1.6 Support Vector Machine

SVM is the most powerful supervised learning algorithm employed for solving both classification and regression problems. It uses hyperplane for classification of objects (Evgeniou and Pontil 2005).

11.2.1.7 Random Forest

RF is the most powerful ensemble classifier technique used for solving classification as well as regression problems (Breiman 2001). But it is more efficient for solving classification problems. As the name suggests this algorithm consists of forest of trees. Gini index is used for splitting process of the decision trees used in RF.

11.2.2 UNSUPERVISED LEARNING

It operates on unlabeled dataset. It is mainly used for clustering operation and for pattern recognition of newly dataset. For training the model it neither requires classified data nor labeled data. K-mean, C-mean, Hierarchical clustering algorithm comes under unsupervised learning.

11.2.2.1 K-Mean Clustering

K-mean clustering is the unsupervised learning which partition data into small clusters based on similarity of various data points (Li and Wu 2012). For a given dataset of items with certain features and values for these features the algorithm will categorize the items into k groups or clusters of similarity. In this clustering to calculate the similarity, different distance metrics such as Euclidean distance, Manhattan distance, hamming distance, and cosine distance are used as measurement. Pseudo code for implementing k-means algorithm is as follows:

Input: k-means algorithm (K number of clusters list of data points)

1. k number of random data points as initial centroids (cluster centers) may be chosen.

2. Repeat until cluster centers stabilize:
- Allocate each point in D to the nearest of the kth centroids.
- Compute centroid by using all the points in the cluster.

11.2.2.1.1   Advantages
- It is simple, easy to implement and to understand.
- It is efficient where the time taken to cluster k-means rises linearly with the number of data points.
- No other clustering algorithms perform better than k-means.

11.2.2.1.2   Disadvantages
- The initial value of k needs to be specified.
- The process of clusters finding may not converge.
- It may not be applicable for discovering clusters which are not hyper spheres or hyper ellipsoids.

11.2.2.2   C-Mean Clustering

In this unsupervised learning algorithm, each data point belongs to a particular cluster having similar features (Bezdek et al. 1984). C-mean clustering is an extension of k-means which discovers the soft clustering. The soft cluster data point belongs to multiple clusters with a certain affinity value toward each which is proportional to the distance from the point to the centroid of the cluster.

11.2.2.3   Hierarchical Clustering

Hierarchical clustering is used for separating one cluster from other clusters in hierarchy form. Individual clusters contain similar data samples. Different probabilistic models are used for distance measurement between each cluster (Patel et al. 2015).

11.2.2.4   Gaussian Mixture Algorithm

The Gaussian mixture algorithm is the most popular soft clustering technique mainly used for computing several types of clustered data. This algorithm is implemented on the basis of expectation maximization (Zhang et al. 2016).

11.2.3   Reinforcement Learning

In this type of learning, the machine learns from the environment. It doesn't require any labeled data. In the absence of training dataset, the machine improves its performance by learning from experience. Reinforcement learning is a type where an agent learns to behave in an environment by performing actions and seeing the results. There is no expected output as in supervised learning. It doesn't require any labeled data. Reinforcement learning system comprises two main components: agent and environment. The agent decides what action is to be taken to perform a task. Reinforcement learning is all about an agent who is put about an unknown environment, and he is going to take a hit and trial method in order to figure out the environment and then come up with an outcome. Q-Learning algorithm is an example of reinforcement learning.

11.2.4 Deep Learning Techniques

DL is part of ANN which consists of multiple layers architecture (Togacar and Ergen 2018) and is mostly used for pattern recognition (LeCun et al. 2015; Tiwari et al. 2020).

11.2.4.1 Auto Encoder

Auto encoder consists of encoder which takes input and gives it to decoder and decoder try to reconstruct the original input. The main purpose of this is dimension reduction from a large noisy dataset (LeCun et al. 2015; Selvathi and Poornila 2018; Tiwari et al. 2020).

11.2.4.2 Sparse Auto Encoders

It is a feed forward auto-encoder which uses back propagation learning algorithm for training the neural network. A sparse auto encoder introduces a sparsity constraint on the hidden layer nodes that penalize activations within a layer. Network learns encoding and decoding that relies on activating a small number of neurons (LeCun et al. 2015; Selvathi and Poornila 2018; Munir et al. 2019).

11.2.4.3 Stacked Sparse Auto Encoder

Stacked spare auto encoder (SSAE) consists of a number of hidden layers which are stack one another based on classifier (LeCun et al. 2015; Selvathi and Poornila 2018; Munir et al. 2019).

11.2.5 Convolutional Neural Network

CNN is based on convolution operation. The layers are divided into convolution, nonlinearity, pooling layer, fully connected, and classification layer. In CNN every node relies on input from a small number of nodes in the previous layer, needing a smaller number of parameters (Fakoor et al. 2013; Munir et al. 2019).

11.2.5.1 Recurrent Neural Network

This type of neural network uses output of the previous layer as an input of the next layer. It has the capability to reduce network complexity by using same parameter at each layer, but it is incapable of processing a large sequence of inputs by using ReLU and Tanh activation functions (LeCun et al. 2015; Hamed et al. 2020).

11.3 METHODOLOGY

A systematic literature review was performed to collect data from different databases such as Science Direct, IEEE, PubMed, Scopus, and Google Scholar resources. For critical covering the most relevant literature contents, the key terms searched included ML tools in COVID-19, ML models predicting COVID-19, COVID-19 diagnosis model by using ML techniques, predicting COVID-19 fatality rates, predicting COVID-19 casualties, and diagnosis of COVID-19 from CT images with ML models. The closely matched data were carefully examined and considered for critical discussion. However, the irrelevant or generalized studies were excluded from our discussion.

11.4 COVID-19 AND ML TECHNIQUES

11.4.1 PREDICTION FOR BETTER HEALTHCARE SERVICE

Hasan (2020) has reported a hybrid model incorporating ANN and Ensemble Empirical Mode Decomposition (EEMD) for predicting COVID-19 epidemic for better healthcare service. The model result was compared with traditional statistical analysis and will be helpful for COVID-19 or other such epidemic prediction. Zhang et al. (2020b) have compared the results of five ML algorithms (logistic regression, RF, k-nearest neighbour, SVM, decision tree). As per the investigation, RF model has achieved best performance for CoV. Ardabili et al. (2020) have reported a comparative analysis of ML with SIR and SEIR models to predict the outbreak of COVID-19. Among the investigated models, MLP and ANFIS models showed promising results. As per the results, the authors suggested that ML is an effective tool to predict such an outbreak.

Jain et al. (2021) have predicted SARS-CoV and SARS-CoV-2 by using several ML models (Naïve Bayes, SVM, AdaBoost, K-NN, gradient boosting, RF, ensembles, XGBoost, and neural networks) with the B-cells dataset. The most accurate result was reported with AUC (0.923), validation accuracy (87.7934%) for SARS-CoV-2 and AUC (0.919), validation accuracy (87.248%) for SARS-CoV. Ghisolfi et al. (2020) have predicted COVID-19 fatality rates on the basis of sex, age, health system capacity, and comorbidities. The SIR model for predicting COVID-19 casualties was also reported by Tutsoy et al. (2020). Iwendi et al. (2020) have reported a fine-tuned RF model boosted by AdaBoost algorithm with the geographical, health, travel, and demographic data of the COVID-19 patients to predict recovery, severity, and possible outcome. This model has an F1 score of 0.86 and accuracy of 94% with the used dataset and revealed a positive correlation between death and gender.

Muhammad et al. (2021) have compared the supervised ML models (logistic regression, SVM, DT, naive Bayes, ANN) by using the COVID-19 infection dataset of Mexico. The methodology to build ML classification models is shown in Figure 11.2. Some 80% of the data set was used for training and 20% was used for testing the models. This study displayed that the NB model has the highest specificity (94.30%), the DT model has the highest accuracy (94.99%), and the SVM model has the highest sensitivity (93.34%).

11.4.2 PREDICTION OF OUTCOMES

Jimenez-Solem et al. (2021) have predicted the risk of death as 0.906 at diagnosis, 0.721 at ICU admission, and 0.818 at hospital admission by ML models. The United Kingdom Biobank SARS-CoV-2 positive cases dataset was used for external validation. In this study, common risk factors are body mass index, age, and hypertension, with top risk features in ICU patients (shock, organ dysfunction). The authors suggested that the ML models may be used for accurate prediction of outcomes in COVID-19 (disease progression and death) at different stages of management.

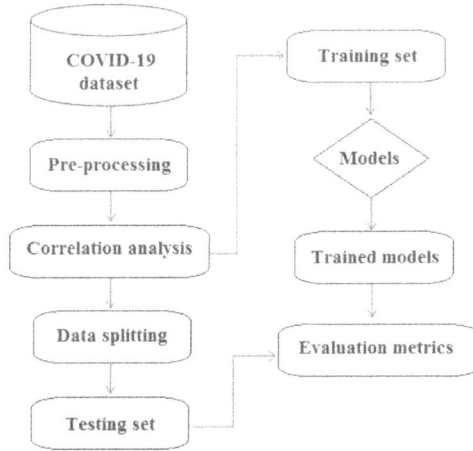

FIGURE 11.2   Methodology to build ML models for COVID-19 infection.

11.4.3   ACCURATE DIAGNOSTIC MODELS

Li et al. (2020) have proposed an accurate diagnosis model on the basis of symptoms and routine test data by using ML techniques to re-analyze reported COVID-19 data. The authors have investigated the correlations between clinical variables (lymphocytes, neutrophils), cluster into subtypes (immune cells, gender), and also classified influenza patients and COVID-19 patients. They have also trained an XG Boost model to attain sensitivity (92.5%) and specificity (97.9%) in discriminating the patients of COVID-19 from influenza patients. However, H1N1 cases were included due to difficulties.

Haque and Abdelgawad (2020) have proposed a CNN model from chest x-ray images to detect COVID-19 patients. For comparative analysis, two more CNN models and three other models (VGG-16, ResNet50, VGG-19) were investigated. All six models were trained, validated with two datasets (small and large). This model performed with 98.3% accuracy, 96.72% precision, 0.983 ROC, and a 98.3 F1-score. The complete system architecture for the detection of COVID-19 with CNN is shown in Figure 11.3. The study will be helpful to control the spread of this virus.

Roberts et al. (2021) have described the ML models for COVID-19 diagnosis from CXR and CT images. The study suggested that none of the reported models are suitable for potential clinical use. Shorten et al. (2021) have described the key limitations (interpretability, generalization metrics, data privacy, and limited labeled

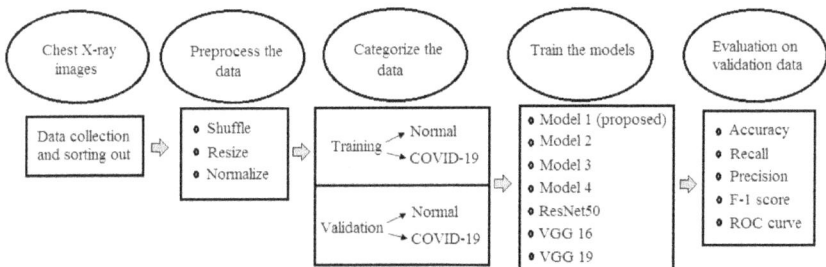

FIGURE 11.3   The architecture for detection of COVID-19 with CNN.

data) of DL in COVID-19 with the availability of big data. They have discussed several aspects such as public sentiment analysis, medical image analysis, ambient intelligence, protein structure prediction, precision diagnostics, and also for drug repurposing. DL technique is also used in forecasting for epidemiology. Hence, the study will be helpful to adopt DL technique for COVID-19 and/or related research.

As we all know, early stage detection/diagnosis is essential to control/prevent the spreading of COVID-19. With this in mind, Silva et al. (2020) have proposed a novel efficient DL technique to screen COVID-19 patients with voting-based approach. The model was analyzed with a cross-dataset study to evaluate robustness. However, the accuracy drops (87.68% → 56.16%) on the best evaluation scenario and suggest improving the model significantly for consideration clinically. Moreover, Shibly et al. (2020) have suggested that the use of DNN techniques coupled with radiological imaging may be useful to identify COVID-19 disease accurately. They have introduced a VGG-16 network-based faster R-CNN framework to detect/screen the patients from chest x-ray images with accuracy of 97.36%, sensitivity 97.65%, and precision 99.28%. So, the proposed model may be helpful to assess COVID-19 initially. The workflow representation with working procedure of the proposed model is shown in Figure 11.4.

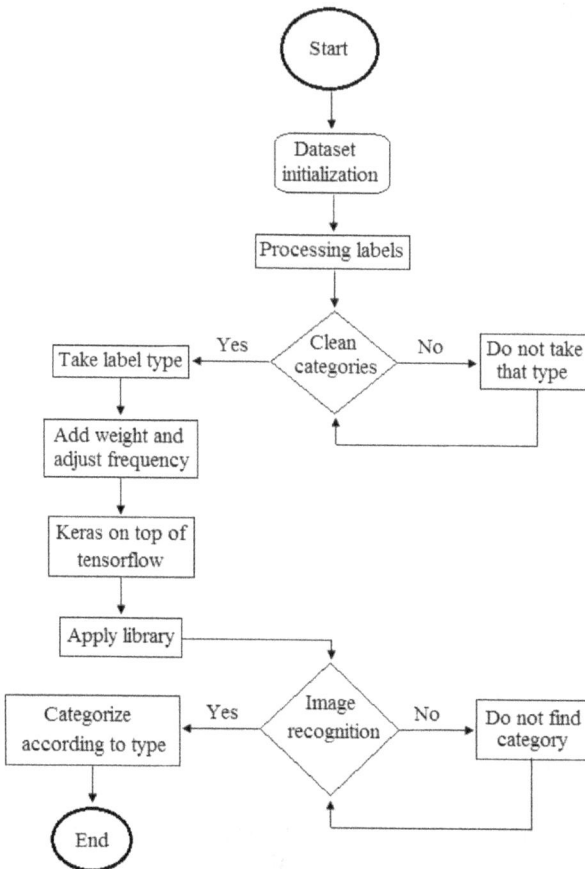

FIGURE 11.4   The workflow representation for the proposed model.

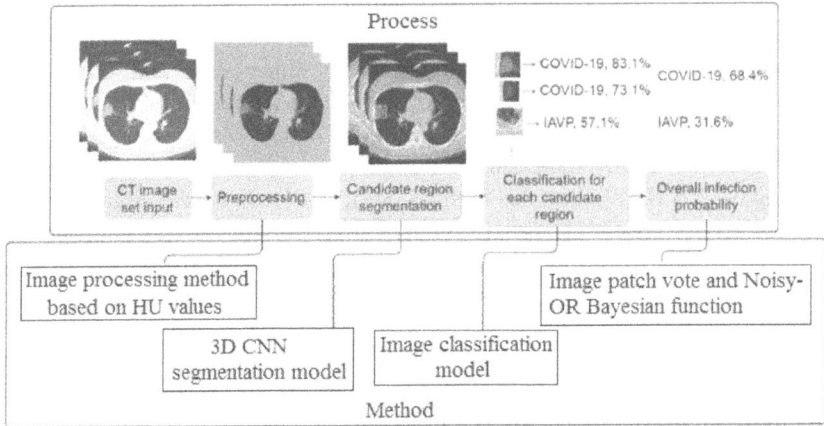

FIGURE 11.5 The process flow chart for the study.

Xu et al. (2020) have reported an early detecting model to identify influenza-A from COVID-19 by pulmonary CT images with DL techniques. The study showed overall accuracy rate of 86.7% with all cases. Hence, the established model was effective for early stage detection in patients. The process flow chart is shown in Figure 11.5.

Khakharia et al. (2020) have developed a prediction system for the COVID-19 pandemic for some densely populated countries. This prediction model has average accuracy of 87.9% ± 3.9% with highest accuracy (99.93%) for Ethiopia. Furthermore, Wang et al. (2020b) have analyzed an RF algorithm to forecast COVID-19 data obtained from Wuhan Fourth Hospital and identified the patients' optimal clinical prognoses. They have chosen 11 clinical parameters (age, Myo, CD8, LMR, LDH, CD45, dyspnea, Th/Ts, NLR, CK, D-Dimer) with AUC (0.9905). The study predicted patient mortality with high accuracy and identified LDH >500 U/L and Myo >80 ng/ml.

11.5 CONCLUSION

Infectious diseases, in particular, are continuously causing seasonal epidemics and pandemics. Hence, the accurate prediction of such diseases is attracting continued interest due to global importance. The uncertainty regarding the growth rate of the recent COVID-19 infection makes it difficult for the healthcare system to adapt according to the increasing requirements. Also, health professionals, certain ages, gender, and races are mostly affected. Some studies have also been reported for the modeling of the recent COVID-19 pandemic in several countries using AI and ML algorithms. The detection and diagnosis of this disease in the early stage is a challenging task. The accurate prediction of the disease will help in providing high-quality healthcare services and may reduce the disease severity and mortality. In this overview, we have discussed different ML techniques for the automotive detection, prediction, and diagnosis of COVID-19 which may help to increase the patient survival rate. Therefore, we hope the study may provide useful information for monitoring such a pandemic as the COVID-19 outbreak in the future.

ACKNOWLEDGMENT

All authors acknowledge their respective institute and university for providing the necessary facilities and support.

REFERENCES

Ahmad, F.K., and N. Yusoff. 2013. Classifying breast cancer types based on fine needle aspiration biopsy data using random forest classifier, in *Proceedings of the 13th International Conference on Intelligent Systems Design and Applications*. 121–25.

Ardabili, S.F., A. Mosavi, P. Ghamisi, et al. 2020. COVID-19 outbreak prediction with machine learning. *Algorithms*. 13:249. https://doi.org/10.3390/a13100249

Arolas, H.P., E. Acosta, G. López-Casasnovas, et al. 2021. Years of life lost to COVID-19 in 81 countries. *Scientific Reports*. 11:3504.

Arumugam, V.A., S. Thangavelu, Z. Fathah, et al. 2020. COVID-19 and the world with co-morbidities of heart disease, hypertension and diabetes. *Journal of Pure and Applied Microbiology*. 14(3):1623–38. https://doi.org/10.22207/JPAM.14.3.01

Bezdek, J.C., R. Ehrlich, and W. Full. 1984. FCM: The fuzzy c-means clustering algorithm. *Computers & Geosciences*. 10(2–3):191–203.

Breiman, L. 2001. Random forests. *Machine Learning*. 45(1):5–32.

Chan, J.F., S. Yuan, K.H. Kok, et al. 2020. A familial cluster of pneumonia associated with the 2019 novel Coronavirus indicating person-to-person transmission: a study of a family cluster. *Lancet*. https://doi.org/S0140-6736(20)30154-9

Dhama, K., S. Khan, R. Tiwari, et al. 2020a. Coronavirus disease 2019-COVID-19. *Clinical Microbiology Reviews*. 33(4):e00028–20.

Dhama, K., S.K. Patel, M. Pathak, et al. 2020b. An update on SARS-CoV-2/COVID-19 with particular reference to its clinical pathology, pathogenesis, immunopathology and mitigation strategies. *Travel Medicine and Infectious Disease*. 37:101755.

Evgeniou, T., and M. Pontil. 2005. Support vector machines: Theory and applications, in *Advanced Course on Artificial Intelligence*. Berlin, Germany: Springer, 249–257.

Fakoor, R., F. Ladhak, A. Nazi, et al. 2013. Using deep learning to enhance cancer diagnosis and classification, in *Proceedings of the International Conference on Machine Learning.*, New York, NY, 28, 1–7.

Fatima, N., L. Liu, S. Hong, et al. 2020.Prediction of breast cancer, comparative review of machine learning techniques, and their analysis. *Journals & Magazines, IEEE Access*. 8:150360–76.

Ghisolfi, S., I. Almås, J.C. Sandefur, et al. 2020. Predicted COVID-19 fatality rates based on age, sex, comorbidities and health system capacity. *BMJ Global Health*. 5:e003094. https://doi.org/10.1136/bmjgh-2020-003094

Hamed, G., M.A.E.-R. Marey, S.E.-S. Amin, et al. 2020. Deep learning in breast cancer detection and classification, in *Proceeding of Joint Euro-US Workshop Appl. Invariance Computing*. Vis. Cham, Switzerland: Springer, 322–33.

Haque, K.F., and A. Abdelgawad. 2020. A deep learning approach to detect COVID-19 patients from chest x-ray images. *AI*. 1:418–35. https://doi.org/10.3390/ai1030027

Hasan, N. 2020. A methodological approach for predicting COVID-19 epidemic using EEMD-ANN hybrid model. *Internet of Things*. 11:100228.

Hassanien, A.E., A. Khamparia, D. Gupta, et al. 2021. Cognitive Internet of Medical Things for Smart Healthcare. https://doi.org/10.1007/978-3-030-55833-8

Ibrahim, A.A., A.I. Hashad, and N.E.M. Shawky. 2017. A comparison of open source data mining tools for breast cancer classification, in *Handbook of Research on Machine Learning Innovations and Trends*. Hershey, PA: IGI Global, 636–51.

Imandoust, S.B., and M. Bolandraftar, 2013. Application of k-nearest neighbor (KNN) approach for predicting economic events: Theoretical background. *International Journal of Engineering Research and Applications*. 3:605–10.

Iwendi, C., A.K. Bashir, A. Peshkar, et al. 2020. COVID-19 patient health prediction using boosted Random Forest algorithm. *Frontiers in Public Health*. 8:357. https://doi.org/10.3389/fpubh.2020.00357

Jain, N., S. Jhunthra, H. Garg, et al. 2021. Prediction modelling of COVID using machine learning methods from B-cell dataset. *Results in Physics*. 21:103813.

Jimenez-Solem, E., T.S. Petersen, C. Hansen, et al. 2021. Developing and validating COVID-19 adverse outcome risk prediction models from a bi-national European cohort of 5594 patients. *Scientific Reports*. 11:3246. https://doi.org/10.1038/s41598-021-81844-x

Jindal, M., J. Gupta, and B. Bhushan, 2019. Machine learning methods for IoT and their Future Applications, 2019 International Conference on Computing, Communication, and Intelligent Systems (ICCCIS), in *IEEE Xplore*. 430–434. ISBN: 978-1-7281-4826-7.

Khakharia, A., V. Shah, S. Jain, et al. 2020. Outbreak prediction of COVID-19 for dense and populated countries using machine learning. *Annals of Data Science*. https://doi.org/10.1007/s40745-020-00314-9

Khamparia, A., P.K. Singh, P. Rani, et al. 2020. An internet of health things-driven deep learning framework for detection and classification of skin cancer using transfer learning. *Transactions on Emerging Telecommunications Technologies*. e3963. https://doi.org/10.1002/ett.3963

Kucharski, A.J., T.W. Russell, C. Diamond, et al. 2020. Early dynamics of transmission and control of COVID-19: a mathematical modeling study. *Lancet Infectious Diseases*. https://doi.org/10.1016/S1473-3099(20)30144-4

Kumar, S., B. Bhusan, D. Singh, et al. 2020. Classification of Diabetes using Deep Learning, International Conference on Communication and Signal Processing, in *IEEE Xplore*. 651–55.

LeCun, Y., Y. Bengio, and G. Hinton. 2015. Deep learning, *Nature*, 521(7553):436–44.

Lenzen, M., M. Li, A. Malik, et al. 2020.Global socio-economic losses and environmental gains from the Coronavirus pandemic. *PLoS One*. 15(7):e0235654.

Li, W.T., J. Ma, N. Shende, et al. 2020.Using machine learning of clinical data to diagnose COVID-19: a systematic review and meta-analysis. *BMC Medical Informatics and Decision Making*. 20:247. https://doi.org/10.1186/s12911-020-01266-z

Li, Y., and H. Wu, 2012. A clustering method based on K-means algorithm. *Physics Procedia*. 25:1104–109.

Mohapatra, R.K., P.K. Das, and V. Kandi. 2020a. Challenges in controlling COVID-19 in migrants in Odisha, India. *Diabetes & Metabolic Syndrome: Clinical Research & Reviews*. 14:1593–94.

Mohapatra, R.K., L. Pintilie, V. Kandi, et al. 2020b. The recent challenges of highly contagious COVID-19; causing respiratory infections: symptoms, diagnosis, transmission, possible vaccines, animal models and immunotherapy. *Chemical Biology & Drug Design*. 96:1187–208. https://doi.org/10.1111/cbdd.13761

Mohapatra, R.K., V.P. Saikishore, M. Azam, et al. 2020c. Synthesis and physicochemical studies of a series of mixed ligand transition metal complexes and their molecular docking investigations against Coronavirus main protease. *Open Chemistry*. 18:1495–506.

Mohapatra, R.K., P.K. Das, L. Pintilie, et al. 2021a. Infection capability of SARS-CoV-2 on different surfaces. *Egyptian Journal of Basic and Applied Science.* 8(1):75–80.

Mohapatra, R.K., S. Mishra, M. Azam, et al. 2021b. COVID-19, WHO guidelines, pedagogy, and respite. *Open Medicine.* 16:491–93.

Mohapatra, R.K., L. Perekhoda, M. Azam, et al. 2021c. Computational investigations of three main drugs and their comparison with synthesized compounds as potent inhibitors of SARS-CoV-2 main protease (Mpro): DFT, QSAR, molecular docking, and in silico toxicity analysis. *Journal of King Saud University – Science.* 33:101315.

Mohapatra, R.K., and M. Rahman. 2021. Is it possible to control the outbreak of COVID-19 in Dharavi, Asia's largest slum situated in Mumbai? *Anti-Infective Agents.* 19(4): 1–2. https://doi.org/10.2174/2211352518999200831142851

Morawska, L., and J. Cao. 2020. Airborne transmission of SARS-CoV-2: The world should face the reality. *Environment International.* 139:105730.

Muhammad, L.J., E.A. Algehyne, S.S. Usman, et al. 2021. Supervised machine learning models for prediction of COVID-19 infection using epidemiology dataset.*SN Computer Science.* 2:11. https://doi.org/10.1007/s42979-020-00394-7

Munir, K., H. Elahi, A. Ayub, et al. 2019. Cancer diagnosis using deep learning: A bibliographic review. *Cancers.* 11(9):1235.

Nicola, M., Z. Alsafi, C. Sohrabi, et al. 2020.The socio-economic implications of the Coronavirus pandemic (COVID-19): A review. *International Journal of Surgery.* 78:185–93.

Panigrahi, N., I. Ayus, and O.P. Jena, 2021. An expert system-based clinical decision support system for hepatitis-b prediction & diagnosis, Chapter 4. https://doi.org/10.1002/9781119792611.ch4

Paramesha, K., H.L. Gururaj, and O.P. Jena, 2021. Applications of machine learning in biomedical text processing and food industry, Chapter 10. https://doi.org/10.1002/9781119792611.ch10

Patel, S., S. Sihmar, and A. Jatain. 2015. A study of hierarchical clustering algorithms, in *Proceeding of Second International. Conference on Computing for Sustainable Global Development (INDIA.com).* 537–41.

Patra, S.S., O.P. Jena, G. Kumar, et al. 2021. Random Forest algorithm in imbalance genomics classification, Chapter 7. https://doi.org/10.1002/9781119785620.ch7

Pattnayak, P., and O.P. Jena, 2021. Innovation on machine learning in healthcare services–an introduction, Chapter 1, https://doi.org/10.1002/9781119792611.ch1

Rana, A.K., A.O. Salau, S. Gupta, et al. 2019. Machine learning methods for IoT and their Future Applications, in *2019 International Conference on Computing, Communication, and Intelligent Systems (ICCCIS)*, IEEE Xplore. https://doi.org/10.1109/icccis48478.2019.8974551

Reddy, R., and T.D. Imler. 2017. Artificial neural networks are highly predictive for hepatocellular carcinoma in patients with cirrhosis. *Gastroenterology.* 152:S1193.

Roberts, M., D. Driggs, M. Thorpe, et al. 2021. Common pitfalls and recommendations for using machine learning to detect and prognosticate for COVID-19 using chest radiographs and CT scans. *Nature Machine Intelligence.* 3:199–217. https://doi.org/10.1038/s42256-021-00307-0

Sah, R., A.P. Khatiwada, S. Shrestha, et al. 2021. The COVID-19 vaccination campaign in Nepal, emerging UK variant and futuristic vaccination strategies to combat the ongoing pandemic, *Travel Medicine and Infectious Disease.* 41:102037.

Selvathi, D., and A. A. Poornila. 2018. Deep learning techniques for breast cancer detection using medical image analysis, in *Biologically Rationalized Computing Techniques for Image Processing Applications.* Cham, Switzerland: Springer, 159–86.

Sharma, H., and S. Kumar, 2016. A survey on decision tree algorithms of classification in data mining. *International Journal of Science and Research,.* 5(4):2094–97.

Shibly, K.H., S.K. Dey, T.-U. Islam, et al. 2020. COVID faster R–CNN: A novel framework to diagnose novel Coronavirus disease (COVID-19) in X-ray images. *Informatics in Medicine Unlocked*. 20:100405.

Shorten, C., T.M. Khoshgoftaar, and B. Furht. 2021. Deep learning applications for COVID-19. *Journal of Big Data*. 8:18. https://doi.org/10.1186/s40537-020-00392-9

Silva, P., E. Luz, G. Silva, et al. 2020. COVID-19 detection in CT images with deep learning: A voting-based scheme and cross-datasets analysis. *Informatics in Medicine Unlocked*. 20:100427.

Singhal, P., and S. Pareek, 2018. Artificial neural network for prediction of breast cancer, in *Proc. 2nd Int. Conf. I-SMAC (IoT Social, Mobile, Anal. Cloud) (I-SMAC)*. 464–68.

Tiwari, M., R. Bharuka, P. Shah, et al. 2020. *Breast cancer prediction using deep learning and machine learning techniques.*

Togacar, M., and B. Ergen. 2018. Deep learning approach for classification of breast cancer, in *Proc. Int. Conf. Artif. Intell. Data Process. (IDAP)*. 1–5.

Tutsoy, O., U. Çolak, A. Polat, et al. 2020. A novel parametric model for the prediction and analysis of the COVID-19 casualties. *IEEE Access*. https://doi.org/10.1109/ACCESS.2020.3033146

Uddin, S., A. Khan, E. Hossain, et al. 2019. Comparing different supervised machine learning algorithms for disease prediction. *BMC Medical Informatics and Decision Making*. 19:281. https://doi.org/10.1186/s12911-019-1004-8

Uzun, Y., and G. Tezel, 2012. Rule learning with machine learning algorithms and artificial neural networks. *Journal of Selcuk University Natural and Applied Science* 1(2):1–11.

Wang, D., B. Hu, C. Hu, et al. 2020a. Clinical characteristics of 138 hospitalized patients with 2019 novel Coronavirus-infected pneumonia in Wuhan, China. *JAMA*. https://doi.org/10.1001/jama.2020.1585

Wang, J., H. Yu, Q. Hua, et al. 2020b. A descriptive study of random forest algorithm for predicting COVID-19 patients outcome. *Peer J*. 8:e9945. https://doi.org/10.7717/peerj.9945

Wu, W., S. Nagarajan, and Z. Chen, 2015. Bayesian machine learning: EEGMEG signal processing measurements. *IEEE Signal Process. Mag*. 33(1):14–36.

Xu, X., X. Jiang, C. Ma, et al. 2020. A deep learning system to screen novel Coronavirus disease 2019 pneumonia. *Engineering*. 6:1122–29.

Zhang, J., X. Hong, S.-U. Guan, et al. 2016. Maximum Gaussian mixture model for classification, in *8th International Conference on Information Technology in Medicine and Education, (ITME)*. 587–91.

Zhang, R., Y. Li, A. L. Zhang, et al. 2020a. Identifying airborne transmission as the dominant route for the spread of COVID-19. *Proceedings of the National Academy of Sciences USA*. 117(26):14857–63.

Zhang, X., H. Saleh, E.M.G. Younis, et al. 2020b. Predicting Coronavirus pandemic in real-time using machine learning and big data streaming system. *Complexity*. 2020, Article ID 6688912, https://doi.org/10.1155/2020/6688912

12 TRNetCoV
Transferred Learning-based ResNet Model for COVID-19 Detection Using Chest X-ray Images

G. V. Eswara Rao and B. Rajitha

CONTENTS

DOI: 10.1201/9781003226147-12

12.1   INTRODUCTION

The new coronavirus disease pandemic, named COVID-19, was identified in Wuhan, China in the December of 2019. The total number of COVID-19 confirmed cases and deaths has been rapidly increasing globally. Following these serious consequences, the World Health Organization (WHO) declared the COVID-19 as a pandemic on March 11, 2020. Since the COVID-19 disease shows a major impact on the respiratory system, chest X-rays (CXRs) and CT scans can help in identifying them easily. Thus, a fast and immediate diagnosis can be done using medical imaging such as CXRs and CT scans, which are used widely. However, CXR image processing has already been proven to be an essential imaging modality while identifying most cases of other respiratory issues. Hence the researchers are widely using this modality for COVID-19 estimation. There are many deep convolutional neural network (DCNN) models proposed during the COVID-19 pandemic. The main scope of deep learning (DL) is widely used in various aspects in terms of medical image inspection, new drug discovery [1], disease detection [2] and diagnosis, and other case study problems of hepatitis virus [3], and COVID-19 prediction.

12.2   ROLE OF CHEST X-RAY IMAGES IN COVID-19 DETECTION

CXRs are utilized as a complementary tool to predict the COVID-19 progression and its severity at different levels. A CXR is cheaper and readily available based on artificial intelligence (AI) techniques. Compared with other approaches, X-rays are easily accessible and achieve the highest performance in automatic diagnosis of the COVID-19 [4]. Particularly in COVID-19 classification, X-rays play a more challenging role to identify COVID-19 in the fight against the pandemic. On the other hand, CXRs are widely used in frontline clinical management during the early outbreak. In addition, different AI classification methods rely on a large-scale CXR dataset to detect the individual patient risk of COVID-19. Furthermore, to improve the DL model accuracy, a well-defined and larger dataset of COVID-19 positive CXRs is required.

This chapter has used the online available standard CXR images and trained on the transferred ResNet model for detection of COVID-19 cases consisting of the categories of Viral and Normal. These CXR images are also used to improve population management by taking immediate diagnosis. Figure 12.1 shows the general workflow for the proposed task.

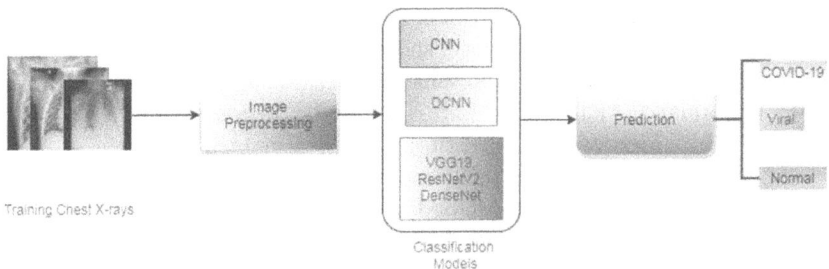

FIGURE 12.1   Overview of the proposed workflow of modern X-ray system for classification of COVID-19.

12.3 MOTIVATION

COVID-19 is a kind of Severe Acute Respiratory Syndrome Coronavirus 2 (SARS-CoV-2), according to Wang et al. [5], and it could lead to acute respiratory distress syndrome and other additional symptoms (i.e. fever, dry cough, body pains, nasal congestion, sore throat, organ failures, etc.). On the other hand, due to the rapid spread of COVID-19 and its long incubation periods and lesser healthcare systems, many countries were unable to manage the infected patients during detection and diagnosis of COVID-19. Ai et al. [6], along with many scientific research institutions and most of the world's governments, have declared that a necessary standard detection system in real-time could be done using the test named: Reverse Transcriptase Polymerase Chain Reaction (RT-PCR). Most of the countries are following this RT-PCR test as an immediate and faster detection kit. However, Kong et al. [7] found that RT-PCR tests often face a high false-negative rate. Moreover, in case the COVID positive cases suddenly increase, these kits are not readily available at all the clinical systems, which could be a reason for the virus spreading. Medical inspection is another clinical complementary method for COVID-19 detection, includes radiography chest images, that is, CXR and CT scan. CT and X-ray images can help in predicting the severity of COVID-19 by identifying the infected regions. Therefore, many AI-aided methods have been proposed and used in the detection of COVID-19 recently. Thus, the main objective of this chapter is to implement a TRNetCoV network model to detect COVID-19 disease with CXR images.

12.4 CHALLENGES IN CHEST X-RAY MODALITY

CXR imaging is widely used for disease classification. This clinical approach also plays an important role in infection recognition, region segmentation, and image acquisition. It also helps in improving the total accuracy and efficiency of the model. Segmentation is a common method for the prediction of COVID-19 severity for developing respiratory systems and modality during pandemics. To extract the lung organs from CXRs is more challenging because the region of interest (ROI) projection onto the soft tissues is a little complicated. Although, a multilevel segmentation method could be proposed to separate the lung organs from the infected regions. However, it is very time-consuming for large-scale training data.

12.5 CONTRIBUTIONS

Our major contributions for this chapter include:

- Studying the state-of-the-art existing DL models aiming to classify the various diseases, which includes COVID-19, viral, normal.
- Proposing a DCNN model that can classify the diseases based on CXR images which is helpful for COVID-19 detection.
- Creating and training the model by fine-tuning to detect the COVID-19.
- Investigating multi-class evaluation by applying hyperparameters in the proposed model.
- Evaluating and comparative analysis of proposed work with existing methods.

This chapter is organized as follows. Section 12.6 presents various existing models to address the COVID-19 detection. Section 12.7 describes some background of deep convolution techniques. Section 12.8 focuses on various preprocessing methodologies, while Section 12.9 presents our experimental setup along with results, and Section 12.10 highlights the complete performance analysis of the proposed system and then ends with a conclusion followed by future remarks in Section 12.11.

12.6   LITERATURE REVIEW

The process of the X-ray inspection method includes three components, such as data review includes (1) high dimensional data analysis [8], (2) pre-trained DCNN models, and (3) detection and classification of diseases [9]. To address the COVID-19 status, several frameworks have been proposed by many scientists. Table 12.1 presents the description of AI-based techniques used in COVID-19 research.

12.7   DEEP LEARNING MODELS

12.7.1   Artificial Neural Networks

Many traditional machine learning models are inspired by the human brain which contains billions of connected neurons and produces the output when the neuron meets a certain activated threshold value. The main property of the biological system is that it is able to learn and reorganize itself from the training experience. It can solve many difficult engineering problems such as disease classification, estimation of parameters, and any other aspects of medical imaging. It can also be used for healthcare services [10].

TABLE 12.1
Description of AI Techniques Used in COVID-19 Research

Acronym Forms	Description	Acronym Forms	Description
CL	Chaotic learning	GANs	Generative adversarial nets
DT	Decision Tree	GRU	Gate recurrent unit
GA	Genetic Algorithm	KNN	K-nearest neighbor
PR	Polynomial Regression	MLP	Multi-layered perceptron
RF	Random Forest	RNN	Recurrent neural network
RL	Reinforcement Learning	SVM	Support vector machine
TL	Transfer Learning	SVR	Support vector regression
CNN	Convolution neural network	DCNN	Deep CNN
DNN	Deep neural network	LSTM	Long short-term memory
GAE	Generative auto-encoder	Mol2Vec	Molecular to vectors
DQN	Deep-Q learning	SEIR	Susceptible infected recovered

12.7.2 Deep Convolution Neural Networks

DCNN is a subdomain of AI that has different transform neurons rather than neural networks. CNN can classify the diseases based on the CXR image dataset. Detecting the disease is usually a difficult task in the area of medicine. These CNNs can save time by automating the pinpoint of detecting the disease. However, the input value is passed to CNN in the form of a two or three-dimensional matrix. In general, DCNN is a network that has two primary components with a set of distinct layers, and each layer has its significance for classifying the disease. The main building blocks are categorized into feature extraction and classification.

12.7.2.1 Feature Extraction

- **Convolution layer:** It has performed some convolution operations during convolution. In this layer, there are two functions that are usually applied over subparts of an input image for feature extraction, such as a matrix called kernel or filter and stride. At each slide, the filter will be moving on input and compute the sum of the products of individual sub-part values. The number of slides and their dimension is determined by stride size. For certain selective features, various filters such as vertical, horizontal, Sobel, and Scharr are usually applied over the input image. Despite these, multiple filter operation is also possible for certain problems.
- **Activation function:** In this part, the output of convolution layer has been passed to the next consecutive layers through a function called activation [11], preferably Rectified Linear Unit (ReLu). The mathematical notation of the function is as follows:

$$f(x) = max(0, x) \tag{12.1}$$

where 'x' is the input value to the node.
- **Padding:** During the feature extraction process, information may be lost as compared with the original input value. Hence, based on selective features, padding will be optional for more remarkable results. In this scene, the input is considered as two dimensions for the summary of convolution will be passed to the pooling process.

Without padding:

$$Input : nXn \tag{12.2}$$

$$FilterSize : fXf \tag{12.3}$$

$$Output : (n - f + 1) X (n - f + 1) \tag{12.4}$$

With padding:

$$Input : mXm \tag{12.5}$$

$$Paddingpissettobe \ 1 \tag{12.6}$$

$$FilterSize : kXk \qquad (12.7)$$

$$Output : (m + 2p + 1) X (m + 2p + 1) \qquad (12.8)$$

where m, n are input size, f, k is the filter size.

- **Pooling:** This is another kind of compression technique to make computation more robust. Given resultant featured input, Max pooling subsampling picks the most prominent value while average pooling takes an average within the given kernel.
- **Dropout:** To minimize the error or overfitting of the model from the training data, some weights will be considered as dropped nodes when having a probability of 0.5, known as a dropout.

12.7.2.2 Classification

This block consists of a set of fully connected layers that takes the group of input features into a one-dimensional vector. It looks at the observed values that are closed to target values by applying some distribution functions.

Softmax Layer: It is a kind of multi-label classifier to distribute the probability of each label. Furthermore, the output of each class label is to be normalizing in the range of (0.1). The standard equation of softmax is defined as follows:

$$\sigma(Z) = {e_i^z} \Big/ {\sum_{j=1}^{K} e_j^z} \qquad (12.9)$$

$$For\, i = 1, 23, \ldots\ldots K and z = (z1,\, z2, z3, \ldots .zk) \in [0,1]$$

12.7.3 Related Work Against COVID-19 Detection

In recent years, a group of DL models was trained on CXR images to identify COVID-19. Among them, the popular DL frameworks proposed for automatic detection of COVID-19 include VGG16, DenseNet201, ResNetV2, MobileNetV2, AlexNet, and XceptionNet. Table 12.2 shows the AI-assisted CXR image detection methods proposed by various researchers for the detection of COVID-19.

TABLE 12.2
AI-assisted CXR Image Detection Methods for COVID-19

Authors	Dataset Size of X-ray Images	COVID-19 Cases	AI-based Deep Models
Wang	13,800	183	COVID-Net
Zhang	1531	100	New DL
Ioannis	1472	224	VGG, MobileNet, Inception
Castiglioni	610	324	ResNet
Loey	306	69	AlexNet, GoogleNet, ResNet
Maghdid	170	60	ALexNet

TABLE 12.3
Various Deep Learning Models Against COVID-19

Clinical Contribution	AI Technologies Based on DL	Model Names
CXR and CT Image Inspection	CNN, DCNN, GANs, TL, Combined ML	U-Net, V-Net, VB-Net, LASSO, LR, RF, VGG, AlexNet, SVM, ResNet

In this way, few models were constructed as image feature extractors based on VGG, AlexNet, GoogleNet, DenseNet, and InceptionResNet. Szegedy et al. [12] and Krizhevsky et al. [13] had also used similar feature extraction methods.

Simonyan et al. [14] had integrated DCNN models built on CXR images, such as the VGG19 model given by Huang et al. [15], DenseNet201, ResNEtV2, and InceptionV3 from Chebet et al. [16].

Later, some of these typical DCNN models –VGG, ResNet50, and InceptionV3 – were improved and recommended for medical image classification on small-scale CXR images for COVID-19. Their results displayed that ResNet50 had achieved 98% accuracy, which was the superior performance among other AI methods they used. Table 12.3 gives more detailed information about various DL models against COVID-19.

12.8   METHODOLOGIES

12.8.1   DATA PREPROCESSING TECHNIQUE

Initially, the collected groups of COVID-19 CXR images could be relatively massive in noise information and this data could sometimes be fake. In the era of social media, filtering fake information is a crucial step in medical imaging. However, AI-based models can be used to identify fake news from online media platforms. As a consequence, this issue can limit the performance of DCNN models in the epidemic prediction. The CXR images are resized to the size of 224x224x3. Then on each image of the dataset, a normalization method is applied, which responds to the model and could benefit in overall performance. Figure 12.2 displays the complete flowchart of data processing stages proposed in this chapter.

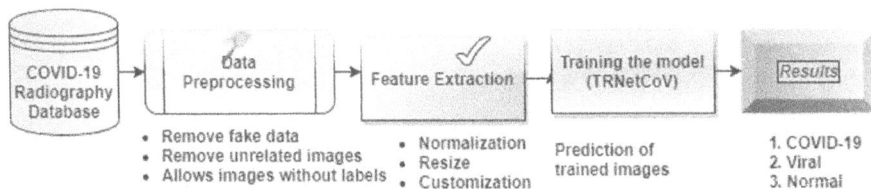

FIGURE 12.2   Steps involved in the preprocessing stage of the proposed work.

12.8.2 Data Augmentation Technique

To build an optimized deep model in the area of medical science, it has to be ensured that the quality of the public dataset be sufficient for training and testing the models. Data augmentation helps in generating such a level of accuracy. To reduce data uncertainty and over-fitting, here in the proposed work, the size of the image training dataset has been increased by applying some image augmentation techniques. For this experiment, different augmentation methods have been developed to increase the amount of data space. More specifically, the image Rescale, Shear_range, zoom_range, horizontal_flip, vertical_flip have been applied with various data processing parameters. For example, during training, all images were randomly rotated by 30 degrees, randomly zoomed by 10–20%, randomly shifted horizontally and vertically by 10% concerning width and height of the image, etc. Additionally, image augmentation expands the size of the small dataset that helps to improve the ability of the model to predict new images.

12.8.3 Proposed Deep Transfer-Based Learning Model

Generally, DL models encourage more number output features from an image; whereas ML-based models still have some limitations in terms of the number of extracted features, preparation of dataset, and overall performance. Therefore DL models have become more accurate approaches for AI-based applications. However, as the model increases the number of layers, the performance and accuracy of a deep trained neural network might degrade due to its vanishing gradient problem. However, residual learning models having more than 150 layers have solved this problem by introducing identity skip connections for a set of convolutional blocks, thus this proposed work used this model. Figure 12.3 presents one such base architecture of the residual learning model.

Here a novel and better-tuned version of deep ResNet architecture called TRNetCoV has been proposed to identify COVID-19 for a large class of disease datasets, such as pneumonia and normal. This new classification model operates based on Shin et al. [18] ResNet with a 50-layer DCNN. This new model will make transfer learning [19] from loaded pre-trained weights of ResNet50 on a small

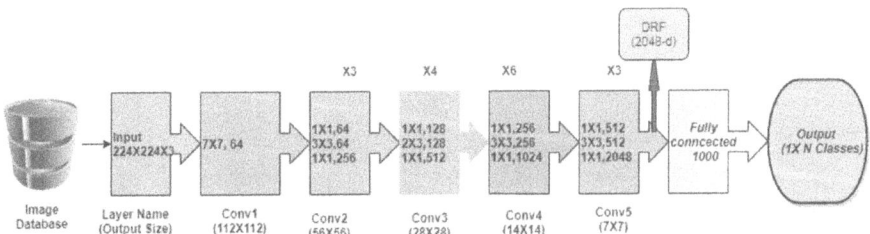

FIGURE 12.3 Basic architecture of residual learning Model. (Modified from He et al. [17].)

COVID-19 dataset. In the proposed work, a pre-trained ResNet50 model consists of the following basic operations.

12.8.3.1 Basic Blocks

From Figure 12.3, the proposed model uses the same basic blocks along with other fine-tuned control parameters as follows:

- **Hinge loss function:** To minimize the loss error from the learning problem, selection of a loss function that will help to reduce the risk. In this multi-label classification, the loss will be controlled and defined as follows:

$$l(y) = max(0, 1 + WyX - WtX) \tag{12.10}$$

where Wt and Wy are the control parameters for the training model.

- **Adam optimizer:** This was adapted to combine the advantages of both RMSprop and AdaGrad, improves the performance over gradient problem. This strategy helps in fixing the updated weight for old weights. All the updating weights will be regularizing by the following rule:

$$wt = wt - 1 - \eta \left(\frac{m^\wedge}{\sqrt{vt + \in}} + \delta wt - 1 \right) \tag{12.11}$$

where indexes wt, $wt-1$ indicate the control parameters on training iterations.

Figure 12.4 demonstrates the overview of the proposed TRNetCoV architecture for classification.

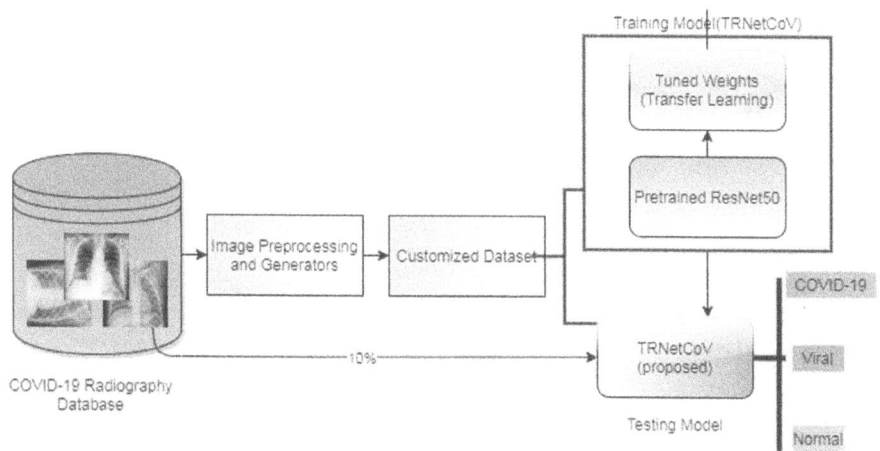

FIGURE 12.4 Demonstrates the TRNetCoV architecture for classification.

TABLE 12.4
Statistics of the Dataset Distribution

Dataset Statistics	COVID	Viral	Normal	Set Size
Number of training images	189	1315	1360	2864
Testing observations	171	1173	1216	2560

12.9   EXPERIMENTAL SETUP AND RESULT ANALYSIS

12.9.1   COLLECTION OF DATASET AND RESOURCES

For experiments, the dataset recently published publicly as COVID-19 Radiography Database and available from the Kaggle [20] website has been used. This open-source dataset has been created with different researchers, doctors, and their collaborators from the University of Dhaka, Qatar University, pad Chest, and other Github resources. All CXR images were collected in the format of portable network graphics with a resolution of 299x299. This database contains a set of 1200 positive COVID-19 cases, 1315 cases of viral, and 1357 normal images.

In this particular experiment, the COVID-19 Radiography Dataset consisting of three categories of CXR images – COVID-19, viral, and normal – has been used. To achieve an efficient evaluation of the TRNetCoV model, the dataset has been separated randomly into two parts, that is, 90% of CXRs were used for training and 10% were considered for both testing and validation. The proposed TRNetCoV has been implemented by using an IDLE as Jupyter notebook, Keras packages, and running on Intel Core i5-CPU 2.50GHz. Table 12.4 shows the complete statistics of dataset distribution.

12.9.2   EXPERIMENT AND RESULTS

The proposed TRNetCoV model had been fine-tuned for 20 epochs, assigned cross-entropy as loss function and batch size is fixed as 32. To minimize the loss, Adam is used as an optimizer with a learning rate of 0.0001. With this experiment, it has been observed that our model was performing better and the same can be seen from Table 12.5.

TABLE 12.5
New Hyperparameters Controls in the Proposed Model

Hyperparameters	Possible Values	Applied Value
Loss function	Binary or Hinge	Categorical Cross entropy
Activation function	Softmax or Tanh or ReLu	ReLu and softmax
Optimizer	Stochastic Gradient descent or Adam	Adam optimizer
Number of epochs	10–1000	20
Batch size	1<BS<3264	32
Learning rate	0.0–1.0	0.0001
Dropout	0.1–0.5	0.4
Output size	1–1000	3

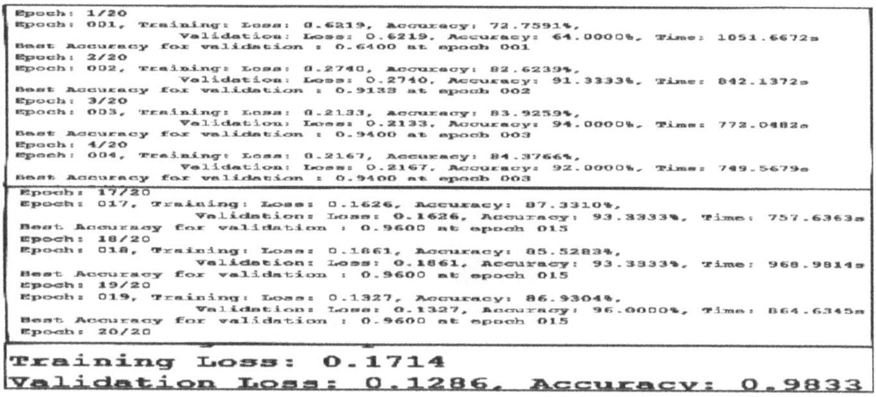

```
Epoch: 1/20
Epoch: 001, Training: Loss: 0.6219, Accuracy: 72.7591%,
              Validation: Loss: 0.6219, Accuracy: 64.0000%, Time: 1051.6672s
Best Accuracy for validation : 0.6400 at epoch 001
Epoch: 2/20
Epoch: 002, Training: Loss: 0.2740, Accuracy: 82.6239%,
              Validation: Loss: 0.2740, Accuracy: 91.3333%, Time: 842.1372s
Best Accuracy for validation : 0.9133 at epoch 002
Epoch: 3/20
Epoch: 003, Training: Loss: 0.2133, Accuracy: 83.9259%,
              Validation: Loss: 0.2133, Accuracy: 94.0000%, Time: 772.0482s
Best Accuracy for validation : 0.9400 at epoch 003
Epoch: 4/20
Epoch: 004, Training: Loss: 0.2167, Accuracy: 84.3766%,
              Validation: Loss: 0.2167, Accuracy: 92.0000%, Time: 749.5679s
Best Accuracy for validation : 0.9400 at epoch 003
Epoch: 17/20
Epoch: 017, Training: Loss: 0.1626, Accuracy: 87.3310%,
              Validation: Loss: 0.1626, Accuracy: 93.3333%, Time: 757.6363s
Best Accuracy for validation : 0.9600 at epoch 015
Epoch: 18/20
Epoch: 018, Training: Loss: 0.1861, Accuracy: 85.5283%,
              Validation: Loss: 0.1861, Accuracy: 93.3333%, Time: 968.9814s
Best Accuracy for validation : 0.9600 at epoch 015
Epoch: 19/20
Epoch: 019, Training: Loss: 0.1327, Accuracy: 86.9304%,
              Validation: Loss: 0.1327, Accuracy: 96.0000%, Time: 864.6345s
Best Accuracy for validation : 0.9600 at epoch 015
Epoch: 20/20
```

Training Loss: 0.1714
Validation Loss: 0.1286, Accuracy: 0.9833

FIGURE 12.5   Training and validation progress of the proposed TRNetCoV model.

Furthermore, Figures 12.5 and 12.6 present the resultant graphs of the proposed model. We computed training and validation accuracy for every epoch which extracts the best accuracy during the forward pass. It also compares the validation loss and training loss at every epoch. The proposed model gave us a better accuracy of 98.33% and validation loss at around 0.12 which can be confirmed by Figures 12.6 and 12.7.

12.10   PERFORMANCE ANALYSIS

12.10.1   METRICS USED FOR PERFORMANCE MEASUREMENT

To assess the performance of the proposed model TRNetCoV for COVID-19 detection, multi-class evaluation criteria techniques have been used. These are average accuracy, sensitivity, specificity, precision, and F1-score. Thus, the equations are different from other classification types in terms of calculation procedures.

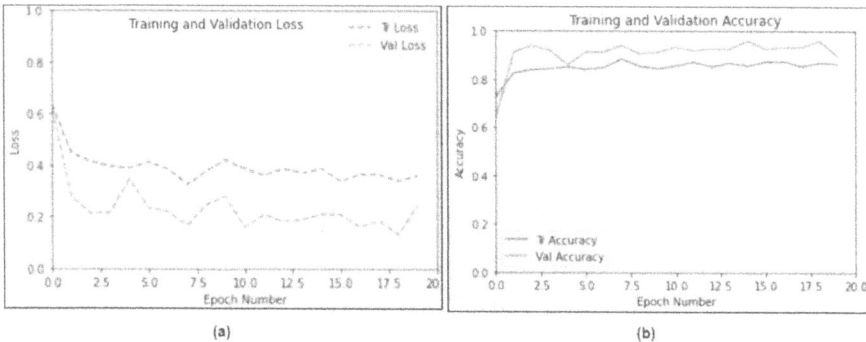

FIGURE 12.6   (a) Loss history of the proposed TRNetCoV model and (b) Accuracy of the proposed TRNetCoV model.

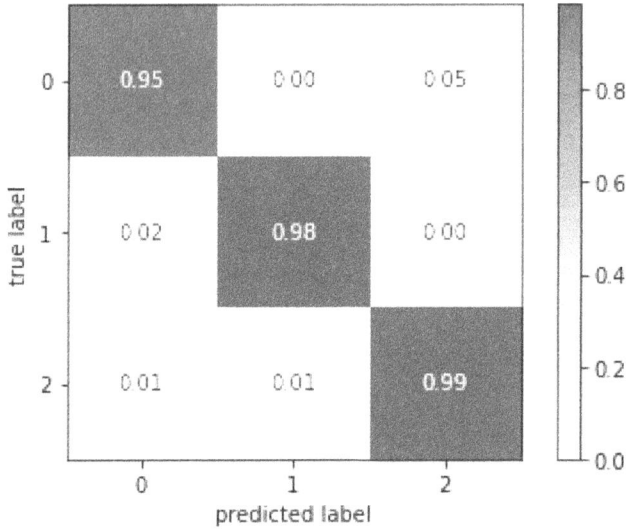

FIGURE 12.7   Confusion matrix of the proposed TRNetCoV model.

The equations of these evaluation multi-class criteria are as follows:

$$Average\ Accuracy = \frac{\sum_{i=1}^{l} \frac{TPi + TNi}{TPi + FPi + TNi + FNi}}{l} \tag{12.12}$$

$$Precision_m = \frac{\sum_{i=1}^{l} TPi}{\sum_{i=1}^{l} TPi + FPi} \tag{12.13}$$

$$Recall_m = \frac{\sum_{i=1}^{l} TPi}{\sum_{i=1}^{l} TPi + FNi} \tag{12.14}$$

$$Specificity = \frac{\sum_{i=1}^{l} TNi}{\sum_{i=1}^{l} TNi + FPi} \tag{12.15}$$

$$F1 - Score = \frac{\left(2 * Precision_m * Recall_m\right)}{Precision_m + Recall_m} \tag{12.16}$$

where,

$TPi = truepositivie, FPi = falsepositive, TNi = truenegative, and\ FNi = falsenegative$

These are referred to the COVID-19 class and other subclasses of non-COVID-19 (viral and normal) and also 'l' represents the set of class labels. Table 12.6 shows the precision and recall values estimated for the proposed model.

TABLE 12.6

Precision and Recall for the Proposed Work

Class	Precision	Recall
COVID-19	0.893	0.974
Viral	0.986	0.979
Normal	0.985	0.979
Total Accuracy	0.95	0.977

TABLE 12.7

Comparative Analysis of Individual Evaluation Performance

Models	COVID-19 Cases	Validation Loss	Accuracy (%)
VGG 19	50	1.05	90.0%
ResNet-18	131	0.15	96.3
ResNet50	189	0.14	98
TRNetCoV (proposed)	189	0.12	98.33

A confusion matrix was obtained for the proposed TRNetCoV model and is presented in Figure 12.7. It is observed that the proposed model predicts true values for most of the classes based on the validation set. Due to the fact of overfitting behavior of DL models, few labels were misclassified. To classify the COVID-19, the proposed model has performed with better accuracy of 98%.

12.10.2 COMPARISON OF THE PROPOSED TECHNIQUE WITH LITERATURE METHODS

The proposed model has been compared with the existing popular DL models. Table 12.7 lists the most recent and most popular relevant studies on the diagnosis of COVID-19 using X-ray image classification methods. From the table, it can be found that the proposed model has gained importance due to its higher accuracy rate and lower validation loss while considering the COVID-19 cases.

12.11 CONCLUSION AND FUTURE WORK

In this chapter, a deep transfer learning framework for COVID-19 detection based on CXR images has been proposed. The proposed model, TRNetCoV, operates using a pre-trained convolution model called ResNet50. To overcome the limitations of CXR image processing as well as to improve the performance of our proposed model, a possible transfer learning method was used to identify the COVID-19 by fine-tuning the weights on each training set of the COVID-19 Radiography Database. This chapter also showed a detailed experimental analysis.

The proposed method in this chapter had provided better performance in terms of higher accuracy and lower validation loss. Thus, it is encouraging to researchers and doctors in detecting and classifying COVID-19 for respiratory issues in less time with higher efficiency.

In the future, this work can be extended to deal with large datasets of COVID-19 CXR images by combining multiple classifiers to achieve a more reliable estimation of disease with wide challenges in the dataset such as image noise, fine and minute classifications between the normal respiratory issues and covid cases, and better pre-processing approaches to avoid illumination changes in the dataset images.

REFERENCES

[1] Paramesha K, Gururaj H L, & Jena O P. (2021). Applications of Machine Learning in Biomedical Text Processing and Food Industry. Machine Learning for Healthcare Applications, 151–67, doi: 10.1002/9781119792611.ch10

[2] Gnter K, Unterthiner T, Mayr A, & Hochreiter S. (2017). Self-normalizing Neural Networks. Advances in Neural Information Processing Systems, 5, 971–80.

[3] Panigrahi N, Ayus I, & Jena, O P. (2021). An Expert System-Based Clinical Decision Support System for Hepatitis-B Prediction & Diagnosis. Machine Learning for Healthcare Applications, 57–75, doi: 10.1002/9781119792611.ch4

[4] Apostolopoulos I D, & Bessiana T. (2003). Covid-19: Automatic Detection from X-Ray Images Utilizing Transfer Learning with Convolutional Neural Networks. Report Number; arXiv, 11617, doi: 10.1007/s13246-020-00865-4

[5] Wang Y, Wang Y, Chen Y, & Qin, Q J. (2020). Unique Epidemiological and Clinical Features of the Emerging Novel Coronavirus Pneumonia (COVID-19) Implicate Special Control Measure. Medical Virology, 92(6), 568–76.

[6] Ai T, Yang Z, Hou H, Zhan C et al. (2020). Correlation of Chest CT and RT-PCR Testing in Coronavirus Disease 2019 (COVID-19) in China. Radiology; Report number: 200642, 296(2), E32–40.

[7] Kon W, Li Y, Peng M, & Kong D. (2020). SARS-CoV-2 Detection in Patients with Influenza-like Illness. Nature Microbiology, 5(5), 675678, doi: 10.1038/s41564-020-0713-1

[8] Patra S S, Jena O P, Kumar G, Pramanik S, Misra C, & Singh, K N. (2021). Random Forest Algorithm in Imbalance Genomics Classification. Data Analytics in Bioinformatics: A Machine Learning Perspective, 173–90. doi:10.1002/9781119785620.ch7

[9] Hemdan E, Shouman M, & Karar M. (2020). COVIDX-Net: A Framework of Deep Learning Classifiers to Diagnose COVID-19 in X-ray Images, Electrical Engineering and Systems Science. 1, 11055.

[10] Pattnayak P, & Jena O P. (2021). Innovation on Machine Learning in Healthcare Services–An Introduction. Machine Learning for Healthcare Applications, 1–15, doi: 10.1002/9781119792611.ch1

[11] Kumar S, Bhusan B, Singh D, & Choubey DK. (2020). Classification of Diabetes using Deep Learning. International Conference on Communication and Signal Processing (ICCSP), 0651–5, doi: 10.1109/ICCSP48568.2020.9182293

[12] Szegedy C, Ioffe S, Vanhoucke V, & Alemin A. (2017). Inception-v4, Inception-ResNet and the Impact of Residual Connections on Learning. AAAI Conference on Artificial Intelligence, 31(1). 4278–4284.

[13] Krizhevsky A, Sutskever I, & Hinton G. (2017). Imagenet Classification with Deep Convolutional Neural Networks. Advances in Neural Information Processing Systems, 60, 84–90, doi: 10.1145/3065386

[14] Simonyan K. & Zisserman A. (2014). Very Deep Convolutional Networks for Large-scale Image Recognition. Computer Vision and Pattern Recognition, 6, 1409–556.

[15] Huang G, Liu Z, & Weinberger K. (2017). Densely Connected Convolutional Networks. IEEE Conference on Computer Vision and Pattern Recognition (CVPR), 4700–08, doi: 10.1109/CVPR.2017.243

[16] Chebet T, Li Y, & Sam Liu Y. (2019). A comparative Study of Fine-tuning Deep Learning Models for Plant Disease Identification. Computers and Electronics in Agriculture, 161, 272–79.

[17] He K, Zhang X, Ren S, & Sun J. (2016). Deep Residual Learning for Image Recognition. IEEE Conference on Computer Vision and Pattern Recognition (CVPR), 770–78.

[18] Shin H.-C. et al. (2016). Deep Convolutional Neural Networks for Computer-aided Detection: CNN Architectures, Dataset Characteristics and Transfer Learning. IEEE Transactions on Medical Imaging, 35, 1285–98.

[19] A, Singh PK, Rani P, Samanta D, Khanna A, & Bhushan B. (2020). An Internet of Health Things-driven Deep Learning Framework for Detection and Classification of Skin Cancer Using Transfer Learning. Transactions on Emerging Telecommunications Technologies, doi: 10.1002/ett.3963

[20] COVID-19 Radiography Database [Online] Available from: https://www.kaggle.com/ tawsifurrahman/covid19-radiography-database [Accessed February 5, 2021].

13 The Influence of COVID-19 on Air Pollution and Human Health

L. Bouhachlaf, J. Mabrouki, and S. El Hajjaji

CONTENTS

13.1 INTRODUCTION

Air pollution can have various health effects either in the short or long term. The danger of acute and chronic breathing and cardiovascular diseases increases with air pollution (Manisalidis et al. 2020). In 2016, the World Health Organization (WHO) stated that 92% of the total population globally breathes substandard air (WHO 2016). This results in significant rates of illness and death especially among the elderly, those with respiratory problems, and young children living in polluted cities (Lelieveld et al. 2015). Air pollution is caused by the occurrence of harmful elements in the air, mostly generated by the actions of humans. These poisonous substances produce a number of events and effects on the various systems and living beings that populate our world; they affect everyone and all sectors (World Bank 2016). It has a high effect on the evolution of plants by inhibiting photosynthesis in the majority of situations, with significant impact on the purification of the air we breathe (Biswal et al. 2021). The accumulation of these substances in the air creates environmental issues whose impact is well noted, such as the destruction of the ozone layer, global climate change, and the greenhouse phenomenon (Menut et al. 2020). The level of these pollutants in the environment is growing at an annual rate of 1%. It is due to the characteristics of some gases like nitrogen dioxide (NO_2), chlorofluorocarbons, carbon dioxide, ozone, and methane, which retain the temperature of the sun in the

DOI: 10.1201/9781003226147-13

235

air, keeping it from getting back into the atmosphere once it has been returned by the ground (Pénard-Morand and Annesi-Maesano 2004; Khomsi et al. 2020).

The main gases that can pollute the air by their high concentration are sulfur dioxide, carbon dioxide, NO_2, and ozone, along with fine dust particles (Sekmoudi et al. 2021). This study focuses on the monitoring of air pollutants that can pollute the air by their high concentration. In this chapter we will focus on monitoring the pollutant NO_2, to analyze the effect of COVID-19 and this air pollutant on human health, as well as examining the level of NO_2 pollutants present in the air, by monitoring the spatial and temporal variability of NO_2 pollution in Morocco from January 2020 to July 2021 using data from MERRA-2 and sentinel 5-P satellites, during the global epidemic and the state of health emergency in Morocco.

13.2   AIR QUALITY AND COVID-19 IN MOROCCO DURING THE STATE OF HEALTH EMERGENCY

Coronaviruses are a family of viruses which cause diseases ranging from the common cold (some of the seasonal variables are coronaviruses) to more severe diseases (such as the respiratory distress of Middle East respiratory syndrome (MERS), severe acute respiratory syndrome (SARS), or COVID-19) (Zhu et al. 2020). The new coronavirus was found for the first time in Wuhan, China (Suresh et al. 2020, Marais et al. 2021). As of March 11, 2020, the WHO called the global situation of COVID-19 a pandemic. Indeed, it evolved rapidly, affecting different regions at different times, becoming a global epidemic, highly contagious. According to the WHO each contaminated person will infect at least three people in the absence of protective precautions, and a person who is contaminated but has no symptoms are able to transmit it to other people (Otmani et al. 2020).

Indeed, in Morocco the first case of coronavirus was recorded on March 2, 2020, and the Moroccan authorities imposed a state of public health emergency on March 20, when the country had only a dozen cases. Since then, the pandemic has followed a controlled trend, with an average daily growth rate of about 5.5%, a low prevalence of less than 1%, and an average case fatality rate of 4% during the containment period (Parrish et al. 2021). After three months of close containment, epidemiology factors favored a progressive de-containment by zone as of June 10, 2020. The number of infections was determined, on the day before the confinement was lifted, at 8508 confirmed cases of coronavirus, including 732 active cases and 211 deaths. This is due to the health situation in the world and in Morocco related to COVID-19. Countries around the world imposed the lockdown which also served to reduce or limit air and road traffic, as well as the decommissioning of several industrial activities. This reduces oil demand and energy consumption (Haddout and Priya 2020). These developments in the transportation sector as well as in oil consumption have a large influence on the quality of the environment, indeed since the beginning of the containment Morocco has experienced a change in the rate of reduction of air pollutants and a significant impact on air quality.

One of the implications is that the implementation of containment to limit the propagation of the virus should significantly change anthropogenic pollutant collections, in terms of both emitted mass and temporal changes. This modification of these issues should change the concentrations of surface pollutants observed in Morocco and also in the world. This has been noted since the start of the lockdown, including by an evaluation of air pollution surveillance measurements (Dirksen et al. 2011).

On the one hand, exposure to the risk of COVID-19 contamination as well as the risk of developing severe forms and of dying are unevenly distributed in the population.. There are disparities in exposure to atmospheric pollution and vulnerability to health effects The same is valid for the health impacts of air quality. We speak of environmental inequalities to describe these differences across socio-economic categories (Khomsi et al. 2021). On the other hand, social inequalities reduce the acceptability and feasibility of measures to limit health risks. For example, compliance with containment was in most cases more difficult for people living in collective housing.

13.2.1 Effect of COVID-19 and Air Pollution on Human Health

Air pollution is the cause of seven million deaths around the world every year, or one in eight early deaths (Metya et al. 2020). Nearly five hundred and seventy thousand children under the age of five die each year from breathing problems associated to air pollution and secondhand smoke (WHO 2016). Children exposed to polluted air have a high risk of developing chronic respiratory problems such as asthma. The effects of air pollution range from difficulty breathing to coughing to worsening asthma and emphysema (Sarfraz et al. 2020). Polluted air can also impair visibility.

Air pollutants have important effects on people's health. Domestic and ambient pollution, such as from cooking ovens and vehicle emissions, contribute to these effects of all environmental health risks, with air pollution having the greatest effect on people's health. It harms and kills in the same way as smoking by increasing the danger of getting respiratory and cardiovascular problems, more than lung cancer. Estimates of the overall health burden of air pollution vary (Tong et al. 2015; Macdonald et al. 2021).

Epidemiological studies have indicated an increase in bronchial symptoms (shortness of breath, chest tightness or pain, difficulty breathing, and whistling noise when breathing) in asthmatic of children with permanent exposure to NO_2. Decreased respiratory function is seen at present levels as well observed in European and North American urban areas (Pénard-Morand et al. 2004).

13.3 MATERIALS AND METHODS

13.3.1 Study Area

Morocco is an African country situated in the far northwest of the continent (Figure 13.1). It has a coastline on both the North Atlantic Ocean to the west and the Northern Mediterranean Sea to the north. The biggest city is Casablanca and the capital is Rabat. Morocco extends over an area of 710,850 km^2 and has a population of more than 36,471,769 (Minister of Mines, Energy and Environment of the Kingdom of Morocco 2019).

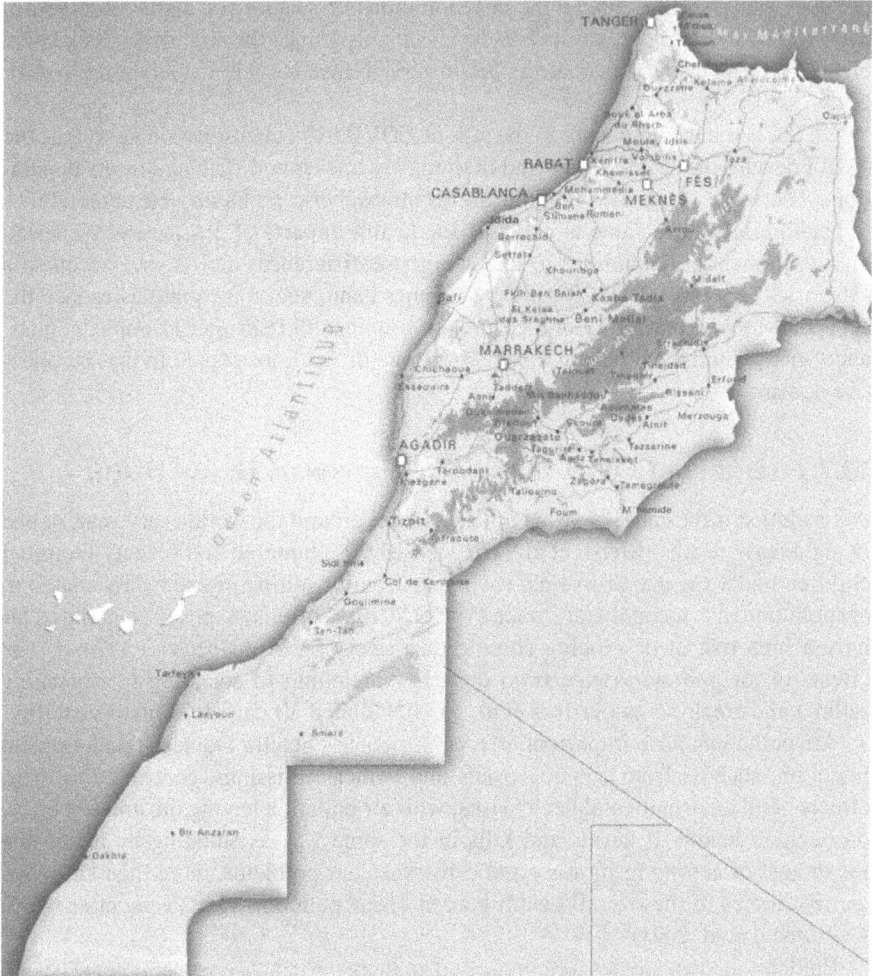

FIGURE 13.1   Map of Morocco.

Most Moroccan industrial units are located at the level of great Casablanca, followed by Fes-Boulemane, Rabat-Sale-Zemmours-Zaers, Tanger-Tetouan, Sous-Massa-Daraa, and Marrakech-Tensift-Haouz.

This assessment is based on monitoring station data analysis both before and after the state of health emergency. This assessment will allow a more detailed analysis of the air pollution situation, including the baseline situation, to draw lessons and make recommendations for limiting post-COVID air pollution (Macd onald et al. 2021).

13.3.2   METHODOLOGY

The ozone-measuring instrument is a Finnish-Dutch image spectrum meter for ozone monitoring (Lokhandwala and Gautam 2020). The instrument is designed to distinguish ozone from other atmospheric species (Ghosh and Ghosh 2020). The high spatial and spectral response of the instrument is important for the analysis of air pollution at the city level (Gelaro et al. 2017). The acquisition of measurements of the stratospheric and tropospheric stages of the earth's atmosphere is the principal aim of the instrument. MERRA-2 is the acronym for Modern Era Retrospective analysis for Research and Applications version 2 (Boersma et al. 2011). MERRA focuses on analyses of the past climate for a variety of weather and climatic periods and situates the NASA Earth Observing System (EOS) suite of images in a climate context (Xu et al. 2008).

OMNO2d stands for OMI and Aura NO_2 Total and Tropospheric Column Filtered (Ghosh and Ghosh 2020). The OMNO2d data is a Level 3 gridded data element in which good quality pixel-level data are averaged and combined into global grids of 0.25-degree x 0.25-degree resolution. This dataset provides the total column of ground-level NO_2 for all atmospheric and cloud fraction conditions below 30% (Duncan et al. 2016; Zambrano-Monserrate et al. 2020).

13.4 RESULTS AND DISCUSSION

Air quality was monitored before, during, and after containment from January 2020 to July 2020.

13.4.1 NITROGEN DIOXIDE MEASUREMENT

NO_2 is formed in the atmosphere from nitric oxide that is liberated primarily by the burning of fossil fuels. It is converted in the atmosphere into nitric acid. Anthropogenic emissions of NO_2 are mainly from combustion (vehicle engines, heating, electricity generation). It is a special chemical substance both in the stratosphere, which is a key component of ozone chemistry, and in the troposphere, where it is a major contributor to ozone production. In the latter, it is generated in different combustion chains and in lightning strikes and is used as an alarm indicator of bad air quality (Wargan et al. 2017; Zhang et al. 2021; Zhao et al. 2021; Jos van Geffen et al. 2020).

13.4.2 SPATIOTEMPORAL EVOLUTION OF NITROGEN DIOXIDE

Spatiotemporal variability of NO_2 pollution in environments in Morocco from January to July.

For the months before the confinement, the quantity of NO_2 (Figure 13.2 (a)) varies between $3.302*10^{15}$ molec.cm^{-2} and $4.952*10^{15}$ molec.cm^{-2} in the Mediterranean and Atlantic coastal areas, then it decreases for the month of March to April and April to May (Figure 13.2 (b)) from $(3.302$ to $1.651) *10^{15}$ molec.cm^{-2}.

It is seen that the variation of NO_2 concentration is high in the coastal areas and especially in the industrial pole of Rabat towards Casablanca and in the northern area Tangier during the month of January to March. And as soon as the month of March starts, we see based on the spatiotemporal figures of the satellite a decrease of variation of concentration of this pollutant in all Morocco; it is quite remarkable in the month April (Figure 13.2 (b)) and it remains weak also compared to the months of January and February. Therefore, we can conclude that during the quarantine,

(a) Spatio-temporal evolution of NO$_2$ Concentration for January to March, 2020

(b) Spatio-temporal evolution of NO$_2$ Concentration for Mars to May, 2020

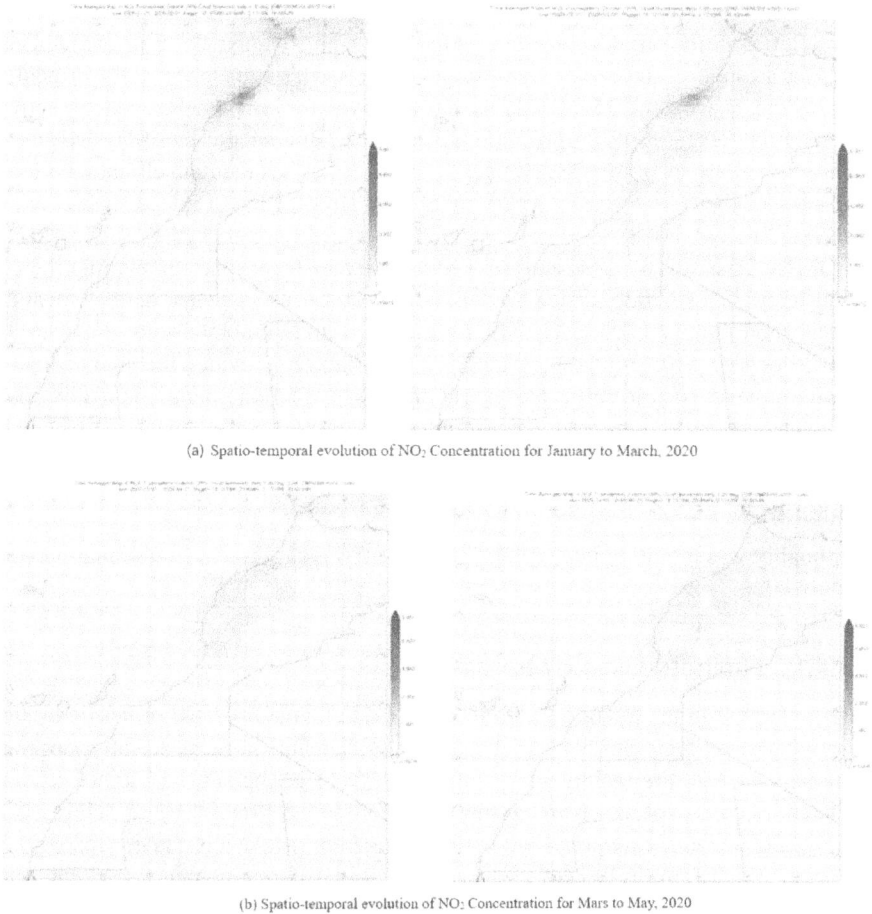

FIGURE 13.2   Spatiotemporal evolution of NO$_2$ concentration in Morocco (a) before lockdown (January to March) and (b) in lockdown (March to May). (From NASA Earth Observatory.)

the NO$_2$ had decreased. This reduction in air pollution has had beneficial effects on people's health and has decreased deaths and saving lives, mostly due to cardiovascular diseases.

In the same way for the months of June and July, it remains low in comparison with the first months (Figure 13.3).

This number represents the number of NO$_2$ molecules in an atmosphere column from the planet's surface to the upper atmosphere, measured upwards one square centimeter of the surface (NASA Earth Observatory, 2021).

The decrease in the concentration of NO$_2$ from 5.25 to 4.25 (10^{15} molec.cm^{-2}) from March to May during the containment (Figure 13.4), which is certainly due to the decrease of anthropogenic emissions. Human activities, due to the strict restrictions imposed by the countries during the lockdown, after the reduction of restrictions in some areas, a gradual increase in the level of pollutants (values of 9.056 *10^{15} molec.cm^{-2}) was observed on (Figure 13.4).

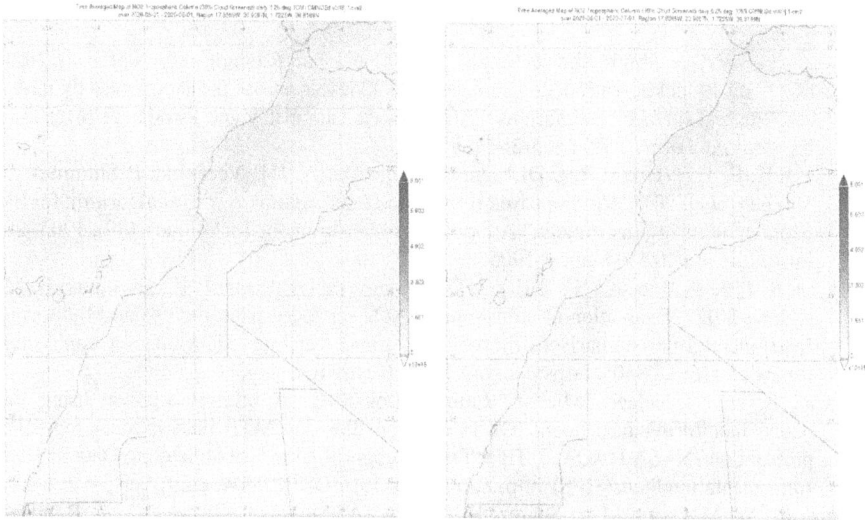

FIGURE 13.3 Spatiotemporal evolution of NO_2 concentration in Morocco after lockdown (May to June). (From NASA Earth Observatory.)

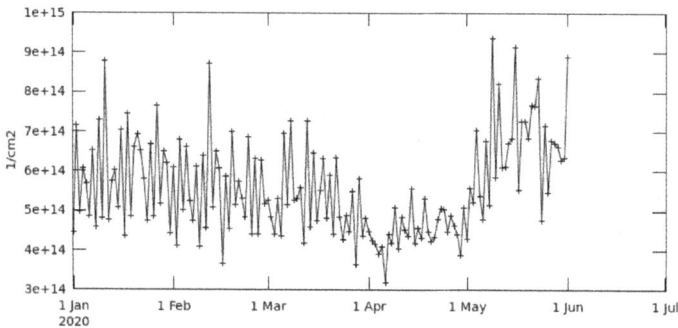

FIGURE 13.4 Time series, area averaged of NO_2 tropospheric column from January to June 2020.

13.5 CONCLUSION

This research presents an evaluation of air monitoring in Morocco during the COVID-19 pandemic from March to June 2020. Satellite data comparing levels of NO_2 concentrations after the shutdown show significant reductions. The satellite data show that, in the confined areas, the average NO_2 levels between March and May 2020 were lower than the June 2020 concentrations after the shutdown. We therefore conclude that the traffic restrictions applied during the quarantine for the COVID-19 pandemic in Morocco were remarkably effective in reducing NO_x emissions. This reduction in ozone precursors reduces ozone.

REFERENCES

Biswal, Akash, Vikas Singh, Shweta Singh, Amit P Kesarkar, Ravindra Khaiwal, et al. 2021. "COVID-19 lockdown-induced changes in NO2 levels across India observed by multi-satellite and surface observations." Atmospheric Chemistry and Physics 21 (6): 5235–51. https://doi.org/10.5194/acp-21-5235-2021

Boersma, K. F., H. J. Eskes, R. J. Dirksen, R. J. Van Der A, J. P. Veefkind, P. Stammes, V. Huijnen, et al. 2011. "An improved tropospheric no2 column retrieval algorithm for the ozone monitoring instrument." Atmospheric Measurement Techniques 4 (9): 1905–28. https://doi.org/10.5194/amt-4-1905

Dirksen, R. J., K. F. Boersma, H. J. Eskes, D. V. Ionov, E. J. Bucsela, P. F. Levelt, and H. M. Kelder. 2011. "Evaluation of stratospheric NO2 retrieved from the Ozone Monitoring Instrument: Intercomparison, diurnal cycle, and trending." Journal of Geophysical Research 116: D08305, https://doi.org/10.1029/2010JD014943

Duncan, Bryan N.; Geigert, Michael; Lamsal, Lok.2016. "A brief tutorial on using the ozone monitoring instrument (OMI) nitrogen dioxide (NO2) data product for SIPS preparation."NASA HAQAST Tiger Team: Supporting the Use of Satellite Data in State Implementation Plans(SIPS). https://doi.org/10.7916/D80K3S3W. Draft Version 2: 1–21.

Gelaro, R., W. McCarty, M. J. Suárez, R. Todling, A. Molod, L. Takacs, C. A. Randles, et al. 2017. "The modern-era retrospective analysis for research and applications, version 2 (MERRA-2)." Journal of Climate 30: 5419–54. https://doi.org/10.1175/JCLI-D-16-0758.1

Ghosh, Shilpi, and Shatabdi Ghosh. 2020. "Air quality during Covid-19 lockdown: Blessing in disguise." Indian Journal of Biochemistry and Biophysics 57 (4): 420–30.

Haddout, S., and K. L. Priya. 2020. "Unveiling the causes of reduction in troposphere no2 in two cities of Morocco during COVID-19 lockdown." Environmental Forensics 21 (3–4): 237–40. https://doi.org/10.1080/15275922.2020.1784313

Khomsi Kenza, Houda Najmi, Hassan Amghar, Youssef Chelhaoui, and Zineb Souhaili. 2020. "COVID-19 national lockdown in Morocco: Impacts on air quality 1 and public health." MedRxiv 20146589. https://doi.org/10.1101/2020.07.05.20146589.

Khomsi, K., H. Najmi, H. Amghar, Y. Chelhaoui, and Z. Souhaili. 2021. "COVID-19 national lockdown in Morocco: Impacts on air quality and public health." One Health 11: 1–13. https://doi.org/10.1016/j.onehlt.2020.100200

Lelieveld, J., J. S. Evans, M. Fnais, D. Giannadaki, and A. Pozzer. 2015. "The contribution of outdoor air pollution sources to premature mortality on a global scale." Nature 525 (7569): 367–71. https://doi.org/10.1038/nature15371

Lokhandwala S. and P. Gautam. 2020. "Indirect impact of COVID-19 on environment: A brief study in Indian context," Environmental Research. 188:109807.

Macdonald, E., N. Otero Felipe, and T. M. Butler. 2021. "A comparison of long-term trends in observations and emission inventories of NO$_x$." Atmospheric Chemistry and Physics 21(5): 4007–23. https://doi.org/10.5194/acp-21-4007-2021

Manisalidis, Ioannis, Elisavet Stavropoulou, Agathangelos Stavropoulos, and Eugenia Bezirtzoglou. 2020. "Environmental and health impacts of air pollution: A review." Frontiers in Public Health. https://doi.org/10.3389/fpubh.2020.00014

Marais, E. A., J. F. Roberts, R. G. Ryan, H. Eskes, K. F. Boersma, S. Choi, J. Joiner, N. Abuhassan, et al. 2021 "New observations of NO2 in the upper troposphere from TROPOMI." Atmospheric Measurement Techniques. 14: 2389–2408, https://doi.org/10.5194/amt-14-2389-2021

Menut, Laurent, Bertrand Bessagnet, Guillaume Siour, Sylvain Mailler, Romain Pennel, and Arineh Cholakian. 2020. "Impact of lockdown measures to combat Covid-19 on Air quality over western Europe." Science of the Total Environment 741: 140426. https://doi.org/10.1016/j.scitotenv.2020.140426

Metya A., P. Dagupta, S. Halder, S. Chakraborty, and Y. K. Tiwari. 2020. "COVID-19 lock-downs improve air quality in the South-East Asian regions, as seen by the remote sensing satellites." Aerosol and Air Quality Research. 20(8):1772–1782.

Minister of Energy, Mines and the Environment of the Kingdom of Morocco. 2020. Qualité de l'air au Maroc pendant l'état d'urgence sanitaire liée au COVID 19. https://www.environnement.gov.ma/fr/134-actualites/3338-qualite-de-l-air-aumaroc-pendant-l-etat-d-urgence-sanitaire-liee-au-covid-19

NASA Earth Observatory. 2021. "Giovanni Parameter Definitions: Nitrogen Dioxide." Atmospheric Composition, Water & Energy Cycles and Climate Variability. https://disc.gsfc.nasa.gov/information/glossary?title=Giovanni%20Parameter%20Definitions:%20Nitrogen%20Dioxide

World Health Organization (WHO). 2016. WHO releases country estimates on air pollution exposure and health impact. Accessed March 5, 2021. http://www.who.int/mediacentre/news/releases/2016/air-pollution-estimates/en/

Otmani, A., A. Benchrif, M. Tahri, M. Bounakhla, E.M. Chakir, M. El Bouch, and M. Krombi. 2020. "Impact of Covid-19 lockdown on PM10, SO2 and NO2 concentrations in Salé City (Morocco)." Science of the Total Environment. 735: 139541. https://doi.org/10.1016/j.scitotenv.2020.139541

Parrish David D., Richard G. Derwent, and Johannes Staehelin. 2021. "Version for publication Long-term changes in northern mid-latitude tropospheric ozone concentrations: Synthesis of two recent analyses." Atmospheric Environment, 118227. https://doi.org/10.1016/j.atmosenv.2021.118227

Pénard-Morand, C., and I. Annesi-Maesano. 2004. "Air pollution: From sources of emissions to health effects." Breathe 1 (2): 108–19. https://doi.org/10.1183/18106838.0102.108

Sarfraz, Muddassar, Khurram Shehzad, and Syed Ghulam Meran Shah. 2020. "The Impact of COVID-19 as a necessary evil on air pollution in India during the lockdown." Environmental Pollution 266: 115080. https://doi.org/10.1016/j.envpol.2020.115080

Sekmoudi, I., K. Khomsi, S. Faieq, and L. Idrissi. 2021. "Assessment of global and regional PM10 CAMSRA data: comparison to observed data in Morocco". Environmental Science and Pollution Research. https://doi.org/10.1007/s11356-021-12783-3

Suresh, Arjun, Diksha Chauhan, Amina Othmani, Neha Bhadauria, Aswin S, Jais Jose, and Nezha Mejjad. 2020. "Diagnostic comparison of changes in air quality over China before and during the COVID-19 pandemic." Research Square 1:1–20. https://doi.org/10.21203/rs.3.rs-30482/v1

Tong Daniel Q., Lok Lamsal, Li Pan, Charles Ding, Hyuncheol Kim, Pius Lee, Tianfeng Chai, Kenneth E. Pickering, and Ivanka Stajner. 2015. "Long-term NOx trends over large cities in the United States during the great recession: Comparison of satellite retrievals, ground observations, and emission inventories." Atmospheric Environment 107: 70–84. https://doi.org/10.1016/j.atmosenv.2015.01.035

van Geffen, J., K. F. Boersma, H. Eskes, M. Sneep, M. ter Linden, M. Zara, and J. P. Veefkind. 2020 "S5P TROPOMI NO2 slant column retrieval: Method, stability, uncertainties and comparisons with OMI." Atmospheric Measurement Techniques 13: 1315–35. https://doi.org/10.5194/amt-13-1315-2020

Wargan, Krzysztof, Gordon Labow, Stacey Frith, Steven Pawson, Nathaniel Livesey, and Gary Partyka. 2017. "Evaluation of the ozone fields in NASA's MERRA-2 reanalysis." Journal of Climate 30 (8): 2961–88. https://doi.org/10.1175/JCLI-D-16-0699.1World Bank and Institute for Health Metrics and Evaluation. 2016. The Cost of Air Pollution: Strengthening the Economic Case for Action. Washington, DC: World Bank.

Xu Pengcheng, Zhixuan Cheng, Qingyi Pan, Jiaqiang Xu, Qun Xiang, Weijun Yu, and Yuliang Chu, 2008. "High aspect ratio In2O3 nanowires: Synthesis, mechanism and NO2 gas-sensing properties," Sensors and Actuators B: Chemical 130(2): 802–08.

Zambrano-Monserrate M. A., M. A. Ruano, and L. Sanchez-Alcalde. 2020. "Indirect effects of COVID-19 on the environment." Journal Science of the Total Environment 728: 138813. https://doi.org/10.1016/j.scitotenv.2020.138813

Zhang Xuguo, Jimmy C. H. Fung, Alexis K. H. Lau, Md Shakhaoat Hossain, Peter K. K. Louie, and Wei Huang. 2021. "Air quality and synergistic health effects of ozone and nitrogen oxides in response to China's integrated air quality control policies during 2015–2019." Chemosphere 268: 129385. https://doi.org/10.1016/j.chemosphere.2020.129385

Zhao Fei, Cheng Liu, Zhaonan Cai, Xiong Liu, Juseon Bak, Jae Kim, Qihou Hu, Congzi Xia, Chengxin Zhang, Youwen Sun, Wei Wang, and Jianguo Liu, 2021. "Ozone profile retrievals from TROPOMI: Implication for the variation of tropospheric ozone during the outbreak of COVID-19 in China." Science of the Total Environment 764: 142886. https://doi.org/10.1016/j.scitotenv.2020.142886

Zhu, Na, Wenling Wang, Zhidong Liu, Chaoyang Liang, Wen Wang, Fei Ye, Baoying Huang, et al. 2020. "Morphogenesis and cytopathic effect of SARS-CoV-2 infection in human airway epithelial cells." Nature Communications 11 (1): 1–8. https://doi.org/10.1038/s41467-020-17796-z

14 Smart COVID-19 GeoStrategies using Spatial Network Voronoï Diagrams

A. Mabrouk and A. Boulmakoul

CONTENTS

14.1 INTRODUCTION

The pandemic looks like a war: people are dying, medical personnel are on the front lines, and authorities are working overtime to tighten control over compliance with protective measures and mandatory health procedures. According to the World

DOI: 10.1201/9781003226147-14

Health Organization (WHO) (World Health Organization 2005), the term pandemic applies when talking about the global spread of a new disease. It occurs when a new virus appears and spreads around the world, affecting a large geographic extent, with no immunity in the vast majority of the population. In the past, pandemics were caused by influenza viruses in animals. Recently, a heretofore unknown agent, the Severe Acute Respiratory Syndrome Coronavirus (SARS) broke out. SARS is the first serious and communicable disease to emerge in the 21st century. The epidemic, which began in China at the end of 2002, erupted around the world in 2003, infecting more than 8000 people and killing nearly 800 people. The SARS virus is spread primarily by droplets through person-to-person contact, although aerosol transmission may also play a role. Nowadays, public health issues have taken on great importance in our society, especially the viral spread in populated areas. This coronavirus, also called COVID-19 (Franch-Pardo et al. 2020; Sun et al. 2020), is a new family of viruses that infects humans. By navigating and moving, infected humans infect other individuals and consequently a transmission caused epidemic outbreaks with almost exponential growth and generated chaos on the planet, where more than a third of the world's population called for containment. This has caused the saturation of health systems, and social and economic disruption. In terms of accountability, the competent national authorities are responsible for managing the national risk of pandemic influenza. Each country is required to develop or update a national preparedness plan for influenza as recommended by the WHO. This management is the solution to reduce the risk of the influenza pandemic spread. For example, during a pandemic alert period, the priority goals of containing the new virus in limited foci or delaying its spread to save time, and then doing everything to contain its spread (Atluri et al. 2018).

On the other hand, this pandemic mobilized scientific research and accelerated the production of knowledge on this virus as well as the means of curing and preventing it. In addition, technologies play a decisive role in ensuring the proper functioning of society in times of containment and quarantine. These technologies can have a lasting impact even after the pandemic (Zhou et al. 2020), (Cherradi et al. 2017; Das and Ghosh 2020). The year 2020, which marks the start of an exciting decade in medicine and science, has allowed the development of many digital technologies. This is artificial intelligence (AI) which uses deep learning; the Internet of Things (IoT) (Pamučar1996; D'silva et al. 2017; Maguerra et al. 2020) with the new 5G; big data analysis; and blockchain technology (Maguerra et al. 2020).

In this work, we propose a set of processes to effectively conduct urgent viral pandemic management operations (Duan et al. 2018). These processes concern the management of confinement/deconfinement at the local or global scale by using spatio-temporal networks of the tessellation/partitioning buffer type (Erwig 2000; Okabe et al. 2008) or of the Voronoï type (buffer, graphs, and polygons) and the structural patterns of complex graphs (Zheng et al. 2011).

This chapter is organized as follows. It starts with an overview of a set of materials and then it presents methods, which are given in Section 14.2. Section 14.3 discusses the different operations of Voronoï spatial diagrams. Section 14.4 shows the results obtained as well as the analysis of these results. Using the interactive smart maps that we developed in this work, the infected areas of the city are visualized and spatial decision support tools are offered to authorities to monitor the pandemic spreading. Finally, in Section 14.5, we draw some conclusions from this study and highlight the future directions of this work.

14.2   MATERIALS AND METHODS

In this section, we develop geoprocessing methods and concepts related to spatial data engineering. These constructions are used for COVID-19 pandemic monitoring. The main constructions come from geographic information systems (GIS), spatial databases, and algorithmic geometry.

14.2.1   Geographic Information Systems and COVID-19 Containment/Deconfinement Operations

Today in the pandemic context, GIS have demonstrated their strength in the management of environmental risks (Zheng et al. 2011; Mabrouk and Boulmakoul 2012; Karim et al. 2017; Mabrouk et al. 2017). During the fight against the pandemic, GIS and spatial tracking technologies are used to spatially control and prevent the transmission of the epidemic, help to allocate emergency space resources, and manage urban data.

In the context of this work, we used a set of functionalities of GIS-software to acquire geospatial data relating to the city (the transport network, roads, hospitals, schools, etc.), and also those related to COVID-19 and especially the information provided by the authorities and the Ministry of Health. Then, these datasets are stored in a geospatial database according to a generic GIS data model (entities, attributes, networks, topologies, raster, etc.), and this to be organized and managed and also in order to be able to use them jointly and make them coherent and harmonized. In addition, we present intuitive ideas for performing containment/deconfinement operations. These operations are based on geoprocessing queries, which concern a city spatial database. In the operations specification, the data was produced from OpenStreetMap and supplemented by digitization, creating the necessary layers (shapefile) of downtown Mohammedia and Tetouan, projected on Merchich Nord EPSG 26191 coordinate system for northern onshore Morocco. To ensure the reliability of the data, the data must be provided by the state departments responsible for urban data and the operations can be carried out by GIS engineers from the Ministry of the Interior.

Based on their spatial characteristics, the integration of this data across different information layers allows us to perform geoprocessing and spatial analysis. This data can then be geovisualized in a cartographic manner in the form of smart maps that show features and their relationships on the earth's surface. This consists of great tools for synthesizing and geovisualizing the underlying geospatial information and performing queries, spatial analysis, and modifying geographic information.

14.2.2   About Geo-Pandemic Data

In this section, we present the geospatial data that we manipulated to accomplish this work. Indeed, the semantic data tables and the spatial queries are presented as follows (Table 14.1–14.3).

TABLE 14.1
Cell Table Attributes

Name	Name of the Location
cell id	Cell identifier (code)
S	Number susceptible individuals
R	Number recovered individuals
I	Number infected individuals
Geom.	Point

TABLE 14.2
Network Table Attributes

Name	Name of the Street
Type	Road type (primary, secondary, residential, motorway)
Geo	Line

TABLE 14.3
Houses Table Attributes

Name	Name of the Street
Type	Road type (primary, secondary, residential, motorway)
Geo	Polygon

Covid_Outbreak makes up the cell layer of COVID-19 virus infection in the city. Each cell is characterized by epidemiological information.

The buffer operation is a common operation in GIS and it is available in PostGIS. ST_Buffer (geometry, distance) takes a buffer distance and a geometry type, and generates a polygon with a limit to the buffer distance of the input geometry as follows:

SPATIAL QUERY 1: MAKE A NEW TABLE WITH A COVID BUFFER ZONE 100M BUFFER ZONE

CREATE TABLE covid_buffer_zone AS
  SELECT ST_Buffer(geo,100): geometry (Polygon,26191) AS geo FROM Covid_Outbreak
  ST_Intersects(geometry A, geometry B) returns the true if geometry A intersects geometry B

The geospatial data concerning the pandemic are processed according to the pipeline presented in Figure 14.1.

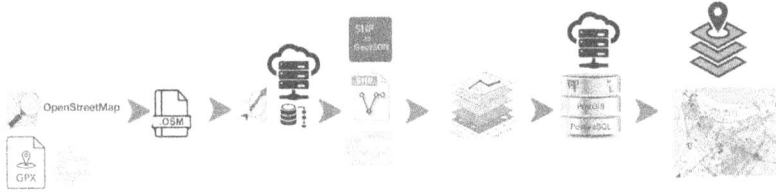

FIGURE 14.1   Pipeline processing.

OSM – > GML – > shapefile – > Qgis– > shapefiles – > postGis – > tables

+ queries – > Qgis – > WEB ‖ svg

14.2.3   GEOPROCESSING BASIC OPERATIONS

The structural strategy implies the use of geometric and topological operations to build problem solving algorithms by means of spatial reasoning (Fabiano et al. 2002; OCG 2002; QGIS 2009; PostGis-Project 2013; Mabrouk and Boulmakoul 2017). Below are some illustrated proposals.

In this pandemic period, during the deconfinement phase, it is essential to ensure the containment of urban areas still affected (infected or sensitive) by the COVID-19 virus. Thus, it will be necessary to extract the dwellings concerned and the road sub-networks which supply them. Operation 1, described below, develops these objectives and the results are shown in Figures 14.1, 14.2, 14.3, 14.4 and 14.5.

14.2.3.1   Operation 1: Continue to Contain Infected Areas

Computation of the network to be confined: Covid_Net

SPATIAL QUERY 2: MAKE A NEW TABLE COVID_NET

```
CREATE TABLE Covid_Net AS
    SELECT *
    FROM Network_City AS net
    JOIN covid_buffer_zone AS covi
    ON ST_Intersects(covi.geo, net.geo)
```

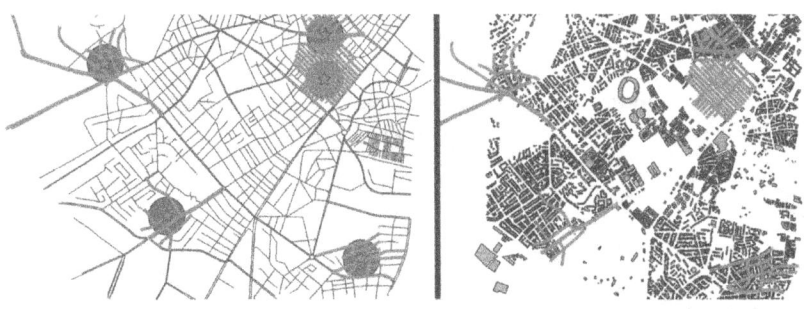

FIGURE 14.2   Covid network layer.

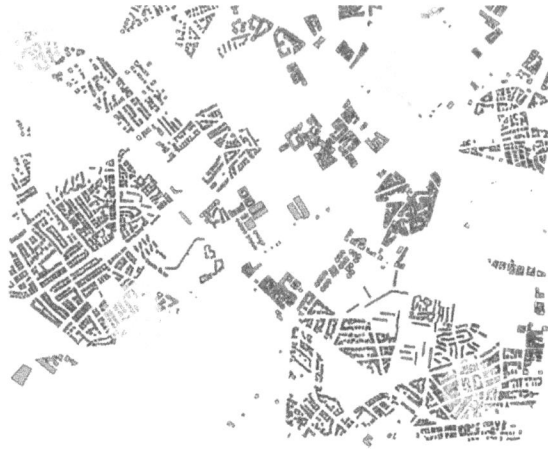

FIGURE 14.3 Confined houses layer.

**SPATIAL QUERY 3: MAKE A NEW TABLE
CONFINED HOUSES**

```
CREATE TABLE Houses_Confined AS
    SELECT *
    FROM Houses_City AS hc
    JOIN covid_buffer_zone AS covi
    ON ST_Intersects(covi.geo, hc.geo)
```

This process performs the deconfinement structures. It defines the green network (uncontaminated) as well as green housing (uncontaminated). The associated processes are described below:

**SPATIAL QUERY 4: MAKE A NEW TABLE
GREEN NETWORK**

```
CREATE TABLE Green_Network AS
    SELECT *
    FROM Network_City AS nc
    JOIN Covid_Net AS covi
    ON ST_Difference (nc.geo,covi.geo)
```

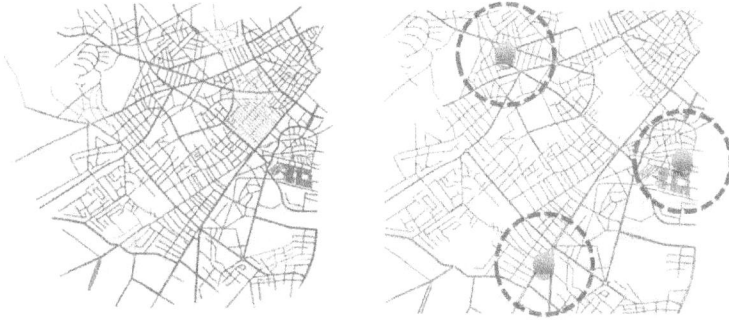

FIGURE 14.4   Green network processing.

SPATIAL QUERY 5: MAKE A NEW TABLE GREEN HOUSING

```
CREATE TABLE Green_House AS
    SELECT *
    FROM Houses_City AS hcity
    JOIN Houses_Confined AS hcovi
    ON ST_Difference (hcity.geo,hcovi.geo)
```

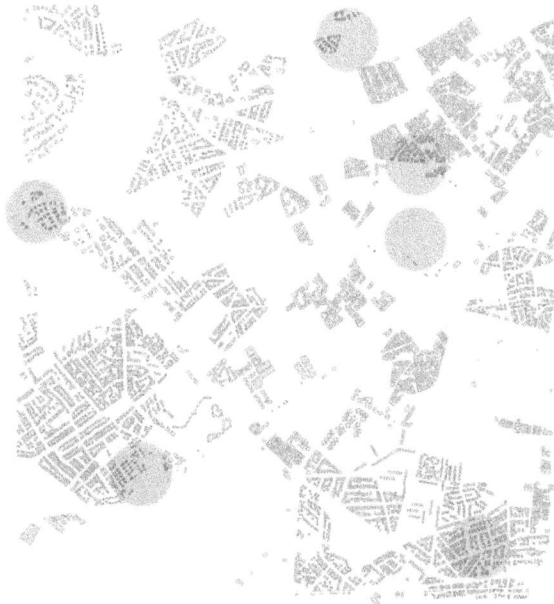

FIGURE 14.5   Green housing processing.

14.2.4   VIRAL INFECTION RISK ANALYSIS BASED ON THE PROXIMITY OF INFECTED AREAS

Individuals' vulnerability to viral infections is based in particular on the systemic approach to risk. A source system and a target system are distinguished. Indeed, the infection environment can be constituted of human targets and virus infection. These two components are connected by the danger flow to the effects of the viruses spread around the infection point.

Based on the work of Mabrouk et al. (2017) and Mabrouk and Boulmakoul (2017), a spatial network N (S, E), which in our context represents roads, pedestrian paths, etc., consists of a node set S to represent interactions, and of a links set E to represent segments of this spatial network. There are two attributes which are defined for each link $(S_i, S_j) \in E$, the viral infection probability P_{ij}^y and the infection consequence C_{ij}^y. Let p be a path consisting of an ordered set of links:

$$A^p = \left\{ \left(S_i, S_j \right)^k \mid S_i, S_j \in S, \; k = 1, 2, \cdots, m^p \right\};$$ (14.1)

In a path p which belongs to the set of available paths, the risk R^p is calculated by using the following formula [2,3]:

$$R^p = \sum_{(i,j) \in A^p} P_{ij}^y C_{ij}^y$$ (14.2)

With P_{ij}^y representing the probability of a danger occurrence and C_{ij}^y representing the consequences on the vulnerable which may result from it given environment elements.

The analysis of the viral infection risk and of the human targets' vulnerability based on the systemic risk approach leads us to conclude that more people get closer to infected people or areas; these targets are more and more in danger (more and more vulnerable). Indeed, if the viral infection probability is higher, then the viral infection risk is higher (Figure 14.6).

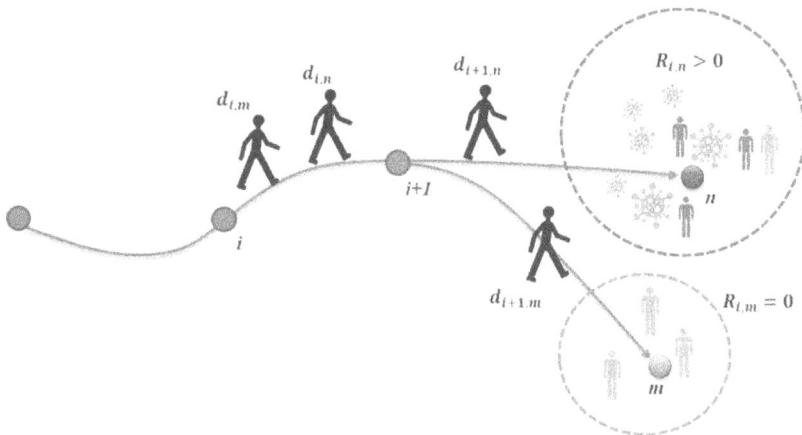

FIGURE 14.6   Viral infection risk analysis based on the proximity of infected areas.

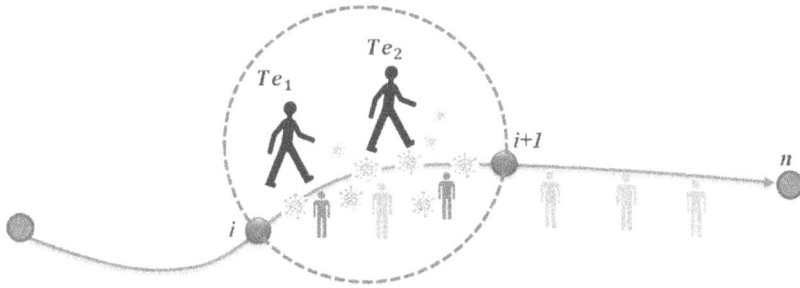

FIGURE 14.7   Viral infection risk analysis based on the duration of exposure.

Let $R_{i,n}$ and $R_{i+1,n}$ and $R_{i,m}$ be the risks assessed respectively on the $p_{i,n}$ and $p_{i+1,n}$ and $p_{i,m}$ paths according to formula (equation 14.2), where $P^v_{i,n}$ and $P^v_{i+1,n}$ and $P^v_{i,m}$ represent the probabilities of viral infection of people heading respectively from node S_i to nodes S_n and m. d_{ij} represents the travel distance between nodes S_i and S_j.

$$d_{i+1,n} < d_{i,n} \Rightarrow P^v_{i+1,n} > P^v_{i,n} \Rightarrow R_{i+1,n} > R_{i,n} \tag{14.3}$$

On the other hand, when the individual changes the direction at node S_{i+1} toward the zone m which is not infected, he moves away from the infected zone n. In fact, the probability of $P^v_{i+1,m}$ infection decreases and consequently the $R_{i,m}$ risk decreases in parallel with the distance of the individual from the infected area.

14.2.5   Viral Infection Risk Analysis Based on the Duration of Exposure

In fact, the exposure time plays a very important role in the change in the risk of viral infection rates. Let T_{e1} and T_{e2} respectively be the travel times between nodes i and i+1 by the two individuals Ind_1 and Ind_2 within an infected zone (Figure 14.7).

Let P_{e1} and P_{e2} be the probabilities of viral infection of individuals Ind_1 and Ind_2 respectively. If the duration of exposure of individual Ind_1 is greater than that of individual Ind_2, then the likelihood of viral infection of individual Ind_1 is greater than that of individual Ind_2. Therefore, the risk of R_{e1} infection of individual Ind_2 is greater than the risk of R_{e2} infection of individual Ind_2.

$$\text{If } T_{e1} > T_{e1} \text{ then } P_{e1} > P_{e2} \Rightarrow R_{e1} > R_{e2} \tag{14.3}$$

14.3   SPATIAL NETWORK VORONOÏ DIAGRAM OPERATIONS

Based on a spatial model of the urban environment, spatial Voronoï diagrams (VDs) provide several spatial operations. They help to calculate the spatial Voronoï accessibility. This provides safe routing and planning of urban displacement and helps to find the shortest and safest routes for people movement and therefore reduces risks and keeps people as far away from harm as possible.

14.3.1 Spatial Network Voronoï Diagrams

The Voronoï tessellation (Figure 14.8) is used to allocate space around a predetermined set of points or generators. It searches for the nearest generator for each point in space. The result is known as the Voronoï diagram (VD). In 1854 the British physicist John Snow used this geometric structure to show that most of the victims of the Soho cholera epidemic lived closer to the infected Broad Street pump than to any other pump (John Snow 1854). The general case in dimension n was defined and studied in 1908 by the Russian mathematician Georgy Fedoseevich Voronoï (or Voronoy) who gave his name to these diagrams. The planar VD (PVD) is defined as a set of polygons or Voronoï regions, Vor={Vor$_1$..., Vor$_n$}, where the polygon Vor$_i$ is given by:

$$Vor_i = \left\{ \forall x \in E \mid d\left(x,\ p_i\right) \leq d\left(x, p_j\right),\ j \neq i,\ j = 1,...,n \right\} \qquad (14.4)$$

Okabe and al. (2008) showed that the Euclidean distance is significantly different from the distance of the shortest path in the urbanized sector. So, in an urban environment, this distance must be calculated on the spatial network. The network Voronoï diagram (NVD) is then defined by the division of the network into Voronoï sub-networks, each of which contains the points closest to each Voronoï generator by traversing the shortest path between these components (Figure 14.8).

For a set of vertices (represent the Voronoï generators) $G = \{g_1,..., g_n\}$ with $G \subseteq S$, the NVD divides a network N (S, E) of vertices S and arcs E, into n Voronoï sub-networks $Vor(1),..., Vor(n)$ with:

$$\text{Vor}(i) = \left\{ \forall p \in P / P\left(pi, p\right) \leq P\left(pj, p\right),\ 1 \leq \forall j \leq n, i \neq j \right\} \qquad (14.5)$$

with $P(v, w)$ represents the weight of the shortest path from v to w in the network N considering v and w two vertices belonging to S.

14.3.2 Spatial Voronoï Accessibility

The NVD divides the spatial network into Voronoï subnets whose nodes and arcs of each of these subnets are associated with a Voronoï generator. Accessibility points provide information on the generator and the distance of the shortest path, associated with each point of the spatial network. The PVD generated by the accessibility

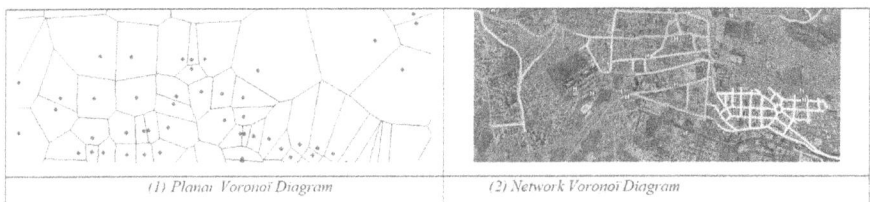

| (1) Planar Voronoï Diagram | (2) Network Voronoï Diagram |

FIGURE 14.8 Spatial Voronoï diagrams.

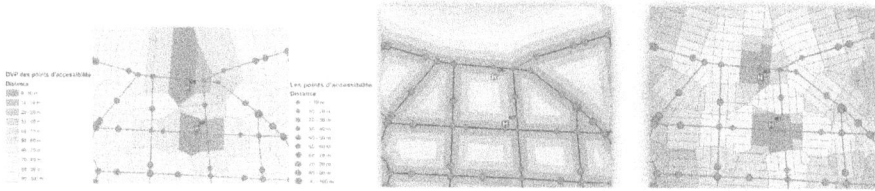

FIGURE 14.9   Generation of spatial Voronoï accessibility areas.

points is a solution to associate, with each set of points surrounding each accessibility point, the Voronoï generators and the distances of the shortest paths to reach these generators. Figure 14.9 shows the polygons of the PVD which are generated by the Voronoï accessibility points. Each polygon contains information about the Voronoï generator, and the shortest path distance from the accessibility point to the Voronoï generator associated with that point.

14.3.3   SPATIAL RELATIONSHIPS AND STATISTICAL EVALUATION OFFERED BY SPATIAL VORONOÏ DIAGRAMS

Mabrouk and Boulmakoul (Mabrouk et al. 2012; Mabrouk and Boulmakoul 2017) propose a spatial object model which constitutes a structure of geographic data layers and data tables. This structure describes spatial objects, their spatial representation (point, line, or polygon), their attributes, their spatial relationships, and their rules by which data is defined, organized, searched, and updated in a geographic information system. The added value of this model lies in its foundation on spatial Voronoï accessibility areas which are defined from a NVD using the PVD.

This model ensures a set of spatial relationships (spatial association, adjacencies, etc.) between all its spatial objects (points, nodes, arcs, Voronoï generators, Voronoï cells, Voronoï spatial regions, etc.). It also offers several spatial and statistical measurements, namely the shortest path distance from the nodes to the generators, and from the generator to the other generators; the length of the spatial network assigned to a generator; the area of a Voronoï spatial region associated with a generator (the catchment area); and the number of places of interest in a Voronoï spatial region associated with a generator. All of these spatial and statistical measures can be combined with weighted attributes of a demographic, economic, or social type. This makes it possible to extract new information on the spatial environment studied, for example the population served by a hospital or the number of pharmacies located in the service area of an hospital.

14.3.4   THE SHORTEST AND SAFEST PATHS BASED ON NETWORK VORONOÏ DIAGRAMS

Mabrouk and Boulmakoul (2017) proposed an approach for routing and planning safe trips in an urban setting. The purpose of this approach is to find the shortest routes for the safe movement of people (Figure 14.10). It helps to reduce risk and

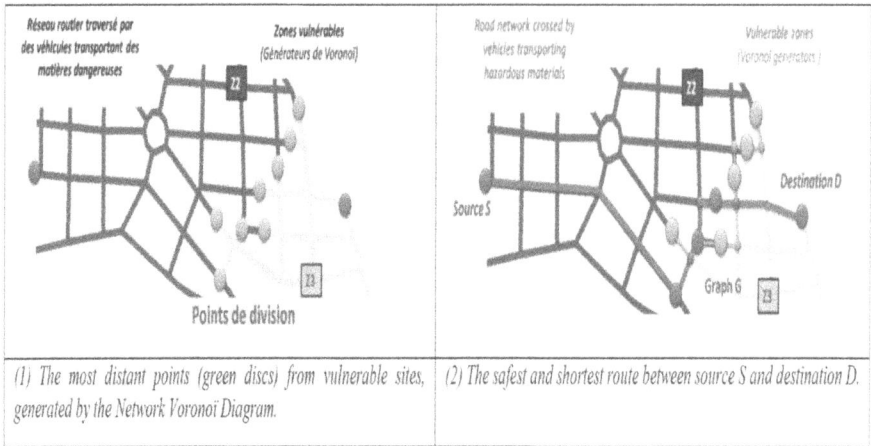

| (1) The most distant points (green discs) from vulnerable sites, generated by the Network Voronoï Diagram. | (2) The safest and shortest route between source S and destination D. |

FIGURE 14.10   The shortest and safest paths in a space environment.

ultimately keep people as far away from harm as possible. Indeed, these authors propose an assessment process based on spatial network modeling, which consists in finding short and safe routes by moving as far as possible from the Voronoï generators (vulnerable sites). These points, called division points, are generated using the NVD (Figure 14.10). They are found at the same distance from every two or more Voronoï generators.

14.4   RESULTS AND DISCUSSION

Analysis of viral infection risk based on space and time parameters (proximity to infected areas and time of exposure to the risk) on the one hand, and a minimum distance to be kept from areas infected by authorities and guiding citizens to travel on safe paths on the other hand, can keep these citizens safe. This minimum distance, according to Erwig (2000) is Euclidean. Okabe et al. (2008) showed that the Euclidean distance is significantly different from the distance of the shortest path in the urbanized sector. So, in an urban environment, this distance must be calculated on the spatial network. Mabrouk and Boulmakoul (2017) improved the computation process through the computation of the spatial Voronoï accessibility. This will allow the calculation of short and safe paths to travel away from the infected areas. Indeed, these authors obtained as results a safe Voronoï spatial graph (Figure 14.12). This graph is made up of a set of short and safe routes for each departure and arrival. These routes include spatial and semantic information that is very useful for the management and planning of citizens' movements in complete safety, namely: Infected areas which are close to the current position of individuals; the time and length of the shortest paths to these contaminated areas; and the distance and time to reach their destinations.

Indeed, the use of this safe Voronoï spatial graph, geoprocessing operations, and recourse to the risk analysis of viral infection will make it possible to choose and

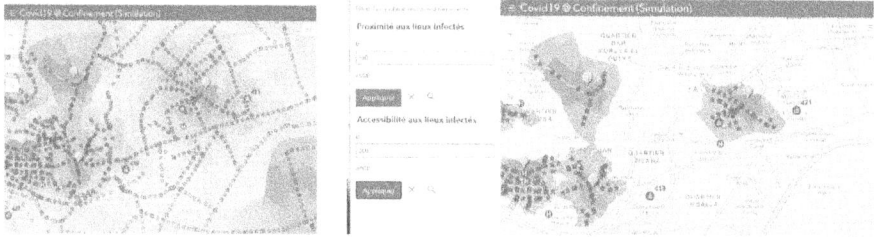

FIGURE 14.11   Interactive map used to isolate infected areas.

implement a set of means and coordinated actions to achieve the objectives of our geostrategy which aims to provide answers to a set of questions that allow citizens to move in a secure urban space far from the flow of danger propagated by areas contaminated by COVID-19. So, we used a set of software components (already developed in the framework of a previous work) and also a set of geoprocessing and geovisualization tools of a GIS system to develop a set of intelligent and interactive maps that allow authorities to isolate infected areas, ensure safe movement and assess different levels of security in relation to infected areas.

14.4.1   Isolate Infected Areas

Using an interactive map that we are developing with the tools and methods described above, we can spatially illustrate the infected areas in the city (Figure 14.11).

It is a spatial decision-making aid that allows the authorities to answer several questions such as: What are the areas to be geographically isolated and in which we must strengthen the control of compliance with protective measures and health procedures? Where should we put barriers to stop the spread of the epidemic in neighboring healthy areas and also to prevent people from accessing these infected areas?

14.4.2   Ensure Safe Travel

Using the tools and methods described above and based on the analysis of the risk of viral infection, we have developed an intelligent map which constitutes a spatial support for decision making (Figure 14.12).

This smart map helps citizens (going to work, schools, etc.), during the period of partial containment, to move safely away from infected areas and to travel the safest paths (green lines). It also allows authorities to organize traffic during this period of containment and prevent citizens from approaching infected areas (Zheng et al. 2011; D'silva et al. 2017).

14.4.3   Evaluate the Various Security Levels Compared to Infected Areas

We have developed an intelligent map that constitutes spatial decision-making support that illustrates the different levels of security in relation to infected areas

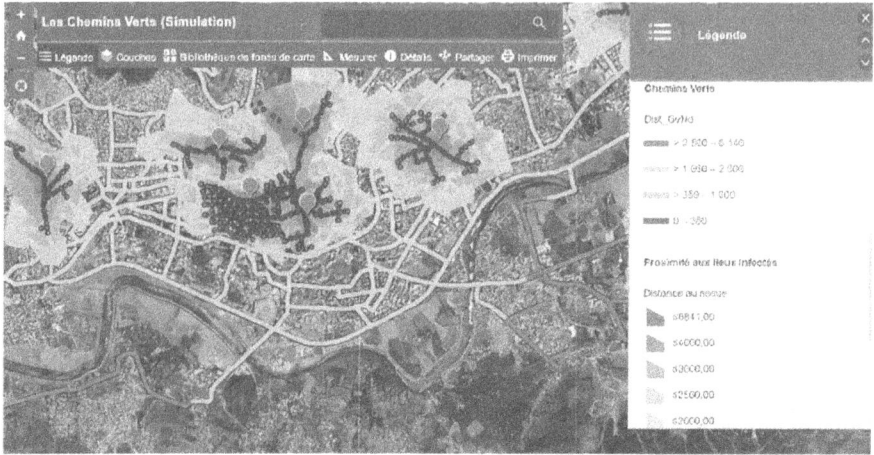

FIGURE 14.12   Interactive map used to find the safest paths (green lines).

(Figure 14.13). This map offers decision-makers the possibility of measuring the risk and consequently of deciding the secure places for the necessary meetings (pick-up points for students, etc.)

A mobile application manipulating the information provided by this spatial support will be able to guide people who move around the city and warn them in real time of infected areas that are found in their proximity, while showing them the distance separating their current geographical position and these infected areas (Figure 14.14). Other services will be added based on the work given in Boulmakoul and Bouziri (2012) and Cassini (1998).

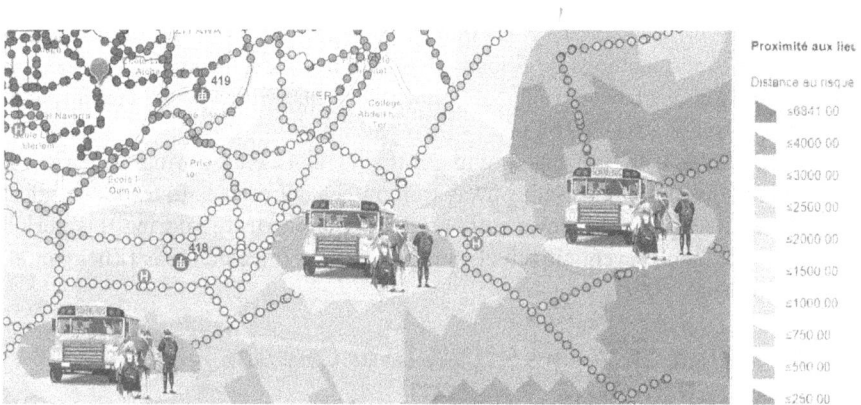

FIGURE 14.13   Interactive map used to evaluate the various security levels compared to infected areas.

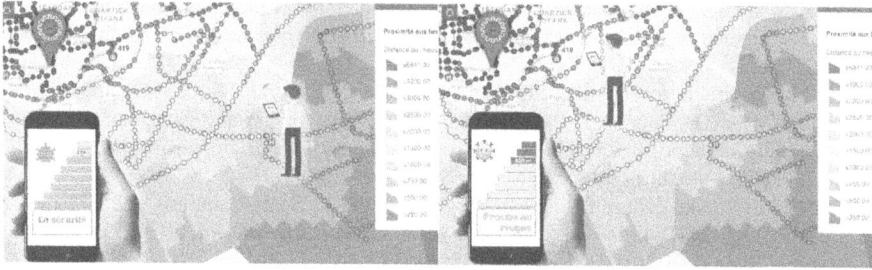

FIGURE 14.14   Mobile application warns in real time of infected areas.

14.5   CONCLUSION

In this chapter we have discussed a set of tools and methods capable of constructing a safe spatial Voronoï graph, and spatially and temporally analyzing the risk of COVID-19 infection. In addition, a set of geoprocessing, geovisualization and intelligent spatial analysis operations will make it possible to choose and implement a set of means and coordinated actions to achieve the objectives of a smart geostrategy which aims to provide answers to a set of questions. Using these methods and tools, we have developed a set of interactive maps that allow citizens to move around a secure urban space far from the risk of COVID-19 contamination and make available to decision makers, during the period of partial containment, a spatial decision-making aid illustrating spatial information on the location and proximity of the infected places, the distance and routes to the nearest infected places, and the security levels of the various infected areas.

REFERENCES

Atluri G., Karpatne A., Kumar V. Spatio-temporal data mining: A survey of problems and methods. *ACM Computing Surveys*, 2018, 51(4): 1–41. https://doi.org/10.1145/3161602

Boulmakoul A., Bouziri A.E. Mobile Object Framework and Fuzzy Graph Modelling to Boost HazMat Telegeomonitoring. In: Garbolino E., Tkiouat M., Yankevich N., Lachtar D. (eds), *Transport of Dangerous Goods. NATO Science for Peace and Security Series C: Environmental Security*. Springer, Dordrecht, 2012.

Cassini P. Road transportation of dangerous goods: quantitative risk assessment and route comparison. *Journal of Hazardous Materials*, 1998, 61(1–3). https://doi.org/10.1016/S0304-3894(98)00117-4

Cherradi G., El Bouziri A., Boulmakoul A., Zeitouni K. Real-Time HazMat Environmental Information System: A micro-service based architecture. *Procedia Computer Science*, 2017, 109: 982–87.

Das M., Ghosh S.K. Data-driven approaches for spatio-temporal analysis: a survey of the state-of-the-arts. *Journal of Computer Science and Technology*, 2020, 35: 665–96. https://doi.org/10.1007/s11390-020-9349-0

D'silva G.M., Khan A., Gaurav, J., Bari S. Real-time processing of IoT events with historic data using Apache Kafka and Apache Spark with dashing framework, *2nd IEEE International Conference on Recent Trends in Electronics, Information & Communication Technology (RTEICT)*, Bangalore, 2017, 1804–09. https://doi.org/10.1109/RTEICT.2017.8256910

Duan P, Mao G, Liang W, Zhang D. A unified spatiotemporal model for short-term traffic flow prediction. *IEEE Transactions on Intelligent Transportation Systems*, 2018, 20(9): 3212–23.

Erwig M. The graph Voronoï diagram with applications. *Networks*, 2000, 36(3): 156–63.

Fabiano B., Curro F., Palazzi E., Pastorino R. A framework for risk assessment and decision-making strategies in dangerous good transportation. *Journal of Hazardous Materials*, 2002, 93: 1–15. https://doi.org/10.1016/S0304-3894(02)00034-1

Franch-Pardo I., Napoletano B., Rosete-Verges F., Billa L. Spatial analysis and GIS in the study of COVID-19: a review. *Science of The Total Environment*, 2020, 739: 140033. https://doi.org/10.1016/j.scitotenv.2020.140033.

Karim L., Boulmakoul A., Mabrouk A., Lbath A. Deploying Real Time Big Data Analytics in Cloud Ecosystem for Hazmat Stochastic Risk Trajectories. *Procedia Computer Science*, 2017, 109: 180–87. https://doi.org/10.1016/j.procs.2017.05.322.

Mabrouk A., Boulmakoul A. Modèle spatial objet base sur les diagrammes spatiaux de voronoï pour la geo-gouvernance des espaces urbains. *Workshop International sur l'Innovation et Nouvelles Tendances dans les Systèmes d'Information*, INTIS, 2012, pp. 105–16.

Mabrouk A., Boulmakoul A. Nouvelle approche basée sur le calcul des itinéraires courts et sûrs pour le transport des matières dangereuses favorisant l'accès rapide aux secours, *The sixth International Conference on Innovation and New Trends in Information Systems*, INTIS, 2017, ISBN : 978-9954-34-378-4, ISSN : 2351-9215.

Mabrouk A. Boulmakoul A., Karim L., Lbath A. Safest and shortest itineraries for transporting hazardous materials using split points of Voronoï spatial diagrams based on spatial modeling of vulnerable zones. *Procedia Computer Science*, 2017, 109: 156–63. https://doi.org/10.1016/j.procs.2017.05.311

Maguerra S., Boulmakoul A., Karim L., et al. Towards a reactive system for managing big trajectory data. *J Ambient Intell Human Comput, Springer Journal.*, 2020, 11: 3895–906, https://doi.org/10.1007/s12652-019-01625-3

OCG. 2002. Open-Geospatial-Consortium. Web map service (1.1.1) implementation specification. http://portal.opengeospatial.org

Okabe A., Satoh T., Furuta T., Suzuki A., Okano K. Generalized network Voronoï diagrams: Concepts, computational methods, and applications, *International Journal of Geographical Information Science*, 2008: 965–94, https://doi.org/10.1080/13658810701587891

Pamučar Dragan, Ljubojević Srđan, Kostadinović Dragan, Đorović Boban. Cost and risk aggregation in multi-objective route planning for hazardous materials transportation—A neuro-fuzzy and artificial bee colony approach. *Expert Systems with Applications*, 1996, 65: 1–15.

PostGis-Project. 2013. Spatial support for postgresql. http://postgis.refractions.net/

QGIS Development Team. 2009. QGIS Geographic Information System. Open-Source Geospatial Foundation. http://qgis.org.

Snow J. The cholera near Golden-square, and at Deptford. *Med Times Gazette*, 1854, 9: 321–22.

Sun Feinuo, Matthews Stephen A., Yang Tse-Chuan, Hu Ming-Hsiao. 2020. A spatial analysis of COVID-19 period prevalence in US counties through June 28, 2020: Where geography matters? *Annals of Epidemiology*, https://doi.org/10.1016/j.annepidem.2020.07.014

World Health Organization. 2005. WHO global influenza preparedness plan: the role of WHO and recommendations for national measures before and during pandemics. https://apps.who.int/iris/handle/10665/68998

Zheng Y., Xiaofang Zhou (Eds). *Computing with Spatial Trajectories*. Springer, 2011, 308. https://doi.org/10.1080/13658816.2012.741688

Zhou Chenghu, Su Fenzhen, Pei Tao, Zhang An et al. COVID-19: Challenges to GIS with Big Data, *Geography and Sustainability*, 2020, 1(1): 77–87, https://doi.org/10.1016/j.geosus.2020.03.005

15 Healthcare Providers Recommender System Based on Collaborative Filtering Techniques

Abdelaaziz Hessane, Ahmed El Youssefi,
Yousef Farhaoui, Badraddine Aghoutane,
Noureddine Ait Ali, and Ayasha Malik

CONTENTS

15.1 INTRODUCTION

Health information systems (HIS) are becoming an increasingly valuable medium for providing healthcare service [1]. Today, a large amount of health data is spread around various websites on the internet. Overchoice and information reliability are some of the challenges a patient may encounter when looking for suitable healthcare providers (i.e. physicians, clinics, therapeutic centers, etc.). Overchoice, also known as "choice overload", is a cognitive disability that occurs when there are too many choices available to consumers. As a result, people find it difficult to make decisions. According to a study conducted on 1000 patients by Software Advice in 2020, 71% of people used online reviews as their first step in finding a new doctor. Internet review sites such as Yelp are having an increasing impact, not only on healthcare providers' reputations but also on the patient decision-making process. These websites offer to their users the possibility of consulting and evaluating a very large number of health professionals [2].

Healthcare provider recommender systems (HPRSs) are viewed in this sense as complementary tools in healthcare decision-making processes [3]. The main goals of these systems are to improve technology usability, reduce process knowledge overload, and find adaptive, trustworthy, and relevant health information [4]. These systems are primarily intended for filtering large amounts of data, which alleviates the problem of choice overload by providing users with relevant items based on their preferences. These preferences can be directly extracted from historical data of users or indirectly by looking into historical data of similar users. The collaborative nature of these systems ensures that the recommendations generated are reliable to some extent [5].

In summary, the major contribution of this work can be enumerated as below:

- The work discusses the background of a HPRS for understanding and developing an efficient system.
- The work highlights all three ways in which a HPRS has been developed, such as a system based on collaborative filtering (CF), a system based on content filtering, and a system based on hybrid manner.
- The work redefines the inspiration for deep study of ML to form a HPRS that eases medicinal facilities.
- The work explores some recently researches in this context and analysis of our work has been done.
- The aime of this work is to test and evaluate other techniques such as co-clustering and the slope one method in the context of the HPRS.

The remainder of this chapter is organized as follows: Section 15.2 highlights the research background related to the proposed system where some existing work done by researchers has been discussed. In addition, Section 15.3 defines the HPRS along with the introduction of HPRS based on CF, HPRSs based on content filtering, and hybrid HPRSs. Moreover, Section 15.4 deliberates the methodology that has been used in the proposed system along with data description, data preprocessing, and proposed solution. Furthermore, Section 15.5 enumerates the ML models where neighbors-based models, latent factors model, slope one based model, co-clustering model, and simple baseline model are explained. In addition, Section 15.6 discusses the evaluation metric and Section 15.7 shows the results. Finally, Section 15.8 concludes and is followed by future work.

15.2 RESEARCH BACKGROUND

Several researches with the aim of recommending healthcare providers have been conducted. Narducci et al. [6] proposed a doctor HPRS based on the semantic relationship between a patient's symptoms and his/her treatment to find a similar patient. Doctors with high ratings will then be recommended. One of the disadvantages of this method is the lack of a strategy for assessing how a patient rates a specific doctor. Archana and Smita [7], proposed a personalized recommender system (PSR) for medical assistance based on keyword extraction. Natural language processing (NLP) technique applied to users' reviews combined with historical feedback are used to predict missing ratings. However, it was unclear which types of factors influenced the patient (i.e. user) rating for a specific doctor. Guo et al. [8] proposed a recommendation system that is based on healthcare data mining techniques to identify key opinion leaders (KOLs) for any specific disease. Waqar et al. [9] built a recommender framework based on the analytic hierarchy process (AHP) model where both subjective and objective parts of a decision-making process can be evaluated. The system's main component is the AHP-based doctor ranking function. Han et al. [10], invented a hybrid family-doctor HPRS. A recommendation list is generated based on different levels of available information about patients such as demographic, interaction, and behavioral data. Zhang et al. [11] proposed a three-module personalized doctor recommendation system called iDoctor. The first module named Sentiment Analysis Module (SAM) is used to estimate the emotional state from user reviews. The user preferences and doctor features from user reviews are directly extracted by the second module named Topic Modeling Module (TMM). Finally, the hybrid matrix factorization module uses the extracted information to predict the rating for doctors. CF techniques such as matrix factorization and neighborhood-based models were used in most of the above studies. However, other models can be used to predict the patient–doctors' missing ratings. [12].

15.3 HEALTHCARE PROVIDER RECOMMENDER SYSTEMS

HPRS is a classical ML application designed to help its user to quickly find relevant information, a product, or a service either by analyzing the evaluations and suggestions provided by other similar users or by exploiting its history. We can qualify them as information filtering systems (IFS) whose main purpose is to face the problem of overload and richness of information available on the web or the e-services platforms [13]. A HPRS aims to provide users with relevant items to choose from. There are three main types of methods for accomplishing this task: CF methods, content-based methods, and hybrid methods.

15.3.1 HPRS Based on Collaborative Filtering

To generate new suggestions, collaborative approaches for HPRSs are methods that are solely focused on previous experiences between users and objects. The user–item interactions matrix stores these interactions [14].

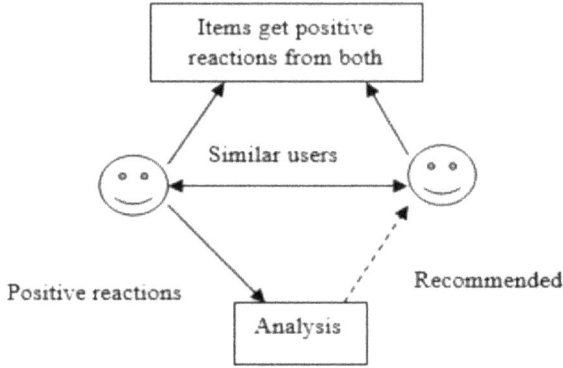

FIGURE 15.1   Collaborative filtering technique.

The first step in CF is to identify users who have similar rating patterns to the new active user, and the second step is to use the ratings of these similar users to make a recommendation for that new user [15]. The filtering process may be one of two types. The first one is user-based CF, in which we want to identify users that are close to a new active user, find their ratings, and then aggregate those ratings to create suggestions for the new user. The second one is item-based CF, in which the similarity of two items is determined based on user reviews of those items. Figure 15.1 shows the working process of CF techniques.

15.3.2   HPRS BASED ON CONTENT FILTERING

Content-based systems create a user interest profile based on the characteristics of objects that the user has previously assessed. It uses keywords to define the item. This method is primarily concerned with data extraction, interpretation, and filtering processes. Two techniques are needed to implement this method of filtering, one to represent the item and the other to create the user profile [16]. Figure 15.2 shows the working process of content-based filtering techniques.

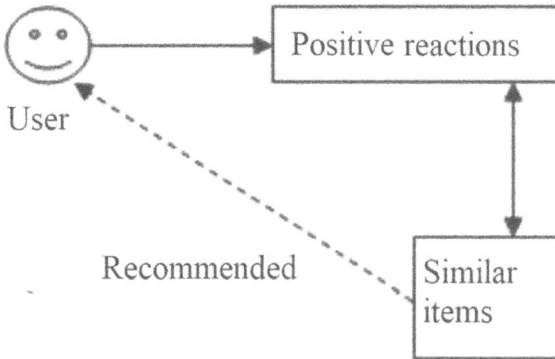

FIGURE 15.2   Content-based filtering technique.

15.3.3 Hybrid HPRSs

Considering the benefits and drawbacks of both of the above methods, it is clear that several systems are focused on their combination, resulting in hybrid filtering systems [17]. In general, hybridization occurs in two stages: first is to create candidate recommendations using CF and other filtering techniques separately and second is to combine these sets of preliminary recommendations using weighting, combining, cascading, swapping, and other methods to produce final recommendations for users [18].

15.4 METHODOLOGY

In this section, the work planning with the internal working process in a proper sequence is discussed, including which kind of data is required by describing them, then it is stated how data get preprocessed and finally proposed solutions are explained.

15.4.1 Data Description

Several review-based HPRSs have been created in recent years to integrate the useful information found in user-generated textual or numerical scale rating feedback into the user modeling and recommendation process [19]. The amount of clientele information in Yelp's database has grown dramatically over the years, and we aim to test the predictive efficiency of various CF techniques on this dataset. There are five json files in this dataset named business, review, user, check-in, and tips. Only three of them were used to construct the dataset, namely: Business.json, which contains business data including location data, attributes, and categories. Categories.json can be used to retrieve category lists and individual category information respectively; this file is used in the filtering process as described in Figure 15.3. The third file is Review.json; it contains full review text data including the ID of the user who wrote the review, the ID of the business the review is written for, the star rating, the review date, and other information.

15.4.2 Data Preprocessing

Since we are interested in healthcare providers' businesses only, the first step of data preprocessing was necessary [20]. Figure 15.3 resumes the preprocessing steps to prepare the data in the right format for the ML-based recommendation algorithms.

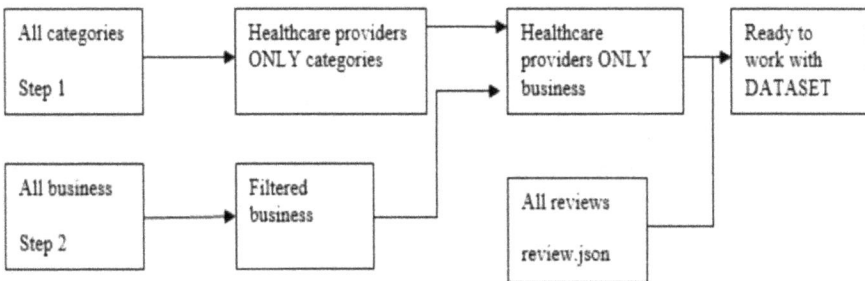

FIGURE 15.3 Data preprocessing steps.

TABLE 15.1
Statistics on Final Dataset

Number of unique healthcare providers	1086
Number of unique users	8344
Number of ratings	+28,000

The first preprocessing step was to extract a list of healthcare providers' business aliases and titles by filtering the categories.json. We aimed in the second step to apply filters on the business.json file to retain only the open businesses and to remove the unnecessary columns. We then build the ready-to-use dataset by combining the files resulting from the two previous steps with the review.json file.

In this study, we limited ourselves to data from the city of Las Vegas only. In order to boost the high sparsity presented by this data, we only keep users who have given many reviews greater than the average number of reviews per user, which is 1.76. (users with only one review are removed). Despite this, the constructed patient-healthcare providers' ratings matrix presents almost 99.7% of sparsity. The challenge was to find the best ML model that can predict the missing ratings with high accuracy. Table 15.1 shows the statistics on final dataset.

15.4.3 PROPOSED SOLUTION

For the establishment of a HPRS based on predictive patient-healthcare professionals rating model, the following approach is proposed. First, data in the form of explicit user ratings of healthcare professionals must be collected and preprocessed. Second, by using the cross-validation technique, we have tested and evaluated the different ML models on the preprocessed data, and we then selected the best performing model. The third step was to tune the hyper-parameters of the chosen model to improve their performance. Finally, we deployed the trained model to construct the intended recommendation system. Figure 15.4 summarizes the different stages of the proposed solution.

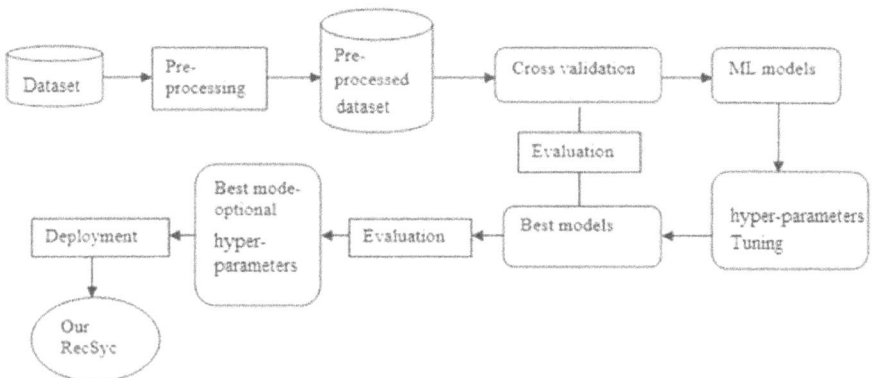

FIGURE 15.4 Flowchart of the proposed solution.

15.5   MACHINE LEARNING MODELS

Systems using the CF technique in a recommendation sense must compare radically different objects like items versus users. The neighbors-based approach and latent factor models are the two key methods for facilitating such comparison. Other methods, such as co-clustering [21] and the slope-one method have been suggested in the literature. In this section, we will describe the ML models we have used to predict missing ratings [22].

15.5.1   NEIGHBORS-BASED MODELS

Recommendations based on neighbors models are done in two main phases: one is the neighborhood formation phase and another one is the recommendation phase.

A similarity between users (user-based approach) or items (item-based approach) is measured during the neighborhood creation process. According to Zhang et al. [23] the two most popular types of similarity measures are Pearson's correlation (PC) coefficient (equation 15.1) and cosine-based similarity (equation 15.2).

$$PC(a,b) = \frac{\sum_{i=1}^{n}(a_i - a')(b_i - b')}{\sqrt{\sum_{i=1}^{n}(a_i - a')^2}\sqrt{\sum_{i=1}^{n}(b_i - b')^2}} \tag{15.1}$$

where a and b are two n-pointed vectors. The mean value of vector a and vector b is represented by a' and b', respectively. In the above equation, PC finds the correlation between the two sets a and b.

$$\cos(\theta) = \frac{\sum_{i=1}^{n} A_i \times B_i}{\sqrt{\sum_{i=1}^{n} A_i^2}\sqrt{\sum_{i=1}^{n} B_i^2}} \tag{15.2}$$

where A and B are two sets of n data points or n feature values. The values of characteristic i in sets A and B are described by A_i and B_i, respectively.

The next step is to predict a rating $\hat{r}_{ui}$ that user u will probably give to item i that he didn't rate yet. One way is to use the calculated similarities and the corresponding ratings. Many variations are possible by adding biases like Z-Score or the user's/item's rating average. In our study, we have tested four variations: KNN baseline, KNN with means, KNN with Z-Score, and the basic KNN

If the approach is user based, then the predicted rating will be calculated as shown in the formula (equation 15.3):

$$\hat{r}_{ui} = \frac{\sum_{v \in N_i^k(u)} sim(u,v).r_{vi}}{\sum_{v \in N_i^k(u)} sim(u,v)} \tag{15.3}$$

Item

	A	B	C	D
1		2.5	3.5	
2	4.0		4.5	
3		1.5		
4				2.0

User (label on left side)

Ratings Matrix (R)

=

1	1.6	0.8
2	0.3	1.0
3	1.2	2.0
4	1.4	0.7

User Matrix (P)

X

A	B	C	D
1.7	0.2	2.0	0.4
1.5	0.6	1.1	0.8

Item Matrix (Q)

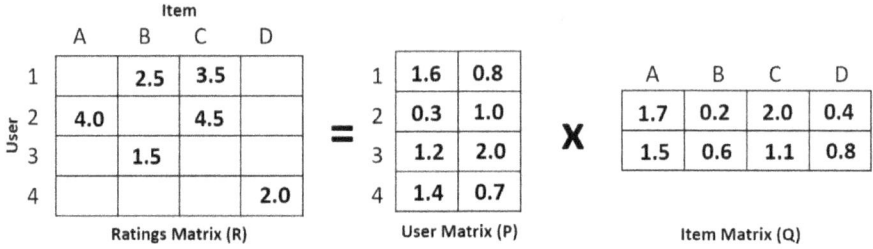

FIGURE 15.5 Matrix factorization technique.

If the approach is item based, then the predicted rating will be calculated as shown in the formula (equation 15.4):

$$\hat{r}_{ui} = \frac{\sum_{j \in N_u^k(i)} sim(i,j) . r_{uj}}{\sum_{j \in N_u^k(i)} sim(i,j)} \tag{15.4}$$

15.5.2 LATENT FACTORS MODELS

Latent factor models are an alternative approach to CF with the objective of uncovering hidden characteristics that explain the explicit data that represent the appreciation of users toward items, which is generally stored as a rating matrix. One of the most common techniques for locating latent factors is matrix factorization [24]. Figure 15.5 explains the principle of this method. In our study, we have tested several matrix factorization methods such as singular value decomposition (SVD), SVD++ and non-negative matrix factorization (NMF).

The prediction of a rating of item i by user u, can be measured easily by calculating the dot product of the two vectors corresponding to q_i and p_u as shown in the formula (equation 15.5):

$$\hat{r}_{ui} = q_i^T p_u \tag{15.5}$$

where,
- q_i: Vector associated with the item i.
- p_u: Vector associated with user u.

15.5.3 SLOPE-ONE-BASED MODEL

The slope-one predictors for rating-based CF algorithms were proposed to minimize overfitting, boost efficiency, and make HPRS implementation easier [25]. They are considered as easy-to-implement methods based on the use of a simple form of regression; a single free parameter is an average difference between the scores of the two items. It has turned out to be much more accurate than linear regression of the scores of one item to the scores of another item in some cases, and it takes half the storage or less [26].

The prediction in this case is defined as (equation 15.6):

$$\hat{r}_{ui} = \mu_u + \frac{1}{|R_i(u)|} \sum_{j \in R_i(u)} dev(i,j) \qquad (15.6)$$

where,
- $R_i(u)$ is the set of relevant elements, the set of elements j rated by u which also have at least one common user with i.
- $dev(i,j)$ is defined as the mean difference between the ratings of item I and those of item j calculated as (equation 15.7):

$$dev(i,j) = \frac{1}{|U_{ij}|} \sum_{u \in U_{ij}} r_{ui} - r_{uj} \qquad (15.7)$$

U_{ij} represents the set of all users who have evaluated the elements i and j.

15.5.4 Co-Clustering Based Model

This unsupervised learning technique allows the simultaneous segmentation of rows and columns of the rating matrix [27]. Thanks to this bi-clustering technique [21], users and elements are assigned certain C_u, C_i clusters and certain C_{ui} co-clusters. Clusters are assigned using a simple optimization method, much like k-means and the predicted rating can be calculated as shown in formula (equation 15.8):

$$\hat{r}_{ui} = \overline{C_{ui}} + \left(\mu_u - \overline{C_u}\right) + \left(\mu_i - \overline{C_i}\right) \qquad (15.8)$$

where,
- $\overline{C_{ui}}$ is the average evaluation of the C_{ui} Co-cluster.
- $\overline{C_u}$ is the average rating of the cluster to which user u belongs.
- $\overline{C_i}$ is the average evaluation of the cluster to which item i belongs.

15.5.5 Simple Baseline Model

The main objectives of this study are to fill in the missing ratings in our patient-healthcare providers' rating matrix and to test the predictive efficiency of nearest neighbor, matrix factorization, co-clustering and slop one method. However, since most CF methods start with a simple baseline model, we will begin by implementing the following models to our data:
- Simple baseline model similar to the model used in [28]. A baseline estimate rating is denoted by b_{ui} and accounts for the user and item effects:

$$b_{ui} = \mu + b_u + b_i \qquad (15.9)$$

Where:
μ is the mean rating of all reviews in the system.
b_u indicates the difference between the average rating of user u and μ.
b_i indicates the difference between the average rating of business i and μ.

- In this model, we take into account the user's mean rating and the mean of the healthcare providers to eliminate any potential bias when forecasting (a consumer has a propensity to give something a higher rating than it deserves).
- Model based on maximum likelihood estimation, a statistical estimator is used to infer the parameters of a normal distribution from a given sample by looking for the values of the parameters maximizing the likelihood function.

15.6 EVALUATION METRIC

The most commonly used evaluation metrics for HPRSs, according to Shani and Gunawardana [29], are RMSE and mean absolute error (MAE). The RMSE is the error metric that we will use in this work, this choice is explained by the fact that this metric uses squared deviations, which means that larger errors tend to get amplified.

RMSE is defined as:

$$RMSE = \sqrt{\frac{\sum \left(\hat{r}_{u,i} - r_{u,i} \right)^2}{n}} \tag{15.10}$$

where,

- $\hat{r}_{u,i}$ is the predicted rating from user u on item i.
- $r_{u,i}$ is the actual rating.
- n is the size of the test set.

We ran a five-fold cross validation RMSE on all of our samples, in which we trained the model on 80% of the data and then tested its accuracy on the remaining 20%.

15.7 RESULTS

Table 15.2 summarizes the results. We have got when testing and evaluating different methods issued from the main models described above.

As shown in Figure 15.6, the user-based KNN model allows to predict the missing ratings with the smallest RMSE; this means that this model is the best among the 11 models tested. The baseline here was used to adjust the data because some users tend to give higher ratings than others, and for some items to receive higher evaluations than others. For this, an estimation (baseline) is calculated using the following formula (equation 15.11):

$$b_{ui} = \mu + b_u + b_i \tag{15.11}$$

with b_{ui} is the estimation (baseline) for an unknown score $\hat{r}_{ui}$ and μ the overall average score. The parameters b_u and b_i respectively indicate the observed deviations of

TABLE 15.2
Summary of Results

Model	Tested Methods	RMSE
Neighbors-based model	User based CF KNN	1.127623
	User based CF KNN + Baseline	1.041687
	User based KNN + Means bias	1.247015
	User based KNN + Z-Score bias	1.244651
Latent factors-based model	SVD	1.139097
	SVD++	1.148156
	NMF	1.151123
Co-clustering-based model	Co-Clustering based on K-Means Algorithm	1.281608
Slope-one-based model	Basic slope-one algorithm	1.175064
Probability-based model	Baseline Only	1.532352
	Maximum likelihood estimation based	2.282016

the user u and the element i from the mean. Other estimations were tested such as Z-Score and means biases.

As described in Figure 15.4, the step of hyper-parameters tuning comes right after the evaluation step. As shown in Table 15.2, the baseline user-based CF KNN was the best model in terms of RMSE value. The main goal of this phase was to find the optimal hyper-parameters of the model. After applying the hyper-parameters

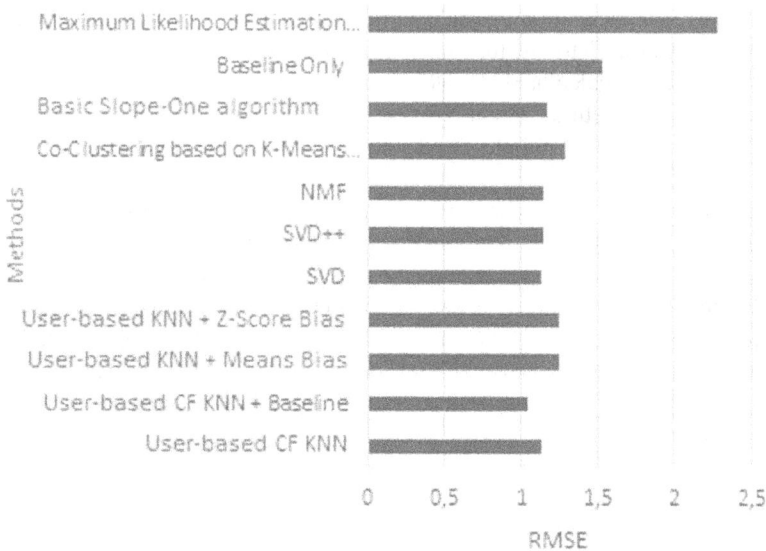

FIGURE 15.6   Performance of tested methods in terms of RMSE.

TABLE 15.3
Some Results of the Hyper-parameters Tuning Phase

Hyperparameter	Values Tested	Optimal Value
Maximum number of neighbors	[2, 4, 5, 10, 15, 20, 25]	4
Similarity method	Mean squared difference, cosine, pearson	Pearson
Approach	User-based, item-based	User-based
Optimization algorithm	Stochastic gradient descent, alternating least squares	Stochastic gradient descent

tuning, the RMSE decreased from 1.041687 to 0.984700. Table 15.3 summarizes some results of this phase.

15.8 CONCLUSION AND PERSPECTIVES

The experiments carried out during the testing and validation phase of the various ML models adopted showed that the neighbors-based models and those based on latent factors generate the recommendations with a minimal error rate compared to the other models. However, we demonstrated in this study that other methods, such as co-clustering and the slope-one method, can be used to solve the same problem of predicting messing values in a patient-healthcare provider rating matrix. Thanks to the hyper-parameter tuning technique, it was possible to improve the performance of the selected model and a recommendation system is finally deployed to address the problem of recommendation of healthcare professionals. However, our system suffers from several limitations, for example, the item side cold start problem and the way similarities are calculated. To overcome these problems, we propose to combine the actual solution with a content-based recommendation system. Another solution is to exploit the written opinions of patients by introducing data-mining techniques and NLP to give more meaning to the rating stars present in the evaluation matrix.

Recommending a healthcare professional is a special and difficult task, and should not be based only on the opinions of similar patients, but on other criteria, such as the service provider's schedule, the patient's health status (emergency or not), and the location (the distance between the patient and the healthcare professional). The quality of the recommendations will be finer and more reliable if additional information about patients and healthcare professionals is available. The more information about the users of the system is available, the more meaningful the similarity calculation will be.

REFERENCES

[1] Haried, P., Claybaugh, C., & Dai, H. (2017). Evaluation of health information systems research in information systems research: A meta-analysis. *Health Informatics Journal*, 25(1), 186–202. https://doi.org/10.1177/1460458217704259

[2] Goyal, S., Sharma, N., Bhushan, B., Shankar, A., & Sagayam, M. (2020). IoT enabled technology in secured healthcare: Applications, challenges and future directions. *Cognitive Internet of Medical Things for Smart Healthcare*, 25–48. https://doi.org/10.1007/978-3-030-55833-8_2

[3] Calero, Valdez A., Ziefle, M., Verbert, K., Felfernig, A., & Holzinger, A. (2016). Recommender systems for health informatics: State-of-the-art and future perspectives. *Lecture Notes in Computer Science*, 391–414. https://doi.org/10.1007/978-3-319-50478-0_20

[4] Aggarwal, C. C. (2016). An introduction to recommender systems. *Recommender Systems*, 1–28. https://doi.org/10.1007/978-3-319-29659-3_1

[5] Sharma, N., Kaushik, I., Bhushan, B., Gautam, S., & Khamparia, A. (2020). Applicability of WSN and biometric models in the field of healthcare. *Deep Learning Strategies for Security Enhancement in Wireless Sensor Networks Advances in Information Security, Privacy, and Ethics*, 304–329. https://doi.org/10.4018/978-1-7998-5068-7.ch016

[6] Narducci, F., Lops, P., & Semeraro, G. (2017). Power to the patients: The HealthNetsocial network. *Information Systems*, *71*, 111–122. https://doi.org/10.1016/j.is.2017.07.005

[7] Archana, B. & Smita, L. (2015). Personalized recommendation system for medical assistance using Hybrid Filtering. *International Journal of Computer Applications*, *128*(9), 6–10. https://doi.org/10.5120/ijca2015906626

[8] Guo, L., Jin, B., Yao, C., Yang, H., Huang, D., & Wang, F. (2016). Which doctor to trust: A Recommender system for identifying the right doctors. *Journal of Medical Internet Research*, *18*(7), e186. https://doi.org/10.2196/jmir.6015

[9] Waqar, M., Majeed, N., Dawood, H., Daud, A., & Aljohani, N. R. (2019). An adaptive doctor-recommender system. *Behaviour & Information Technology*, *38*(9), 959–73. https://doi.org/10.1080/0144929X.2019.1625441

[10] Han, Q., Ji, M., de Troya, I. M. de R., Gaur, M., & Zejnilovic, L. (2019). A Hybrid Recommender System for Patient-Doctor Matchmaking in Primary Care. *ArXiv: 1808.03265 [Cs, Stat]*. http://arxiv.org/abs/1808.03265

[11] Zhang, Y., Chen, M., Huang, D., Wu, D., & Li, Y. (2017). iDoctor: Personalized and professionalized medical recommendations based on hybrid matrix factorization. *Future Generation Computer Systems*, *66*, 30–35. https://doi.org/10.1016/j.future.2015.12.001

[12] Puri, D., & Bhushan, B. (2019). Enhancement of security and energy efficiency in WSNs: Machine Learning to the rescue. *2019 International Conference on Computing, Communication, and Intelligent Systems (ICCCIS)*. https://doi.org/10.1109/icccis48478.2019.8974465

[13] Gulyani, V., Dhiman, T., & Bhushan, B. (2020). Introducing machine learning to wireless sensor networks. *Deep Learning Strategies for Security Enhancement in Wireless Sensor Networks Advances in Information Security, Privacy, and Ethics*, 1–22. https://doi.org/10.4018/978-1-7998-5068-7.ch001

[14] Ricci, F., Rokach, L., & Shapira, B. (2015). Recommender systems: Introduction and challenges. *Recommender Systems Handbook*, 1–34. https://doi.org/10.1007/978-1-4899-7637-6_1

[15] Bhushan, B., & Sahoo, G. (2019). ISFC-BLS (intelligent and secured fuzzy clustering algorithm using balanced load sub-cluster formation) in WSN environment. *Wireless Personal Communications*. https://doi.org/10.1007/s11277-019-06948-0

[16] Soni, S., & Bhushan, B. (2019). Use of Machine Learning algorithms for designing efficient cyber security solutions. *2019 2nd International Conference on Intelligent Computing, Instrumentation and Control Technologies (ICICICT)*. https://doi.org/10.1109/icicict46008.2019.8993253

[17] Gaur, J., Goel, A. K., Rose, A., & Bhushan, B. (2019). Emerging Trends in Machine Learning. *2019 2nd International Conference on Intelligent Computing, Instrumentation and Control Technologies (ICICICT)*. https://doi.org/10.1109/icicict46008.2019.8993192

[18] Erritali, M., Hssina, B., & Grota, A. (2021). Building recommendation systems using the algorithms KNN and SVD. *International Journal of Recent Contributions from Engineering, Science & IT (IJES)*, 9(1), 71. https://doi.org/10.3991/ijes.v9i1.20569

[19] Chen, L., Chen, G., & Wang, F. (2015). Recommender systems based on user reviews: The state of the art. *User Modeling and User-Adapted Interaction*, 25(2), 99–154. https://doi.org/10.1007/s11257-015-9155-5

[20] Jindal, M., Gupta, J., & Bhushan, B. (2019). Machine learning methods for IoT and their Future Applications. *2019 International Conference on Computing, Communication, and Intelligent Systems (ICCCIS)*. https://doi.org/10.1109/icccis48478.2019.8974551

[21] George, T., & Merugu, S. (2005). A Scalable Collaborative Filtering Framework Based on Co-Clustering. *Fifth IEEE International Conference on Data Mining (ICDM'05)*, 625–28. https://doi.org/10.1109/ICDM.2005.14

[22] Sil, R., Roy, A., Bhushan, B., & Mazumdar, A. (2019). Artificial Intelligence and Machine Learning based Legal Application: The State-of-the-Art and Future Research Trends. *2019 International Conference on Computing, Communication, and Intelligent Systems (ICCCIS)*. https://doi.org/10.1109/icccis48478.2019.8974479

[23] Zhang, S., Yao, L., Sun, A., & Tay, Y. (2019). Deep learning based recommender system: A survey and new perspectives. *ACM Computing Surveys*, 52(1), 1–38. https://doi.org/10.1145/3285029

[24] Montesinos-López, O. A., Montesinos-López, A., Crossa, J., Montesinos-López, J. C., Mota-Sanchez, D., Estrada-González, F., Gillberg, J., Singh, R., Mondal, S., & Juliana, P. (2018). Prediction of multiple-trait and multiple-environment genomic data using recommender systems. *G3 Genes|Genomes|Genetics*, 8(1), 131–47. https://doi.org/10.1534/g3.117.300309

[25] Goel, A., Bhushan, B., Tyagi, B., Garg, H., & Gautam, S. (2021). Blockchain and machine learning: Background, integration challenges and application areas. *Emerging Technologies in Data Mining and Information Security*, 295–304. https://doi.org/10.1007/978-981-15-9774-9_29

[26] Lemire, D., & Maclachlan, A. (2008). Slope One Predictors for Online Rating-Based Collaborative Filtering. *ArXiv:Cs/0702144*. http://arxiv.org/abs/cs/0702144

[27] Malik, A., Gautam, S., Abidin, S., & Bhushan, B. (2019). Blockchain Technology-Future of IoT: Including Structure, Limitations and Various Possible Attacks. *2019 2nd International Conference on Intelligent Computing, Instrumentation and Control Technologies (ICICICT)*. https://doi.org/10.1109/icicict46008.2019.8993144

[28] Koren, Y. (2008). Factorization meets the neighborhood. *Proceeding of the 14th ACM SIGKDD International Conference on Knowledge Discovery and Data Mining - KDD 08*. https://doi.org/10.1145/1401890.1401944

[29] Shani, G., & Gunawardana, A. (2011). Evaluating Recommendation Systems. In F. Ricci, L. Rokach, B. Shapira, & P. B. Kantor (Eds), *Recommender Systems Handbook* (pp. 257–297). Springer US. https://doi.org/10.1007/978-0-387-85820-3_8

Index

For Product Safety Concerns and Information please contact our EU
representative GPSR@taylorandfrancis.com
Taylor & Francis Verlag GmbH, Kaufingerstraße 24, 80331 München, Germany

www.ingramcontent.com/pod-product-compliance
Lightning Source LLC
Chambersburg PA
CBHW060343220326
41598CB00023B/2796

9 781032 127644